D0922113

Human Simulation for Nursing and Health Professions

Linda Wilson, PhD, RN, CPAN, CAPA, BC, CNE, is Associate Clinical Professor and Assistant Dean for Special Projects, Simulation, and Continuing Nursing Education Accreditation at the College of Nursing and Health Professions, Drexel University. Dr. Wilson completed her BSN at College Misericordia in Dallas, Pennsylvania, and her MSN in Critical Care and Trauma at Thomas Jefferson University in Philadelphia. She completed her PhD in Nursing Research and Theory Development at Rutgers, The State University of New Jersey in Newark.

Dr. Wilson has also obtained a Postgraduate Certificate in Pain Management from the University of California, San Francisco, and completed the National Library of Medicine/Marine Biological Laboratory, Biomedical Informatics Fellowship, and the Comprehensive Workshop and Graduate Course at Harvard-MIT's Institute for Medical Simulation.

Dr. Wilson served as the President of the American Society of Perianesthesia Nurses (2002–2003) and has served as an ANCC Commission on Accreditation site surveyor since 2000. She has lectured extensively, both nationally and internationally, on simulation, technology, informatics, perianesthesia, and pain management.

Dr. Wilson is the Project Director/Primary Investigator for SimTeam: The Joint Education of Health Professionals and Assistive Personnel Students in a Simulated Environment, a US$128,000, two-and-a-half-year project funded by the Barra Foundation Inc. Dr. Wilson is also the Project Director/Primary Investigator for the Faculty Development: Integrating Technology into Nursing Education and Practice Project, a near US$1.5 million, 5-year project funded by the Health Resources and Services Administration, Department of Health and Human Services (Grant No. 1 U1KHP09542–01–00).

Leland "Rocky" Rockstraw, PhD, RN, is Associate Clinical Professor of Nursing and Assistant Dean for Simulation, Clinical & Technology Academic Operations, Drexel University College of Nursing and Health Professions in Philadelphia, Pennsylvania. A native of Rhode Island, he is a graduate of University of Nebraska, Central Michigan University, University of Southern Alabama, and Drexel University School of Education. In 2006, Dr. Rockstraw completed his PhD in Educational Leadership Development and Learning Technologies. He completed a Biomedical Informatics Fellowship from the National Library of Medicine and Marine Biological Laboratory in 2004. He has attended Harvard's Institute for Medical Simulation Comprehensive Undergraduate Course as well as the Graduate Course.

Under his tenure at the college, he has led the creation of a new centralized college-wide department that provides support in information technology, online learning technologies, web design, clinical and simulation practice, and "just-in-time technology education" to the faculty, the staff, and the students.

Dr. Rockstraw has presented nationally on a variety of nursing, health sciences, simulation, management, and learning resource center topics. He has assisted numerous academic institutions in developing programs in the use of human patient simulation, standardized patient, and handheld technology and has traveled to the foothills of the Himalayas in India to introduce the technology. He serves on the Pennsylvania Workforce Investment Board, Pennsylvania Center for Health Careers Clinical Education Task Force. Dr. Rockstraw is a co-investigator for the Faculty Development: Integrating Technology into Nursing Education and Practice Project, a near US$1.5 million, 5-year project funded by the Health Resources and Services Administration, Department of Health and Human Services.

Human Simulation for Nursing and Health Professions

Linda Wilson, PhD, RN, CPAN, CAPA, BC, CNE

Leland Rockstraw, PhD, RN

Editors

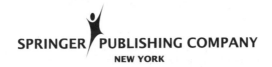

SPRINGER PUBLISHING COMPANY
NEW YORK

Springer Publishing Company, LLC
11 West 42nd Street
New York, NY 10036
www.springerpub.com

Acquisitions Editor: Allan Graubard
Composition: Newgen Imaging Systems

ISBN: 978-0-8261-0669-8
E-book ISBN: 978-0-8261-0670-4

11 12 13 14 15/ 5 4 3 2 1

The author and the publisher of this Work have made every effort to use sources believed to be reliable to provide information that is accurate and compatible with the standards generally accepted at the time of publication. Because medical
science is continually advancing, our knowledge base continues to expand. Therefore, as new information becomes available, changes in procedures become necessary. We recommend that the reader always consult current research and specific
institutional policies before performing any clinical procedure. The author and publisher shall not be liable for any special,
consequential, or exemplary damages resulting, in whole or in part, from the readers' use of, or reliance on, the information contained in this book. The publisher has no responsibility for the persistence or accuracy of URLs for external or
third-party Internet web sites referred to in this publication and does not guarantee that any content on such web sites is,
or will remain, accurate or appropriate.

Library of Congress Cataloging-in-Publication Data
Human simulation for nursing and health professions/editors, Linda Wilson,
Leland Rockstraw.
    p. ; cm.
  Includes bibliographical references and index.
  ISBN 978-0-8261-0669-8   978-0-8261-0670-4 (e-book)
  1. Nursing—Study and teaching. 2. Simulated patients. 3. Active
learning. I. Wilson, Linda, 1962– II. Rockstraw, Leland.
  [DNLM: 1. Education, Nursing—methods. 2. Health Occupations—education.
3. Patient Simulation. 4. Problem–Based Learning—methods. WY 18]
  RT71.H76 2012
  610.73076—dc23   2011028443

Printed in the United States of America by Bradford & Bigelow

This book is dedicated to all my family, friends, and colleagues who have helped me through this simulation called life. To Dr. Gloria F. Donnelly and Dr. Mary Ellen Glasgow, thank you for all your inspiration, support, encouragement, patience, and opportunities. To H. Lynn Kane, Helen "Momma" Kane, and Linda Webb, thank you for your amazing friendship and for being my family. To my friend and colleague Rocky Rockstraw, thanks for everything. To Fabien Pampaloni, thank you for your endless help and support. To Hector Bones, thank you for keeping me healthy and strong. To Lou Smith, Evan Babcock, and Steve Johnson, thanks for your friendship and support. To all the contributors in this book, thanks for helping make a dream a reality. To our wonderful standardized patients who make the simulation experience unforgettable, you all deserve an Oscar. And last, but not least, to the memory of Dr. Kathleen Kinney Falkenstein, a treasured colleague and a good friend.

Linda Wilson, PhD, RN, CPAN, CAPA, BC, CNE

This book is dedicated to all who have made this exciting and laborious task of writing/editing "real"; to my family—my partner Jorge, my daughter Savannah, my sister Jodi, and my father— without their support, I would not be who I am today; to my colleague and friend Linda Wilson, a friend in every sense of the word; to my niece, Melissa Baker, for her editorial and writing style; to all the chapter authors, wow, what a group of like-minded individuals can accomplish (both within this book as well as individually across the world); to the actors who bring "life" and "real" patient experiences to our future health care givers; to our students who trust us to guide them through this difficult path we call an education; and to you, the reader—it is my hope that you digest this information, make it better, and add to the body of knowledge of this exciting "arm" of health care education I call simulation.

Leland "Rocky" Rockstraw, PhD, RN

Contents

Contributors

Alejandro Martinez Arce, RN
Virutal Hospital Valdecilla
Santander, Spain

Mary Ellen Bednar, BSN, RN, CPAN
Virtua Memorial Hospital
Mt. Holly, NJ

Maria Benedetto, PT, DPT
Drexel University
Philadelphia, PA

Lewis Bennett, MSN, CRNA
Drexel University
Philadelphia, PA

Stephanie Brooks, MSW, LSW
Drexel University
Philadelphia, PA

Jean Forsha Byrd, MSN, RN, CEN
Community College of Philadelphia
Philadelphia, PA

James R. Carlson, MS, PA-C
Rosalind Franklin University of Medicine and
    Science/The Chicago Medical School
Chicago, IL

Robert J. Chapman, PhD
Drexel University
Philadelphia, PA

Ferne Cohen, MSN, CRNA
Drexel University
Philadelphia, PA

Ronald Clay Comer, DSW, MA, BA
Drexel University
Philadelphia, PA

John Cornele, BSN, RN, CEN, EMT-P
Drexel University
Philadelphia, PA

Fran Cornelius, PhD, RN, CNE, BC
Drexel University
Philadelphia, PA

Sukhtej Dhingra, PhD
Education Management Solutions
Philadelphia, PA

Gloria F. Donnelly, PhD, RN, FAAN
Drexel University
Philadelphia, PA

Robert Feenan, CNA
Drexel University
Philadelphia, PA

Alberto Alonso Felpete, RN
Virutal Hospital Valdecilla
Santander, Spain

Gayle Gliva-McConvey
Eastern Virginia Medical School
Norfolk, VA

Jorge L. Gomez-Diaz, MSN, RN, CNOR
Kennedy Health System
Washington Township, NJ

Mary Gallagher Gordon, MSN, RN, CNE
Drexel University
Philadelphia, PA

Robert Hargraves, BA
Jefferson Medical College
Philadelphia, PA

Souzan Hawala-Druy, MPH
Howard University
Washington, DC

Mary H. Hill, DSN, RN
Howard University
Washington, DC

H. Lynn Kane, MSN, MBA, RN, CCRN
Thomas Jefferson University Hospital
Philadelphia, PA

Laurie L. Kerns, MS
Education Management Solutions
Philadelphia, PA

Denise LaMarra, MS
University of Pennsylvania
Philadelphia, PA

Margery A. Lockard, PhD, PT
Drexel University
Philadelphia, PA

Jose M. Maestre, MD, PhD
Virutal Hospital Valdecilla
Santander, Spain

Catherine Jean Morse, MS, CRNP, CCRN
Drexel University
Philadelphia, PA

Nina Multak, MPAS, PA-C
Drexel University
Philadelphia, PA

Amy Nakajima, MD
Sound Care Medical Center
Ottawa, Ontario, Canada

Carol Okupniak, MSN, RN
Drexel University
Philadelphia, PA

Michael J. Onori, BA
Drexel University
Philadelphia, PA

Fabien Pampaloni, BSN, RN
Drexel University
Philadelphia, PA

Pilar Hernandez Pinto, MD
Virutal Hospital Valdecilla
Santander, Spain

Glenn D. Posner, MDCM, FRCSC, MEd
Sound Care Medical Center
Ottawa, Ontario, Canada

Racine Henry, MS
Drexel University
Philadelphia, PA

Amy Flanagan Risdal, MFA
Uniformed Services University
Bethesda, MD

Leland Rockstraw, PhD, RN
Drexel University
Philadelphia, PA

Kathy Ryan, MD
Drexel University
Philadelphia, PA

Karen Saewert, PhD, RN, CPHQ, CNE
Arizona State University
Phoenix, AZ

Mary Ellen Smith, PhD, RN, ACNS-BC
Drexel University
Philadelphia, PA

Linda Webb, MSN, RN, CPAN
Cooper University Medical Center
Camden, NJ

Joanne Weinschreider, MS, RN
University of Rochester
Rochester, NY

Sarah Wenger, PT, DPT, OCS
Drexel University
Philadelphia, PA

Susan E. Will, MS, RNC
Johns Hopkins Hospital
Baltimore, MD

Linda Wilson, PhD, RN, CPAN, CAPA, BC, CNE
Drexel University
Philadelphia, PA

In addition, Melissa A. Kaniecki, BA, from Bristol, RI, made her own significant contribution as an Editorial Reviewer.

Foreword

When I was eight years old, someone gave me a small oak roll top desk with cubbies and two secret hiding places. My parents placed it in my room where I pretended for hours that I was a teacher preparing my lessons or entering grades in my students' report cards; I was Beatrix Potter writing a new children's book; I was the school principal counseling a student who had misbehaved. When I was a doctoral student pursuing a PhD in Child and Adolescent Development, I studied children's play and noted the power that pretending has to transform language and action. Fast forward four decades and all of my pretend scenarios have come true—I am a teacher, an author, and an academic administrator. Without that roll top desk as the prop to fuel my imagination, who knows where I would be?

Today there is an explosion in the use of simulation in nursing and health professions education. The contributors to this text are experts in this format of teaching. They are the designers of the learning spaces, the authors of simulation cases and evaluation methods, and the experts who program the human patient simulators and who teach the patient actors to enact the clinical scenarios. They are the faculty who give students feedback and who glean feedback from the aggregate simulation reports so that teaching can be improved. They are faculty who are preparing undergraduates to enter the health workforce and the graduates who are diagnosing, prescribing, and implementing care. Simulation is changing the format and quality of clinical education, and students who have experienced this form of learning will tell you that it builds confidence, knowledge, and skill that contribute to safe and excellent patient care.

Medical education has used objective, structured clinical experiences (OSCEs) to teach diagnosis and treatment skills to physician students for at least 30 years. Patient actors called "standardized patients" were trained to evaluate the skill level of physician students in physical examination, communication, and patient teaching scenarios. In 2002, the nursing faculty of Drexel University elected to include, as a permanent part of all curricula, simulation with standardized patients. The results were so compelling that the college soon built its own digital-video standardized patient laboratory and recently completed outfitting an additional 2,200 square feet for all types of simulation exercises, including the use of computerized mannequins programmed for serious illness parameters or birthing scenarios; the use of a simulation board room to teach group and family therapy, leadership, and to simulate ethics boards. Every clinical program in Drexel's College of Nursing and Health Professions has incorporated simulation experiences into the curriculum, including nursing, physician assistants, physical therapists, nurse anesthetists, and mental health therapists. Most recently, the faculty have incorporated assistive personnel into scenarios to promote team building and effective communication. We are also working with students from the theater and scriptwriting departments for scenario construction, effective prop room management, and creating film clips that can raise the level of distraction during simulations.

I consider this as a "handbook" on the design, evaluation, and practice of simulation for clinical education. If you are a faculty member with concerns about how your students will make the transition from student to professional, use simulation in your curriculum and learn for yourself that *pretending is simulation for life but simulation is pretending for the delivery of exquisite clinical care.*

Gloria F. Donnelly, PhD, RN, FAAN
Dean and Professor
Drexel University
College of Nursing and Health Professions
Philadelphia, PA

CHAPTER 1

Building a Human Simulation Laboratory

Leland J. Rockstraw

INTRODUCTION

*L*ights, camera, action! This battle cry has its history in filming, and I remember wanting to call this out to alert our standardized patients (SPs) or actors as we began to film our health professional students. However, careful planning in the building of a human simulation laboratory (SP simulation) is needed to ensure efficient use, proper professional and actor flow, and clinical education and assessment of participants; then you will be ready to call out "lights, camera, action." In addition to planning the physical layout, understanding the recording software and hardware as presented in chapter 2 will give the reader great insight. This chapter will outline a practical approach in understanding the following key factors to consider in designing a human patient simulation (HPS)/SP laboratory: forming a design team; function and utilization; work flow as it relates to participants, actors, and professional staff; simulation-specific considerations; utilities; and a virtual walkthrough of any future human simulation laboratory. For the ease of the reader, this author uses the following definitions:

- SP—denotes the focus of human simulation specifically to SPs or standardized actors who have historically been used for the education and assessment of clinical competence of the health care provider.
- Participant—a person participating as the customer in the SP experience; this customer can be a health care student, a bedside provider, and in some cases a non–health care professional.
- Encounter—refers to a single participant scenario (simulated experience) that includes not only the actual simulated encounter but also the pre-encounter and post-encounter work.

FORMING A DESIGN TEAM

In building a human simulation/SP laboratory, development and organization of the design team will help provide a deeper and fuller understanding of all considerations of planning and result in building a high-quality and efficient simulation center. The

qualifications and experience of the design team members should include prior simulation experience in the areas of SP simulation and health science examination room
layout construction and/or use. They should also understand the intended use in the
areas of (a) skills practice, (b) education, and (c) assessment, the ability to translate ideas
and visions into a functional image and floor plan, the ability to capture audiovisual of
the participant's experience in both general filming and skill specific, and the general
construction (electric, plumbing, and finishing) of any construction project.

Design team members should include you (the customer with a dream), an SP simulation consultant, a project manager, an architect, a general contractor, a plumbing and
electric contractor (if the general contractor does not have the expertise), an audiovisual
consultant, and an information technology consultant. Individual traits for each team
member should include the following:

- *Customer with a dream*—instrumental in understanding the vision of the stakeholders
  of the SP laboratory; that is, its administrators, faculty, future participants (students),
  and flow.
- *SP simulation consultant*—understands the programmatic use of SPs in the area of
  participant instruction, assessment, and workload, which will aid in educating other
  design team members.
- *Project manager*—responsible for planning, executing, and closing the simulation
  laboratory project. The key to ensuring the collaboration of all team members in the
  areas of design, construction, networking, and telecommunication considerations
  such as scheduling and meeting deadlines and purchasing, receiving, and storing
  equipment and hardware.
- *Architect*—trained and licensed in planning and designing buildings, as well as in
  supervising the construction, electric, and plumbing specifications. This role will
  assist the project manager in closing the project.
- *General contractor*—works with the project manager and is responsible for the overall construction, renovation, and demolition of a space or building. They lend their
  expertise to the planning and implementation phase and the responsibility of following up on the customer's "punch list" to ensure the project is completed to the
  specifications within the building plans.
- *Electric and plumbing contractor*—lends expertise in the areas of electric and plumbing
  work.
- *Audiovisual consultant*—creates a design as it relates to audiovisual capturing, which
  includes camera, microphone, and speaker placements; cabling requirements, rack
  elevations and wring; and computer-aided drafting. He or she also provides technical assistance to all members of the design.
- *Information technology consultant*—a specialist in the use of computers, telecommunications, and storing, retrieval, and transmitting information. Experience in networking
  is strongly suggested.

This team is generally organized by the project manager; however, the customer
may need to inform the project manager of their desire to be an active member of the
design team. From design and through building, weekly or bimonthly meetings are held
to discuss issues, provide clarifications, and ensure all team members are "on the same
page" of the design and building. It is during these meetings that the dream begins to
transform into a reality, and the customer gains valuable insight that will aid well into
the future daily management and operations of the simulation laboratory.

FUNCTION AND UTILIZATION

There are three main methods of health care simulation. SPs (the use of actors to simulate patients in a standardized manner) promote practice and assessment of individual skills such as interpersonal communication, verbal and physical assessment of the patient, and diagnostics reasoning, which is the focus of this chapter and book. Other simulation methods include HPS, or use of full body-length computerized mannequins to promote teamwork; communication between team members; crisis resources management; and task trainers, which are focused, skill-specific simulations such as central line placement, surgery, and other types of invasive high-risk procedures. Many simulation centers are also providing hybrid simulations that will blend any combination of the three methods previously mentioned.

Functionality of simulation laboratories refers to the ability to use the space in certain modalities. Early and frequent discussion with end users (administration, faculty, and future participants) will assist in the design of a simulation center's functionality that will last into the foreseeable future. Some simulation centers serve a single discipline, such as nursing, physician assistant, or medicine, and others serve multiple disciplines; it is important to understand participant disciplines, population sizes, and proposed percentage of use during the planning for annual projection (calendar or academic), and projected growth within the given discipline(s) and participants is vital. Planned use of simulation or examination rooms in educational and assessment can include (a) encounters with SPs (patient–provider interaction and communication skills), (b) task trainers (procedures such as central lines), (c) hybrid encounters (SP and task trainer), and (d) nonsimulation uses (such as skills training or educational practice). Functionality also refers to access and egress of participants, actors, and professional staff, and access to support areas such as offices, observation areas, classrooms, debriefing rooms, break rooms, storage, and bathrooms. Further discussion of space functionality will be provided with room diagrams in the following sections of space and work flow, and detailed room diagrams will be presented in chapter 2.

Space utilization refers to the use or traffic of participants, many times demonstrated as a percentage. Generally, a use rate of 75% is considered to be at capacity (Seropian, 2008). Utilization planning by discipline and population size will aid in the design phase to ensure adequate space of the simulation examination rooms as well as support space (such as classroom and debriefing space). For example, if you were to run a 1-hour encounter for 40 participants, you would be able to accomplish this in 4 hours with 10 examination rooms versus 10 hours with 4 examination rooms. Scheduling of simulation rooms and additional space will become complex, and time spent in understanding and projecting space utilization will ensure adequate space is created for simulation and clinical.

The following space and work flow sections and figures are added to aid the reader in understanding the concept of designing an HPS center. The floor plan presented is one of many possible configurations and may not fit into your current plan for simulation centers; nonetheless, the figures are included to aid in understanding work flow for participants, actors, and professional staff. Any design plans for an HPS center should include a deliberate approach to participant, actor, and professional staff work flow.

SPACE AND WORK FLOW FOR PARTICIPANTS

The typical SP simulation laboratory mimics a provider's office with examination rooms, a reception room, and hallway work stations with patient charts and computers. Space design and participant access to patients should also mimic "real-life" providers' offices, which have both a professional and a medical feel. Generally, participants would be brought into the reception room and stationed in front of a preassigned examination room to familiarize themselves with a pre-encounter case study that will assist them as they prepare to conduct a patient interview and physical examination.

On entering the room, the participant should see and have access to the patient, the medical supplies, and the equipment, as well as the typical examination tables found in a provider's office. The size of examination rooms may dictate placement of furniture and recording equipment and collaborative discussions with the simulation, and the health care construction consultant will be instrumental in the design of examination rooms. Strategic placement of mirrors will assist with providing multiple recording angles in any given room; collaborative discussion between the simulation and the audiovisual consultants is vital to ensure proper placement while providing the professional environment of examination rooms.

During the post-encounter period, participants may be required to complete exercises such as patient care notes, electronic medical records access, surveys, or assessment examinations at stations outside each examination room. The reception area allows for staging a proctor as a receptionist to monitor activity, as well as offering a relaxing seating area if the participant is participating in multiple encounters. The goal of participant flow is twofold: to provide the typical direction that participants would enter and leave patient examination rooms, and to ensure that the flow does not cross or come in

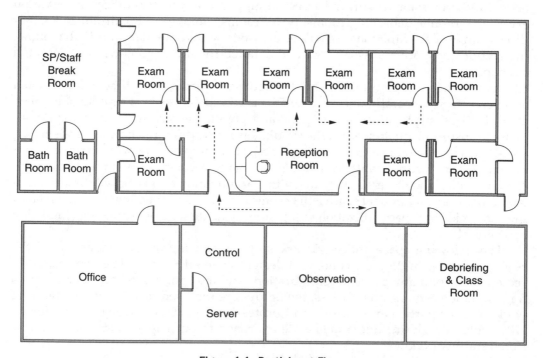

Figure 1.1 *Participant Flow.*

contact with actor flow. See Figure 1.1 for a graphical representation of participant flow into and out of the simulated patient examination rooms.

SPACE AND WORK FLOW FOR ACTORS

The human simulation center should provide the actor with (a) a backdoor access to patient examination rooms, (b) an area to change into patient gowns, and (c) an area to relax between encounters and during breaks. Space design for actor access should allow entry and egress to or from the simulated patient examination rooms without crossing the flow of participants, thus enabling the actor to travel to and from examination rooms and changing rooms, to prepare rooms with health care supplies and equipment, and to gain access to faculty observers. This back door access allows for the free flow work of the actors while protecting the integrity and feel of a "real provider's office" for the participant. Generally, patients (actors) would never be viewed by providers performing room preparation or faculty consultation, and neither would health care students have faculty standing directly outside examination rooms observing student patient interactions, thus having the separate space for actors and faculty will aid in providing for a "real feel."

On entering the room, the actor should have access to medical supplies and equipment from cabinets within the examination room for participant use during the simulation encounter. Easily removable instructional charts and case studies can be posted on the examination room door as called for by the case encounter forms. Restocking of examination gloves, medical linen, and medical supplies and equipment can be easily accomplished between cases and during breaks via the actors' work flow without interrupting the participants' encounter.

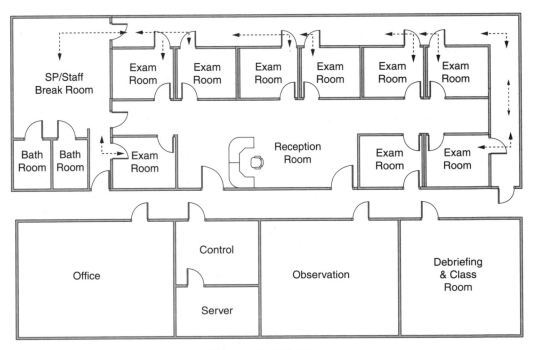

Figure 1.2 *Actor Flow.*

During the post-encounter period, actors would document participants' performance using a computer-generated checklist, which is typically completed immediately after the participant leaves the room; the immediate completion of this checklist allows for the actors' immediate recall of observed performance and offers the participant a respite before returning to the examination room for feedback. Additional information regarding participant evaluation can be found in chapter 4. An actor "office drawer or cabinet" will allow storage of the actors' personal belongings, as well as copies of the case encounter for referencing between encounters. See Figure 1.2 for a graphical representation of actor flow into and out of the simulated patient examination rooms.

SPACE AND WORK FLOW FOR PROFESSIONAL STAFF

The work flow of professional staff will differ as they support and come in contact with participants, patient actors, and faculty. Space design should allow for professional staff access to and from patient examination rooms the same as participants and patient actors. During the pre-encounter period, professional staff may be called on to assist participants in finding appropriate examination room assignment, interpretation of case studies outside the patient examination room, and in calming the nerves of the participant before entrance. In addition, professional staff may be called on to assist actors in room preparation, obtaining the needed case-specific medical supplies or equipment, or answering case-specific questions. The multidimensional work flow allows the greatest access to both participants and actors while protecting the integrity of the simulation experience.

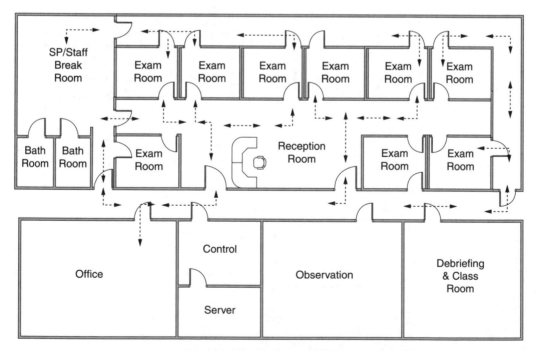

Figure 1.3 *Professional Staff Flow.*

During and after the simulation encounter, the professional staff will need access to the reception area (to assist the proctor or participants), the control room (to monitor filming), the observation room (to assist faculty and other observers), and the office space. The multidimensional aspect of work assistance that professional staff offers both participants and actors could have the professional staff in many rooms of the human simulation center. Proper planning will assist in the effective and efficient use of the space, and professional staffing needs may decrease the actual required full-time equivalents. Space design can also allow for assisting more than one group of participants; that is, appropriate professional staff can work with participants within the simulation suite reception room and then exit and attend to a participant in the classroom or observation area(s). See Figure 1.3 for a graphical representation of professional staff flow into and out of the simulated patient examination rooms.

SIMULATION-SPECIFIC CONSIDERATIONS

The SP experience is one of the three methods of simulation. Planning for effective use of simulation centers may require designs that create multiple methods simulation laboratories, combining SPs, HPSs, and task trainers. Individual specifications such as creation of a new simulation center building versus renovation of the current space, physical size and participant population (current and projected), and funds will affect the size, the level of audiovisual recording installation, and the types of capital equipment used. Familiarization with textbooks, networking, visiting existing simulation centers, and attending health care simulation conferences will greatly assist in the planning and creation of a simulation center that will meet the current and future simulation needs of any institution.

UTILITIES

Understanding utilities such as lighting, electric, plumbing, medical gases, and suction; how sound will affect recording; and security, server, and storage space is important in the design of any simulation center. With construction of an SP simulation center, decisions may be made as a cost-saving measure; because one of the outcomes of construction is to offer a "real-feel" environment, careful considerations should be made to construction costs. Lighting and plumbing and medical gases are expensive line items in any simulation budget. Lighting and plumbing are important in designing the SP laboratory; however, for simulation centers exclusively built for SP simulation, medical gases (such as oxygen and medical air) are typically not required, thus eliminating one expensive line item from the construction budget. Care should be taken in any line item deletions in the planning phase to ensure that no future use plans would change the focus of the simulation laboratories, thereby creating a need for expensive remodeling. Lighting and soundproofing rooms should be explored from the patient examination view as well as audiovisual. The ability to alter lighting and to turn off lights greatly aids the provider in eye examination; however, the ability to provide quality filming is diminished with decreased lighting. Training the SP on what a safe and competent eye examination should feel like will decrease the effects of poor quality recording during eye examination. Installation of sinks in examination rooms with hot and cold water is an additional expense but a great investment toward the creation of a real environment and instruction and the reinforcement of infection control techniques. The adequate soundproofing of examination rooms proves beneficial for both patient assessment and recording of audio. The use of soundproof wall material from the floor, past drop ceilings, to meet the flooring structure of the ceiling assists greatly in preventing sound and noise from traveling between examination rooms and altering the quality of the recorded sound. The deliberate placement of microphones directed toward patient sitting and lying areas and away from noisy air ducts and speakers is suggested.

In the design of space, the storage space should be centrally located to aid with quick and easy access before and between encounters, and while restocking the simulation center at the end of the day. Multiple wide doors will allow for the easy storage of large medical equipment, such as examination tables, if you desire to transform an examination room into a simulated office or community waiting room. Examination rooms should contain space to allow storage of routine medical supplies, and bulk storage of medical supplies can be provided in the storeroom.

In the age of digital media, the placement of the control room and server space is not critical to the proximity of the simulation examination rooms for recording and monitoring of simulation encounters; however, care should be given to the distance of the control room if the expectation of the professional staff working in the control room includes providing assistance to other areas within the simulation center.

Security of space, computers and servers, medical equipment, and audiovisual data requires careful consideration during space planning. Door locks, electronic door card swipes, and electric monitoring of space may be determined by current institutional capabilities and policies. The recording of confidential data (audiovisual) may require additional security measures for students (Family Educational Rights and Privacy Act) as well as planned research activities (Institutional Review Boards and Health Insurance Portability and Accountability Act). The review of all applicable guidelines will help with the understanding and required measures in providing the appropriate level of security for space, equipment, and recorded encounters.

A VIRTUAL WALK-THROUGH

Envision it as a health care professional student. You are scheduled to participate in an SP encounter to measure your competence and skill obtainment in patient interview and assessment techniques. You arrive 15 minutes before the schedule at the simulation center's classroom dressed in your finest professional attire and crisply pressed white laboratory coat, with your tools of practice (a pen light, a stethoscope, a tuning fork, a reflex hammer, and an iPod with electronic references). Your professor greets you warmly and spends 20 minutes providing a prepatient briefing and objectives of today's visit to the simulation center. Approximately 5 minutes before your scheduled start time, you are escorted to the reception room and find your assigned examination room: 7. You take note of the door sign, which provides an introduction to your case, information about the patient you are scheduled to meet, a reminder of the objectives for the simulation experience (you make a note to thank your professor for this reminder), and a note on the time allowed. At the work station just to the left of the door sign, you note that there is a wall computer with access to your patient's electronic medical record; you spend a few minutes looking up laboratory values and results of earlier performed medical tests. There is an announcement overhead, which states "attention in the simulation center, you my now begin your encounter."

It's time. You confidently knock and enter the patient's examination room. You encounter a 55-year-old patient lying on his left side in a fetal position, moaning in pain, asking for your help to make him feel better; something in the back of your mind says, "Take note of this, I think this: might be important." You introduce yourself to your patient, and while you are washing your hands, you ask the patient to share with you the reason behind his visit today to the provider's office. You sit down and begin to implement the interview skills and techniques of interpersonal communication, obtaining the current information related to the chief complaint and pertinent past medical history, and a focused physical examination. You find yourself growing alarmed with the patient's chief complaint of severe left flank pain and plan your assessment skills and diagnostic reasoning accordingly. Suddenly, there is an announcement that you have 5 minutes remaining to complete your encounter; you are surprised how quickly 35 minutes have passed and are confident that you have determined that your patient's chief complaint is related to possible pancreatitis. You finish your patient encounter by educating him with the additional laboratory tests you would like to accomplish and a possible hospital stay, and ask again if he has any questions. You shake his hand and explain that you will return shortly; as you exit the room, an overhead announcement states, "Attention, the encounter is now over; please exit the examination rooms." You nailed this one perfectly. You sit on one of the couches in the reception room and talk excitedly with one of your fellow students, being careful not to share any confidential patient information. Approximately 5 minutes later, you are invited back into examination room 7 and immediately notice that your patient is smiling and stands and shakes your hand as you enter the room. The feedback begins as you close the door and sit down across from an SP actor trained to provide targeted advice on your verbal and physical assessment skills. The 5 minutes allotted for feedback passes quickly. When the overhead announcement is made to exit the simulation center, you smile as you recall your answer to the actor's quire, "What led you to focus your assessment on possible pancreatitis?" and you reply that it was his position on the examination table as you entered that began your targeted assessment.

CONCLUSIONS

The creation of an HPS center may begin with a dream; however, it ends with deliberate planning and designing. You begin to share this dream with a group of professionals trained and experienced in designing, planning, and constructing simulation centers is critical in ensuring effective and efficient space utilization. Designing a space that promotes the practice and objective assessment of a functional SP simulation center with state-of-the-art audiovisual capturing apparatus, medical equipment, and furniture will aid in the transformation of your dream into a reality. The creation of a learning laboratory that is clinically safe not only allows the participant to practice to the edge of her comfort zone, but also offers a sort of safety net in taking calculated risks in that your patients are not patients, but only actors playing patients, and your decisions (right or wrong) will not harm them. Your experience in the simulation laboratory will aid in your learning, practice at patient interview and physical assessment skills, and diagnostic reasoning.

REFERENCES

Seropian, M. (2008). Simulation facility design 101: The basics. In R. R. Kyle, Jr. & W. B. Murray (Eds.), *Clinical simulation: Operations, engineering, and management* (pp. 177–185). Burlington, MA: Academic Press.

SUGGESTED READING

Jeffries, P. R. (2007). *Simulation in nursing education—From conceptualization to evaluation.* New York: National League of Nursing.

Kyle, R. R. (2008). *Clinical simulation—Operations, engineering and management.* Burlington, MA: Elsevier.

CHAPTER 2

Hardware and Software

Sukhtej S. Dhingra and Laurie L. Kerns

INTRODUCTION

*H*uman simulation laboratories offer a safe, practice-based learning and teaching environment. The effectiveness of this environment is an important consideration for any organization. The quantitative representation of the learning outcomes provides significant insight into the needs and design for improved simulation and evaluation techniques over time. These factors define the needs for hardware and software tools to assist any simulation laboratory to meet its objectives. The best systems use the latest Internet-based information technology (IT) and audiovisual recording solutions. The functional capabilities of these systems include learner-focused teaching and training along with efficient operation and administration needs of the laboratory. This chapter presents the unique functions that these tools provide for effective learning, as well as the important space design considerations for efficient operations and administration of the simulation laboratory.

LEARNING AND TEACHING SYSTEMS FOR SIMULATION LABORATORIES

An immersive experience is the ultimate goal for a human simulation laboratory, and simulating a real-life situation is a challenge in itself. Creating a controlled environment that includes other external systems, such as recording and evaluation tools, presents complex design decisions and implementation hurdles. The need to capture this experience demands careful planning and proper selection of hardware and software solutions. Generally, these tools include software application solutions to capture the training and assessment of the simulation, as well as a hardware solution to capture and facilitate the playback of the simulation experience. These systems also provide the means for efficient operations and administration of the simulation laboratory. The required level of details for the immersive experience drives the selection and configuration of these tools.

This chapter presents the definition of the needs for the simulation training and assessment and how the design of a well-equipped simulation laboratory then offers the best educational tool for the learners. The ease of use as well as the flexibility offered by these tools to meet the demands of simulation is the measure of any successful simulation laboratory.

SIMULATION LABORATORY DESIGN

Simulation laboratories are designed within the scope of scenarios conducted for training and evaluation. The education and practice provided by the simulation session is driven by the settings—as a clinical training center or competency and continuing assessment center. The combination of the two is generally the norm given the cost of building and operating such a facility.

Human simulation laboratories typically conduct three forms of simulation: human patient, hardware based, and software based. Each form requires specific system functionality to capture the experience and to achieve the learning objectives. Human patient simulation includes actors and standardized patients (SPs) that provide evaluation for human communication and behavioral learning. Hardware-based simulation use sophisticated electronic and mechanical simulators—full-body or task trainers—to provide tools for skills training in a safe environment. Software-based simulation may use virtual reality to provide tools to train and assess clinical knowledge and decision-making skills.

Human simulation laboratories also allow scene-based simulations, where the space is remodeled to depict the required scene for participants to experience and learn. This staging of a simulated scene requires the flexibility and reuse of equipment for different situations. An alternative that is gaining popularity is to create one setting for the space—like operating room, intensive care unit, multiple-bed hospital room, and so forth—to allow for more focused scene settings. All of these variations require hardware and software tools to be adaptable and compatible with the needs of the simulation.

Another factor that plays an important role in defining the needs for hardware and software tools is the facility layout. The size of the laboratory as well as the demand for administration defines the specific needs for the solution that will provide the most effective and efficient operations.

The following sections provide details on the hardware and the software tools that should be considered, as well as the space needed and the layout design for the facility. These tools do not have to be commercially available tools; they can be procured and designed within the resources available in an organization. For example, the learning management system (LMS) can be customized to achieve the training and assessment needs of the laboratory. Also, consulting with your organization's IT/information system and multimedia/audiovisual group can provide many tools for immediate needs. It is important to acknowledge the need for a multidisciplinary team to evaluate and to recommend the final design. The description here is limited to the generic design considerations and the minimum requirements that the implemented technology will provide the most benefit for the learners.

LEARNING AND TEACHING SYSTEM

The rapid growth in hardware technology and application software makes it difficult to provide a design solution that can adapt and use these advancements. The compatibility of the solution to be supported and upgraded with time should be a consideration in the design during the buildup stage. The focus should be on the currently available technology and software tools that are engineered to suit the design requirements. For early adopters, it is paramount that the technology is reviewed and perceived as the most progressive and that it will be backed by the manufacturer and supported by the vendor.

Another design challenge stems from selecting multiple systems, using diverse technology, to be engineered as an integrated solution. These systems include audiovisual, IT, information system, simulators, and LMSs. An option here is to explore commercially engineered solutions that can provide a packaged yet customizable solution. An alternative would be to partner with solution integrators who will collaborate, design, and implement an integrated solution for your laboratory. The last option may be the most expensive option as it requires independent project analysis and design. The first option is suited for one to start small, with limited implementation, and then expand on the basis of the emerging needs and lessons learned. The commercial solution provides the best option to gain from the integrator's experience, to explore all design options, and to select the best viable integrated solution.

The hardware and the software selection will also be dependent on the expected utilization of the simulation laboratory. The expected number of learners and departments using the laboratory will drive the hardware and software functionality to cater to the operational and administrative needs of the laboratory. Redundancy and high availability of these solutions should be considered in the planning stages to offset the heavy demand phases and the near-future growth expectation. This expectation will drive the final configuration of the systems deployed in the laboratory.

The following sections present the hardware and the software tools to consider in supporting the simulation laboratory. The software solution is described first, which will be used throughout the laboratory. A web-based solution provides access flexibility via any network-connected PC workstation. This allows laboratory operations to be managed by any staff member from anywhere in the simulation laboratory. The next section presents the descriptions of the hardware—audiovisual, system control, and presentation tools—that are required on the basis of the physical layout and the space considerations of the rooms. The description is limited to the technology tools available for learning and teaching. The operational workflow management is an important factor in selecting these technology tools. The hardware tools are focused on IT, audiovisual recording and streaming, and laboratory intercom and public address systems. Descriptions do not include content-specific tools like high-fidelity mannequin simulators, specific task trainers, and so forth.

LEARNING MANAGEMENT SYSTEMS

LMSs in the context of the simulation laboratory are defined as an application for managing the learning content, the learner training, the learner evaluation, and the laboratory operations. The IT-based solution provides access via the web and has a password-protected user access that is based on assigned rights controlled by a simulation administrators. The system offers multiple task-oriented functions to manage the complete learning process by the teaching faculty and the laboratory administrative staff. The system also provides functions for operational needs as laboratory scheduling, calendar management, operational reports, utilization statistics, and laboratory inventory. All these functional tasks are defined as the user's role in the system and allow team collaboration to create and manage the information.

The following functions broadly define the system requirements of any learning management application for a simulation laboratory.

1. Role definition and access management—the ability to define roles for the users, including learners and default access permission to the information stored in the system. This role definition then allows the administration of user classification and session scheduling for the laboratory. Examples of such roles include faculty, observer, instructor, learner, actor, and so forth. The user access permission adds another layer of security in terms of the access—read, write, or edit—to the information stored within the system. For example, access to learner evaluation reports could be restricted to only the faculty involved with that simulation and would be off limits to the learner or the actor.

2. User management—the ability to manage the user information in the system. This entails managing user profiles, including updates, and authenticating user access to the system. Given the number of users expected to participate in the simulation activity, it is recommended that the system be integrated with the institution's centralized user directory authentication system (sometimes referred to as *active directory* or *Lightweight Directory Access Protocol user directory authentication*). The system will keep the history of the user (e.g., graduating class) to allow context-based reporting and statistical analysis. Automatic communication with the user—via e-mail, text messaging, telephone, and so forth—regarding simulation sessions, learning activity, and reports is a desired but optional feature of the system.

3. Simulation scenario management—the ability to manage the simulation scenario content, including reference materials, educational outcome objectives, and program and course curriculum objectives. The system provides a placeholder for scene definition, scene enactment details, participant scripts, scenario management paths, scenario distraction paths, and alternative scenario endings (optional). This information then provides a standard reference to evaluate and to compare the simulation effectiveness and learning outcomes for targeted learner groups.

4. Calendar management—the ability to manage the simulation laboratory schedule and to maximize laboratory utilization. The system allows laboratory administrative staff to manage users and laboratory resources efficiently to conduct simulation. The system should offer communication features like e-mail, text messages, and so forth, to inform and to accept reservations from users to use laboratory resources. Even laboratory resources—simulators, medical devices, and so forth—should be scheduled and managed within the system.

5. Assessment item management—the ability to define and to use question items and evaluation checklists to assess learning and simulation effectiveness. The capability to manage an item library, including questionnaire checklist items, scoring criteria for evaluation, and survey feedback from a simulation session, is an important function of the system. The information captured will present the user with statistical reports on the performance of the learner groups and learning outcome assessment of the simulation.

6. Reports management—the ability to create score reports and analytical statistics for learning performance and resource utilization. The system offers predefined learner- and system-specific reports for automated publishing and distribution. The system will also have the capability to export raw data from any reference—date, user, scenario, and so forth—for further analysis by the user.

7. Advanced features and integration modules—the ability to offer additional advanced features and integration modules to expand the laboratory operations. These features

are driven by the needs of the simulation laboratories. Some examples of such advanced features include actor online training modules, simulation course management, laboratory inventory management, assistance in managing external clients for simulation training, and so forth.

8. Besides built-in functions, LMS systems should have integration capability to synchronize information with other systems used in the laboratory. These integration modules include data interface to high-fidelity patient simulators, task trainers, and so forth. This information exchange allows the LMS to store a complete information history of the simulation and allows the user to review all aspects of the simulation for debriefing and postanalysis. The desired integration is limited to the functions made available by the simulator manufacturer and the capability of the system integrator to incorporate the interfaces in the system design.

The functional modules described above provide the framework for any simulation laboratory to manage laboratory functions. These functions may already be available in the organization. However, the synergy of a comprehensive single system will provide optimum effectiveness to the operations and administration.

LMS system features primarily focus on information-based data saved in a relational database on a server. However, multimedia graphical information and digital video recording with web streaming have added an important technology dimension that is essential for any simulation laboratory.

DIGITAL VIDEO RECORDING AND WEB-STREAMING SYSTEM

Digital video recording is defined as the recording of videocamera images by a digital video capture device. These are cameras with built-in recording capability—a camcorder, combination of camera and digital recording device, or web camera and PC recorder. A camera with built-in recording capability offers convenience but limits the user with respect to camera specification and recording capacity. A second option of matching any camera with any digital video recorder provides the flexibility on camera specification—light sensitivity, zoom, and pan–tilt–zoom—and digital video recording format—resolution, storage capacity, and streaming capability. The cameras are also available with different signal output formats—analog or digital—that will then be matched with the digital video recorders (DVR) with analog inputs or digital media storage. Although the video recorder is generally always referenced in context of camera view, there is also a microphone audio that is recoded in sync with the video.

The selection of the digital video recording system should be driven within the confines of the available technology of videocameras and recording devices. Recent advances and emerging technology need to be supported by the manufacturer and the industry. Another factor is the proprietary formats of the video recording and the limitation to the distribution via the Web or storage devices like USB flash drives and CDs and DVDs. If possible, the recording format should be accepted as a standard open source in the video recording and streaming industry.

In addition to the specification of the devices, the physical form factor of these devices needs to be considered to provide a distraction-free simulation experience for the learners. The room layout design should take this into consideration for installation and operation needs. The camera locations should be unobstructed during the scenario and should provide a clear view of the scene for effective video recording and debriefing. Also, the space and its layout will drive the number of microphones to be used to capture the conversation in the room.

All video recordings saved in the digital format are cataloged and made available for distribution by the web-streaming system. The current technology of database-driven video indexing—referenced against time, date, scenario, participant, and instructor—is critical for the easy search and retrieval of the video recordings. The access depends on the user's role and the access permission assigned by the laboratory, where it is either restricted to specific users within the laboratory or available for everyone online via the web. The web streaming over the Internet then involves support of the institution's network support team to allow secured user access to the video archive via the web.

The confluence of evaluation and video information stored in digital format and rendered on demand over any network-enabled device becomes an important operational need for any teaching and learning system implemented in the simulation laboratory.

SYSTEM LAYOUT DESIGN FOR SIMULATION LABORATORY

The simulation laboratory is a safe, practice-based learning center for the user. This experience can be enhanced and more effective with proper planning of the laboratory space design. For a center with specific needs, this task is easier as the focus of the design is to replicate real-life situations. However, this one-purpose design will be restrictive if multifunction simulation and training space is desired.

Day-to-day operation of the simulation laboratory needs to be reviewed before the acceptance of the space design. The separation of learners from other users and administrative staff is important to provide a perception of real-life experience for the learners. The complete experience for the learner from entry to the simulation laboratory to the last simulation activity should mimic closely the needs of the simulation scenario. Efforts should be taken during scheduling to spread the simulation time schedule to minimize interaction between multiple simulation activities for different learner groups. All this can be achieved by careful planning of the space layout and the expected user flow in the space during any simulation.

The following sections describe the technology tools on the basis of generic physical locations in the simulation laboratory. The physical layouts are rooms that provide specific simulation functions in the laboratory. The description provides examples of room types and technology requirements pertinent to the simulations conducted in the room. These should be used as guidelines to incorporate the tools as deemed necessary for the space design. Also, it is important to consider the capacity of the tools to change with any transformation of the physical space to provide flexibility and multifunctional capability.

Control Room

This room serves as the command center for the laboratory during any activity. The layout and the location of this room should allow convenient access from all parts of the laboratory. The room will require the maximum technology tools to assist in the operations of the laboratory. It will host a centralized video display wall to monitor all cameras in the laboratory. Communications equipment such as an intercom, overhead paging, public address, and a security monitor need to be designed and installed to make this a one-person operation. It should be noted that the control room not only serves as the administration of the laboratory but also provides (space permitting) control of simulator equipment in the laboratory. This is designed as a separate designated area within the room and should not interfere with the laboratory operation command center.

Hospital Simulation Room (With Control Room)

This will be designed to reflect a specific functional area such as an ER, ICU, or hospital room—within any hospital. The decision on the final layout should depend on the number of rooms in the laboratory and the expected usage of the room type. Special attention to details will allow the learners to be immersed in the learning experience. The simulators and trainers installed in the room need to be wired for remote control and ideally located in a control room adjacent to this room (Figure 2.1). Multiple cameras (minimum of three) should be installed to capture the activity with all its learners. If possible, a one-way mirror window should be installed to allow direct viewing from the control room. A raised platform in the control room will allow viewers to have an overhead view of the simulation activity. All cables to control simulator and training equipment should be hidden or covered for safety and realism. The room should also have a large TV display panel for learners to review laboratory results (content controlled from the control room), reference information, electronic health records, and activity documentation tracking. The display can also be used to stream, LIVE, the activity in the room for group viewing and review.

The control room will have complete control of the simulation room. It should have the capability in which the instructor can switch the power off in the simulation room, manage air-conditioning, and provide the "voice of god" via the overhead speaker. The user can use an intercom to communicate with the simulation participant regarding, for example, laboratory results, department calls, and so forth. The room will be equipped with display panels to review and to control the cameras in the simulation room. The start and stop of video recording will also be controlled from a workstation connected to the digital video recording system in this room.

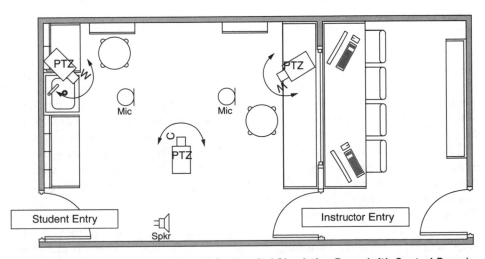

Figure 2.1 *Conceptual Layout Design for Hospital Simulation Room (with Control Room).*

Clinical Simulation Room

This room will be a simulation of a physician clinic room (Figure 2.2). The room should be equipped with at least two cameras to capture the facial expression of the learner and the patient actor (SP). An overhead speaker connected to the paging system from the central control room will allow the operational staff to manage the session schedule. A workstation placed in the room will be used by the patient actor to provide evaluation/feedback on the learner's performance. The room can also have one-way mirror windows for direct observation.

Just outside the room, next to the student entry door, another workstation should be placed on either a wall-mounted cabinet or a small desk to allow the learner to document the follow-up postclinical information in the LMS. The security of the workstation at this location will be either through a cabinet lock or storing the workstations/laptops at another location.

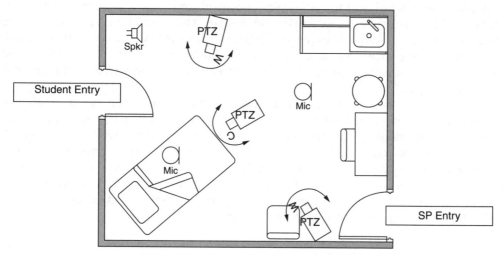

Figure 2.2 *Conceptual Layout Design for Clinical Simulation Room.*

Nursing Ward/Multiple-Bed Room

This may simulate a multiple bed hospital room to recreate recovery room or a practice room. The open layout design will also allow rearranging the room for other group learning sessions. Given the flexibility an open space offers, it creates the challenge for the placement of audiovisual hardware to capture the experience. The cameras should be placed on specific bed locations with localized microphones unless there is a specific need to have cameras and microphones for all beds. Also, the system should include a touch panel with preprogrammed configurations to allow the operator to mark different sets of cameras to record one activity. In such cases, the video recordings from the camera set will be mapped to a particular activity.

For more flexibility in using the system, cameras can be installed on track rails, which will permit mobility to position the camera anywhere on the track. Additional cameras will be required to capture the general view of the room to accommodate

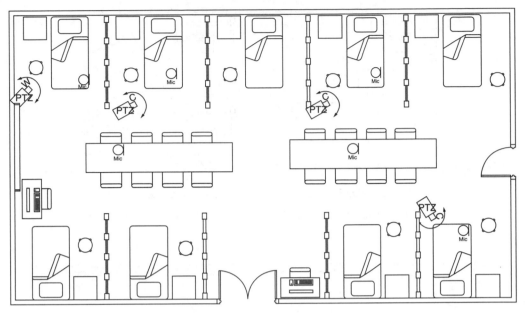

Figure 2.3 *Conceptual Layout Design for Nursing Ward—Multiple Hospital Beds.*

group learning or multiple-activity sessions. Additional functionality with overhead paging speakers and an instructor-led public address system can be added to facilitate the operations within the room (Figure 2.3).

In addition, a space should be designated with a desktop workstation for access to the LMS. This area can be setup with workbenches that can be used for group discussions as well as have laptops placed to access online resources. A projector with screen should also be available for group reviews and presentations.

Problem-Based Learning Room

This room provides a combination of simulation and conference room setup to allow team-based learning. One section of the room permits a few team members to participate in a simulation activity while others are observing from the other section. The instructor-led training allows the instructor to control the pace of the sessions and to provide pertinent break points to discuss the simulation activity. The room is equipped with cameras and microphones to capture both sections of the room. The system will allow users to capture either side's events in parallel or as a single event as desired (Figure 2.4).

Home Care Health Room

This room is set up for home care—apartment, home room—to allow home care training and evaluation. The cameras will be placed with discretion to record all activity, and a standard work space in the room can have a computer workstation to access the LMS system. Options to control the power, the air-conditioning, and other effects can be installed and monitored from the central control room (Figure 2.5).

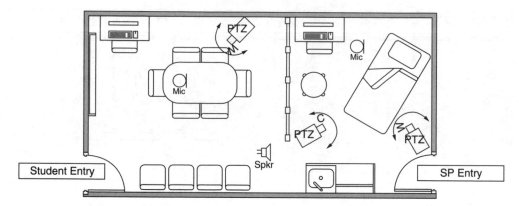

Figure 2.4 *Conceptual Layout Design for Problem-Based Learning Room.*

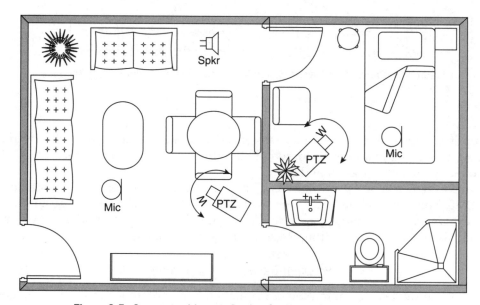

Figure 2.5 *Conceptual Layout Design for Home Care Health Room.*

Procedure Training Room

This is a multifunctional room with designated work spaces as individual training stations. These stations include task trainers and virtual reality (computer-based) simulation stations. The stations will be equipped with recording cameras, as well as capture—if possible—the activity from the instrument. The learner's actions and the instrument display activity should be recorded for synchronized playback to allow for evaluation and feedback.

Conference/Debriefing Room

This is a multifunctional room that will have standard conference and multimedia presentation capability. The projection system is linked to LMS and a web-streaming system to allow participants to observe any room in the laboratory. Cameras installed in this room can be used to record the debriefing session, which is then mapped with the simulation activity. An override control function needs to be installed to disable camera viewing and recording of this room for private meetings.

All technology present in the room will be managed via a central control—either touch screen panel or wall push button—located in the room. This will control all audio-visual channels, computers, projections, audio speakers, and so forth. If required, this room can also be equipped with a videoconferencing capability, which can be used for remote meetings as well as distance learning. The system is also programmed to allow camera feeds from any simulation room to be transmitted for viewing at the remote location via the video conference system.

Observation Rooms

These rooms serve as places to observe the simulation activity from any room in the laboratory. The layout can be multifunctional to serve as a conference/meeting room as well as a small classroom. Besides this, the room will have multiple observation work-stations and a large video display panel. These display devices will be connected to the LMS and the web-streaming system to select and view any simulation room within the laboratory. The users can then perform independent, activity-based observation as well as have group observation of any activity. These rooms can also be used for postactivity individual reviews and debriefings.

If the room shares a common wall with any simulation room, it is recommended that a one-way mirror window be installed to allow direct observation. The audio from the simulation room can be heard on an installed speaker or headphone ports near the mirror window.

Waiting/Staging Area

Multiple rooms should be made available to stage groups in the simulation laboratory. The groups will include actors and SPs, various learner groups, faculty, and observers. The needs will be driven by the simulation schedule, and care should be taken to prevent accidental meetings of these groups. All these rooms should have overhead paging speakers for public address. The actor and SP staging area should have work-stations to access the LMS system. This will also help to host training sessions for new members of the group. The learner staging area could be monitored via videocamera for security and managing the activity schedule. Some rooms can be equipped with a video display panel for use as a classroom, a session briefing and debriefing area, and/or a self-study area.

Server Room

This will be "another" closet besides the network and telecommunication closet for the simulation laboratory. The room's location and design should be in compliance with the organization's data center code. Uninterrupted electrical supply and air-conditioning needs are paramount in providing a successful back-end support to the laboratory operations. This room hosts computer servers and audiovisual equipment racks to support the LMS and the web-streaming system. The access to the room needs to be secured to avoid an unauthorized access to the data servers. Special needs to monitor and provide uninterrupted service—temperature sensors, power surge protectors, and battery backup—should be planned and implemented as per the requirements.

Security System

This should be an important consideration for the simulation laboratory, especially if the location is close to open areas within the building such as a cafeteria, student lounge, and so forth. The system can be part of the organization's security system or an independent system for the laboratory. The system will include secured access—keycard, pin lock—for restricted entry as well as security camera monitors with a minimum of 72 hours recording time. Special multiplexed viewing stations can be placed in the central control room and near the administration offices for general observation.

Reception

The entry way to the laboratory can provide the start of the simulation experience or a waiting room for the learner. A digital signage screen with a sign-in kiosk will allow learners and visitors to assimilate with the laboratory and get automated assistance to register and get instructions to proceed to a staging area. This assistive technology tool can maintain the visitor log and provide useful laboratory utilization information. A security camera and a key card access control will be required for the security of the operational staff, especially if the area will not be continuously staffed.

Hallways and Corridors

All hallways should be equipped with proper overhead paging speakers to allow efficient work flow management. The ability to monitor the space using cameras and the ability to make announcements from the control room will allow one member of the operations staff to manage multiple activities in the laboratory. Intercoms should be placed at various places for users to communicate with the operations staff.

Administration Offices

These rooms are typical office rooms with standard desktop workstations to allow access to the LMS and the web-streaming system. Depending on the layout, a security camera display in one of the offices will allow monitoring of the laboratory from one location. An overhead paging system connected with the rest of the laboratory will allow the staff to be aware of and direct the laboratory activity.

Distance Learning

As part of providing training and assessment tools using simulation, the laboratory can be equipped for long-distance learning. Along with the LMS and the web-streaming system, the capability to conduct telemedicine or videoconferencing passive learning activity will be an added benefit. Clinical rooms can be equipped with a recording technology to record telephone conversations between a learner and a remote patient or colleague. Also, in multiple campus settings, remote learners can watch any simulation and participate in the debriefing using the videoconferencing system installed in the conference and debriefing room.

Mobile/Portable Recording System

This will provide an in situ video recording capability to push the learning opportunity beyond the physical confines of the simulation laboratory. The system is portable and works independently of the simulation laboratory systems. The user will be able to take the system to any location to conduct simulations. All recordings are available within the system for instant debriefing and playback. Once the system is brought back to the simulation laboratory, recordings can be transferred and synced with the systems in the laboratory. Multiple units may be made available depending on the usage as well as added to the system with growing demand.

CONCLUSIONS

A simulation laboratory provides an effective learning and teaching method as well as serves as an experience to remember for the learners. The reinforcement of this learning with video feedback and quantitative evaluation provides enhanced education and practical experience. The return on investment from a well-designed solution that will provide a safe learning environment as well as an opportunity to improve the learning techniques is a major factor to consider when deciding to purchase such a system. It is important to understand the learning outcome needs and to match those with the available technology to provide a safe and effective learning environment using simulation laboratories.

SUGGESTED READING

Bradley, P. (2006). The history of simulation in medical education and possible future directions. *Medical Education, 40,* 254–262.

Errichetti, T., & Dhingra, S. S. (2008). *Instructional technology planning for medical simulation labs.* Exton, PA: White Paper Education Management Solutions.

Jeffries, P. R. (2007). *Simulation in nursing education—From conceptualization to evaluation.* New York: National League of Nursing.

Kyle, R. R. (2008). *Clinical simulation—Operations, engineering and management.* Burlington, MA: Elsevier.

Salas, E., Wilson, K. A., Burke, C. S., & Priest, H. A. (2005). Using simulation-based training to improve patient safety—What does it take? *Journal on Quality and Patient Safety, 31*(7), 363–372.

CHAPTER 3

What Is a Standardized Patient?

Michael J. Onori, Fabien Pampaloni, and Nina Multak

The clinical competence of health care providers is achieved in the educational environment through the standardization of training and assessment, and standardized patients (SPs) are commonly utilized to accomplish this goal. An SP is an individual who has been trained to portray a patient in a consistent manner and has the capability to present a variety of health care issues. Simulation training with SPs enables nursing, medical, and other health profession students to develop their clinical and interpersonal skills in a controlled environment before encountering actual patients in a clinical setting.

HISTORY OF THE SP

The concept of a programmed patient was first introduced in 1963 by neurologist and medical educator Dr. Howard S. Barrows from the University of Southern California. The term *standardized patient* was coined in the late 1970s by Geoffrey Norman, a Canadian psychometrician. Around the same time, Dr. Paula Stillman, a pediatric clerkship director at the University of Arizona, contributed to the development of an assessment instrument. This tool was used to assess both the content and process of simulated medical experiences to give accurate and useful feedback to the students. It was not until the early 1980s that the SP concept was actually used as a recognized educational tool for teaching and assessment using simulated patients in health care institutions around the world (May, 2008; Wallace, 1997).

An SP, also known as a simulated patient or patient instructor (Austin, Gregory, & Tabak, 2006), is an individual trained to portray a patient with a variety of health-related conditions. An SP can portray an individual with both physical and behavioral issues, providing a realistic experience for students in a controlled setting. In addition to medical conditions, an SP may also present an ethical dilemma or an event with a focus on communication skills. This allows a student to have the opportunity to develop their interpersonal and clinical skills in a safe environment. Some of these skills include patient interview and assessment, team collaboration, psychotherapeutic intervention, and patient education. Although these are only a few of the basic teaching tools for the student, SPs are carefully trained to provide scenarios with a high degree of realism, effectively mimicking actual encounters with a patient in a hospital or some other clinical venue.

DESIGNING A SCRIPT

The first step in standardizing training begins with case scenario development. Cases that are used in preparing an individual for their role can either be real or fictional. Of course, the name of the patient in an actual case would be changed. Cases can be designed for one person and may also be developed for a group of SPs playing a family of sorts, such as in psychotherapy encounters. Nevertheless, it is very important that the individual(s) playing the role remains standardized throughout the encounter to give each student the same opportunity to practice their skills with little or no deviation from the script. This includes using the same opening line, exactly as written, and the behavioral affect as well. Cases can range from having a simple headache to more complex cases such as appendicitis or congestive heart failure. Most cases also include past medical history, social and family history, medications, allergies, and other information that may be pertinent to the overall characteristics of the role the SP is playing. Also, there may be one or two challenging questions that the SP gives the student to see how he or she responds. On the basis of whether a student is in their first year of school or last year, the complexity of a case is adjusted to fit their present learning skills.

RECRUITING STANDARDIZED PATIENTS

SPs can be recruited locally to support a health care simulation training program. Retirees, hospital volunteers, actors, and students can be effectively trained to portray patients of varying age groups. Labor laws prevent employment of minors for pediatric cases. Standardization of patient encounters occurs through the use of SPs, who are not known to the examinees. Use of faculty members or other students in a student's training program may introduce bias on the part of the SP, who may be asked to grade the student.

Competency, Assessment, and Grading

Clinical skills are more effectively evaluated with the use of SPs than with traditional multiple-choice assessment. SPs rate each student on the content of an encounter according to an established grading rubric, generally developed by the faculty in the student's educational training program. If the student encounter is part of a high-stakes examination, the grading criteria are established by a group of professionals in the field.

Health care provider students may encounter SPs in a single-station session or in multiple station sessions. An Objective Structured Clinical Examination (OSCE) is used commonly to assess competence in clinical skills. An OSCE is a circuit-like examination with several 5- to 10-minute stations. At each station, a student encounters an SP or other simulated modality requiring a skill to be performed (Harden & Gleeson, 1979). In some health care disciplines in North America, SPs are utilized in OSCEs for which successful completion enables the student to graduate, to proceed to the next step in their health care training, or to gain licensure (Felbush, 2002).

At the conclusion of each individual SP encounter, the student leaves the examination room and the SP completes the grading portion of the encounter, which consists of checklist items or rating scales, typically completed on a computer that is provided in each examination room. The student evaluation primarily focuses on interpersonal and physical examination skills. With regard to the interpersonal skills, some of the items may include the following: Did the student have good eye contact (>50%)? Did he/she introduce him or herself (name and professional title)? Did they use terminology understandable to the patient (three-strike rule)? Did the student interrupt the patient when in conversation? Did the student show empathy or encouragement toward the patient during the encounter? In reference to the physical examination portion of the encounter, some of the items listed would be as follows: Did the student wash their hands before doing the physical examination? Did the student listen to the patient's lungs bilaterally in the appropriate locations? Did the student check the patient's blood pressure in different positions? Did the student do a heart examination? Did the student use a drape to cover the patient during examination to protect the patient's modesty? Some of the checklist items may also ask if the student was well-versed in educating the patient on a particular subject. For example, did the student talk about the importance of taking medication as prescribed and that quitting smoking now would greatly reduce certain risks?

A note to mention here, other than the case materials taught, is that the SP is well-trained in physical examination techniques by professional staff. This grading process of both interpersonal and physical examination skills can be used as part of the student's actual grade or as a tool to improve their skills as they continue to move forward in their education.

FEEDBACK

The final phase in an SP encounter is the feedback session. This is probably the most important and rewarding part of the total simulated encounter for both the student and the individual(s) playing their prospective roles. Once the student and the SP have completed their postencounter documentation, the student returns to the examination room for feedback, which is given from a patient's perspective. SP feedback is provided following an encounter by students who are in formative training. Students who are involved in summative or high-stakes evaluation may receive feedback from a medically trained rater or faculty member. Postencounter feedback from an SP may consist of many different facets that took place during the encounter. The main focus discussed here is whether the student made the SP feel comfortable during the encounter. The conversation between students includes both positive and constructive feedback. The SP should discuss what the students did well and what they could work on the next time. Both positive and constructive feedback should be followed with examples. Regardless of what feedback is given to the student, it should always be done with a smile. They are there to learn from the experience, not to be reprimanded for not doing a good job.

Generally, sessions are digitally recorded, enabling the student to view their performance at a later time. Also, quality assurance takes place during these encounters. If there was a problem or disagreement between the student and the SP, the recording can be viewed by staff or faculty to make any corrections needed. An encounter at random may be watched and graded from another room by either faculty or another SP to assure that both the viewer and SP in the encounter are in tune with each other.

The SP program is an excellent training modality for anyone in health care education. Although these encounters are all simulated with actor patients from different ages, backgrounds, cultures, and so forth, these experiences with students are as close to real encounters as possible. Interpersonal, clinical, and communication skills included in an effective SP training program will likely reduce medical error and increase patient satisfaction and compliance with medical treatment, assuring clinically competent providers. The rewards of standardized patient programs are far reaching.

REFERENCES

Austin, Z., Gregory, P., & Tabak, D. (2006). Simulated patients vs. standardized patients in objective structured clinical examinations. *American Journal of Pharmaceutical Education, 70*(5), 1–7.

Felbush, K. C. (2002). *USMLE Step 2* (3rd ed.). Baltimore, MD: Lippincott, Williams and Wilkins.

Harden, R. M., & Gleeson, F. A. (1979). Assessment of clinical competence using an objective structured clinical examination (OSCE). *Medical Education, 13*, 39–54.

Holmboe, E., & Hawkins, R. (Eds.). (2008). *Practical guide to the evaluation of clinical competence.* Philadelphia, PA: Mosby/Elsevier.

May, W. (2008). Training standardized patients for a high-stakes clinical performance examination in the California consortium for the assessment of clinical competence. *Kaohsiung Journal of Medicine, 24*(12), 640–645.

Wallace, P. (1997). Following the threads of an innovation: The history of standardized patients in medical education. *Caduceus, 13*(2), 5–28.

CHAPTER 4

Development of Evaluation Measures for Human Simulation: The Checklist

Karen J. Saewert and Leland J. Rockstraw

INTRODUCTION

*T*he challenges associated with clinical evaluation mirror those faced when doing evaluations in general (Krichbaum, Rowan, Duckett, Ryden, & Savik, 1994). Although there have been advances and improvements in clinical evaluation practice, the underlying difficulties of past decades remain and include the following: (a) inherent bias and subjectivity of evaluation based on direct observation; (b) subjectivity of a performance-based process situated in the authentic or simulated environment, where it is subject to the influence of the clinical milieu, actions of others, and responses of patients; and (c) different learning and clinical evaluation situations for each student, which are created by the ever-changing clinical milieu, challenging our ability to evaluate students in the same way, on the same bases, or under the same circumstances (Saewert & Yarbrough, 2009).

Evaluation of health care professional students has historically been limited to written testing and observation in the clinical setting. Evaluation using written testing is considered more objective because it gives the evaluator the ability to use statistical analysis to determine overall test and test item validity and reliability, in addition to being able to evaluate the difficulty of the individual test items. Although observation in the clinical setting is intended to be conducted by qualified health care professionals and educators, the objective quantification of the observation presents a challenge and calls into question the validity of clinical evaluation. Patient care and communication may distract the observer as well, and the inability of the evaluator to directly experience the student's performance of skills (e.g., palpation and auscultation) contributes to the subjectivity of the evaluation.

The use of standardized patients for formative assessment and summative evaluation is a recent trend in the education of health care professional students. The use of standardized patients allows for the development and evaluation of the student's skills in communication, psychomotor performance, and decision making (Decker, Sportsman, Puetz, & Billings, 2008), for formative assessment or for summative competency evaluation. The ability to objectively measure students' performance of clinical skills lets us identify those health care students who are able to provide safe and effective patient care, as well as those with clinical skills deficiencies, for whom referral to remediate those deficiencies is indicated (Boulet, Smee, Dillon, & Gimpel, 2009).

This chapter presents strategies for evaluating the health care professional student in the areas of communication, history-taking, physical assessment, and diagnostic reasoning (differential diagnosis), using a standardized patient environment. We discuss the development and use of a checklist as the tool of measurement. In this chapter, the term *actor* is used to denote the standardized patient.

THE CHECKLIST

A checklist, often used to evaluate an expected student behavior, can be used (a) to clarify for the learner the expected steps or required performance criteria, (b) to assess the performance of a variety of psychomotor skills, and (c) to conduct formative and summative evaluations (Jeffries & Rogers, 2007). Actor training and preparation, as well as assessment of the health care professional student by the actor and by a qualified health care professional or educator, are the intended purposes of the checklist discussed in this chapter. The use of the checklist in standardized patient simulations aids the actors in their performance of health care professional student observation and in the documentation of the student's communication, history-taking, and physical assessment skills. The checklist also aids the faculty in assessment and evaluation of diagnostic reasoning skills. As the standardized patient encounter, intended learning objectives, and scenario are being developed, great care in creation of the checklist early on will greatly assist the evaluation of the health care professional student. Careful attention to linking checklist items to intended learning objectives will assist the actor in case training (see chapter 5), in implementing the human patient simulation encounter (see chapter 7), and in observing and recalling the health care student's behavior so that it is possible for the actor to accurately compare the behavior to checklist items and complete the checklist. It is considered good practice to allow actors the opportunity to rehearse filling out the checklist as a separate skill from their case performance, to provide instruction and coaching, to enhance completion of the checklist, and to relate the checklist to what was actually observed. Principles for checklist coaching include filling out the checklist immediately after the encounter, encouraging the actor to anchor each checklist item to a specific action observed, reminding the actor that checklist accuracy becomes more difficult with each additional encounter, identifying the more challenging items on the checklist, and encouraging checklist item completion before the actor offers written comments (Wallace, 2006).

The checklist should be organized by sections that identify the skills to be observed and documented. For this chapter, the skills sections addressed are as follows: (a) communication skills, (b) history-taking, (c) physical assessment, and (d) diagnostic reasoning (differential diagnosis). The communication skills section should include items to assess verbal communication, interpersonal behavior, and culture-specific speaking skills. The history-taking section typically includes items the student is expected to ask during the course of taking the patient's health history. The physical examination section of the checklist includes actions and maneuvers the student is expected to perform during the course of a physical examination. The diagnostic reasoning section allows the student to demonstrate his or her informed and reasoned opinion of the patient's presentation after carefully reflecting on the data collected during the history-taking and physical examination. The diagnostic reasoning section of the checklist should be scored by a qualified health care professional or educator who has relevant knowledge and experience that is related to the clinical competency being evaluated.

When completing a checklist, actors may indicate whether each item was done or not done (Checklist 4.1). Some checklists may provide an additional response option of "Done, but not done correctly" (Checklist 4.2). Checklist items may also reflect assessment of the level of performance and may include the following: Unacceptable, Marginal, Needs Improvement, Good, Very Good, and Outstanding (Checklist 4.3). Examples of checklist items are shown in Checklists 4.1 to 4.3, following a discussion of each skill section.

Checklist Items for Communication Skills

One of the most important factors in patients' compliance in clinical practice is a positive health care professional–patient relationship. Communication skills—both verbal and nonverbal—and interpersonal skills are included in the communication skills section of the checklist. When developing a checklist, it is important to pay attention to details, including establishing a professional relationship (introducing oneself, shaking hands, asking permission to perform the interview and physical examination); being aware of facial expressions; sitting down, facing, and leaning in toward the patient; nodding the

Checklist 4.1

Component	Category	Item	Done	Not Done	Comments

Checklist 4.2

Component	Category	Item	Done Correctly	Done Incorrectly	Not Done	Comments

Checklist 4.3

Component	Category	Item	Level of Performance						Comments
			Unacceptable	Marginal	Needs Improvement	Good	Very Good	Outstanding	

Checklist 4.4 *Sample Items: Communication and Interpersonal Skills*

Component	Category	Sample Item: Did the student...	Done	Not Done	Comments
Communication Skills	Arrival	Knock before entering the room?			
	Introduction	Introduce self, including name and title?			
	Appearance	Appear professional in dress, grooming and hygiene?			
	Interaction	Make comfortable eye contact?			
	Attitude	Present a respectful and nonjudgmental attitude?			
	Privacy Concern	Provide for privacy during the physical examination?			
	Verbal Interactions	Allow time for response to questions without interrupting?			
		Ask open-ended questions?			
		Use lay terminology?			
	Style	Place you at ease?			
		Communicate information to you in a calm and non-alarming manner?			
	Responsiveness	Ask you if you had any questions?			
		Answer your questions in a prompt and thorough manner?			
		Answer your questions in a thorough manner?			

head periodically; and attempting not to appear stiff. In the evaluation of the health care professional student, the actor will document communication and interpersonal skills by completing checklist items like those shown in Checklist 4.4.

Checklist Items for History-Taking Skills

The history-taking portion of the standardized patient checklist guides the student in the task of obtaining information needed for diagnostic reasoning and making differential diagnoses. Development of the case presentation assists the actors in providing clinical information pertinent to the illness being portrayed. Typically, there should be only one main clinical problem modeled, rather than numerous clinical problems, because of the time constraints of a human patient simulation encounter. The checklist items in the section on history-taking skills should focus on assessing the student's ability to direct questions. Specific questions include the following: history of present illness; site, onset, duration, intensity, quantity, and quality of symptoms; aggravating and alleviating factors; and associated manifestations. The student should then be positioned to combine history-taking with subsequent physical assessment information to begin to generate hypotheses that will lead to accurate diagnoses. In the evaluation of the health care student, the actor will document history-taking skills by completing checklist items like those shown in Checklist 4.5.

Checklist 4.5 *Sample Items: Cardiovascular History-Taking*

Component	Category	Sample Item: Were you asked	Done	Not Done	Comments
Cardiovascular History Taking	Identifying Information	Your name?			
		Your age or date of birth?			
	Work History	About work history?			
	Symptoms	About shortness of breath?			
		About chest pain (i.e., location, quality, severity, radiation)?			
		About relieving or alleviating factors?			
		Where you asked about aggravating factors?			
		About chest pain at rest?			
		About heartburn?			
	Past Medical History	About previous hospitalizations?			
		About past surgical history?			
		About family health history?			
	Lifestyle Practices	About diet?			
		About exercise?			
		About lifestyle stresses or stress in general?			

Checklist Items for Physical Assessment Skills

During development of the case that will be modeled, consider giving written documentation from case studies to assist the actor to model the illness being portrayed as you prepare the physical examination component of the checklist. We recommend measurement of each physical assessment skill, broken down by components (see the cardiovascular physical assessment items below for examples). For brevity here, the checklist items for physical assessment skills that we present focus on the cardiovascular system. Additional systems that should be included in the physical assessment portion are digestive, endocrine, excretory, immune, integumentary, muscular, nervous, reproductive, respiratory, and skeletal systems. In the evaluation of the health care student, the actor will document the student's cardiovascular physical examination skills through the completion of checklist items like those given in Checklist 4.6.

DIAGNOSTIC REASONING SKILLS WORKSHEET

Diagnostic reasoning can be defined as the student's ability to diagnose a health problem correctly and to recommend appropriate therapy. Consideration of the student's problem-solving abilities and differential diagnosis abilities is an important part of measuring a student's competence to provide safe, quality health care. On the basis of the information gained by the student through the student's skillful history-taking and physical assessment, a hypothesis of one or more differential diagnoses may be proposed. Students can further demonstrate the development of their diagnostic reasoning

Checklist 4.6 *Sample Items: Cardiovascular System Physical Exam*

Component	Category	Item	Done Correctly	Done Incorrectly	Not Done	Comments
Physical Exam	While the patient is sitting	Assess blood pressure				
		Check pulses—Listen to the carotids then palpate carotids, radial, posterior tibial, and dorsalis pedis pulses				
		Examine for dependent edema				
	Have the patient lie down on the exam table	Assess for jugular vein distention				
		Palpate for PMI, heaves, and thrills				
		Listen of all four cardiac fields				
	Have the patient sit up again	Listen to all four cardiac areas				
		Have the patient lean forward and listen at base				
		Listen to the lungs				
		Assess for tenderness at costochondral margins				

Checklist 4.7 *Sample Items: Cardiovascular System Physical Exam*

Based on the data collected from the patient chart, interview and physical examination, please **list five differential diagnoses** with the most likely one first, and use the most exacting disease terminology. Remember to directly link the second problem with the first.
1.
2.
3.
4.
5.
Based on the differential diagnoses, please **list five diagnostic tests** and group similar tests. Remember to list simple, noninvasive and less expensive tests and only include more invasive tests if they are crucial to the diagnosis.
1.
2.
3.
4.
5.

competence by correlating diagnoses with appropriate diagnostic testing procedures. Diagnostic tests can include sputum, blood, and urine tests; x-rays; ultrasounds; and other procedures. A sample diagnostic reasoning skills worksheet may include the following, as shown in Checklist 4.7.

DATA AND RESULTS REPORTING

The basic styles of performance measurement and the methods by which to collect, interpret, and publish data are addressed in chapter 9, where reports and measurements are presented in broad terms. Purposes and types of data collection are considered; methods of data collection and assessment instruments are described; and analysis, interpretation, and dissemination of findings are outlined.

BEYOND THE GOALS OF HUMAN SIMULATION

Is the use of human simulation a teaching and learning strategy, or is it an evaluation tool? Health care professional education programs need to identify their philosophy about the use of human simulation for assessment (formative) or evaluation (summative) purposes (Leighton & Johnson-Russell, 2011). Leighton (2009, p. e57) recommended that a number of questions be addressed in these discussions:

■ Is the simulation laboratory better suited to facilitating learning or to evaluation of students? Is it possible to do both?
■ Is it fair to test students in a human simulation situation if they have not had significant exposure to simulated clinical experiences?
■ Are faculty members all competent in their roles? How is the faculty competence variable controlled, for evaluation purposes?
■ How do we account for the variety of student responses and interventions that are inherent in simulations?
■ Are we sending mixed messages when we tell students that simulation is a safe environment to learn in but then use that same environment for their evaluation?
■ Do we test students in the traditional clinical environment? Is it then fair to test in the simulation laboratory also?
■ If the focus is on testing in the simulation lab, will the experience become one about performing, rather than about learning?
■ What can you learn about your students in the simulation environment, even without formally evaluating or testing them?
■ If we say that most of the learning occurs in debriefing, can we fairly evaluate students before that debriefing occurs?

The human simulation itself must also be evaluated, for making adjustments and revisions to enhance the effectiveness of the human simulation experience and activity and to provide insights for its future application (Leighton & Johnson-Russell, 2011). Evaluating the human simulation activity should occur systematically during all phases—design and development, implementation process, and learning outcomes—as noted in Jeffries and Rogers (2007). As simulations gain wider use in curriculums, efforts to evaluate their effectiveness need to expand (Elfrink, Kirkpatrick, Nininger, & Schubert, 2010). Increased use of simulation as an educational tool in health care professional education, gaps in the evaluation of simulation as a pedagogical strategy, limited availability of formal evaluation tools specifically designed to evaluate simulations, and a paucity of studies that objectively evaluate the outcomes of simulation use suggest that there is a need for research to be conducted in this area in order to strive for higher levels of evidence in simulation evaluation (Harder, 2010; Kardong-Edgren, 2010).

CONCLUSIONS

The use of clinical evaluation methods in the simulation environment is relatively new, and the challenges faced parallel those of evaluations in general. However, the use of standardized patients in formative assessment and summative evaluation is beginning to remedy these challenges by introducing objective measurement of students' performance of clinical skills. Checklists used by actors (standardized patients) are and should be used to clarify expected performance criteria for the learner, appraise psychomotor skills, and perform formative and summative evaluations (Jeffries & Rogers, 2007). Use of a checklist of expected student outcomes, as presented in this chapter, aids in the standardization of evaluations of students; with proper training of actors, it will strengthen the objectivity of the measurement of outcomes. Although the styles of checklist will vary depending on the learning objectives desired and the outcomes being measured, the data collected will add to meaningful measurements of student performance, course outcomes, and the effectiveness of the human simulation experiences.

REFERENCES

Boulet, J. R., Smee, S. M., Dillon, G. F., & Gimpel, J. R. (2009). The use of standardized patient assessments for certification and licensure decisions. *Simulations in Healthcare: The Journal of the Society for Simulation in Healthcare, 4*(1), 35–42.

Decker, S., Sportsman, S., Puetz, L., & Billings, L. (2008). The evolution of simulation and its contribution to competency. *Journal of Continuing Education in Nursing, 39*(2), 74–80.

Elfrink, V. L., Kirkpatrick, B., Nininger, J., & Schubert, C. (2010). Using learning outcomes to inform teaching practices in human patient simulation. *Nursing Education Perspectives, 31*(2), 97–100.

Harder, B. N. (2010). Use of simulation in teaching and learning in health sciences: A systematic review. *Journal of Nursing Education, 49*(1), 23–28.

Horn, M., & Carter, N. (2007). Practical suggestions for implementing simulations. In P. R. Jeffries (Ed.), *Simulation in nursing education: From conceptualization to evaluation* (pp. 59–72). New York: National League for Nursing.

Hovancsek, M. T. (2007). Using simulation in nursing education. In P. R. Jeffries (Ed.), *Simulation in nursing education: From conceptualization to evaluation* (pp. 1–9). New York: National League for Nursing.

Jeffries, P. R., & Rogers, K. J. (2007). Evaluating simulations. In P. R. Jeffries (Ed.), *Simulation in nursing education: From conceptualization to evaluation* (pp. 87–103). New York: National League for Nursing.

Kardong-Edgren, S. (2010). Striving for higher levels of evaluation in simulation. *Clinical Simulation in Nursing, 6*(6), e203–e204.

Krichbaum, K., Rowan, M., Duckett, L., Ryden, M. B., & Savik, K. (1994). The clinical evaluation tool: A measure of the quality of clinical performance of baccalaureate nursing students. *Journal of Nursing Education, 33*(9), 395–404.

Leighton, K. (2009). What can we learn from a listserv? *Clinical Simulation in Nursing, 5*(2), e59–e62.

Leighton, K., & Johnson-Russell, J. (2011). Innovations in facilitating learning using simulation. In M. J. Bradshaw & A. J. Lowenstein (Eds.), *Innovative teaching strategies in nursing & related professions* (5th ed., pp. 239–264). Sudbury, MA: Jones and Bartlett.

Saewert, K. J., & Yarbrough, S. S. (2009). Evaluation of clinical performance. In N. Ard & T. M. Valiga (Eds.), *Clinical nursing education: Current reflections* (pp. 92–101). New York: National League for Nursing.

Wallace, P. (2006). *Coaching standardized patients for use in the assessment of clinical competence.* New York: Springer Publishing.

SUGGESTED READING

Jeffries, P. R. (Ed.). (2007). *Simulation in nursing education: From conceptualization to evaluation*. New York: National League for Nursing.

Kyle, R. R., & Murray, W. B. (Eds.). (2008). *Clinical simulation: Operations, engineering and management*. Burlington, MA: Academic Press.

McNelis, A. M., Jeffries, P. R., Hensel, D., & Anderson, M. (2009). Simulation: Integral to clinical education. In N. Ard & T. M. Valiga (Eds.), *Clinical nursing education: Current reflections* (pp. 145–164). New York: National League for Nursing.

Wallace, P. (2006). Coaching standardized patients for use in the assessment of clinical competence. New York: Springer Publishing.

CHAPTER 5

Standardized Patient Training

Robert Hargraves

INTRODUCTION

*T*he purpose of this chapter is to discuss the training of standardized patients (SPs) in terms of what, who, why, and how: What is an SP? Who is an appropriate candidate for hiring as an SP? Why use SPs instead of real patients? Once hired and trained, how can SPs be effective tools in the instruction and training of Medical Professionals? After reading this chapter, you will have a full understanding of the importance of complete and proper training of SPs so that they can become the valuable tools of instruction and education they are meant to be.

What is an SP? How many times has this question been asked to SP trainers across the globe? The easiest answer is "an SP is a person trained to pretend to be sick for the instruction of medical students." The most common response to this answer is "oh, you mean like in that 'Seinfeld' episode where Kramer and the dwarf were arguing over which venereal disease they had!" This reaction is, while amusing, not the reaction a trainer wants to hear from anyone.

If you look at the Association of Standardized Patient Education web site, the page that describes SPs says the following:

DEFINITION OF AN SP

An SP is a person trained to portray a patient scenario, or an actual patient using their own history and physical exam findings, for the instruction, assessment, or practice of communication and/or examining skills of a health care provider. In the health and medical sciences, SPs are used to provide a safe and supportive environment conducive for learning or for standardized assessment. SPs can serve as practice models, or participate in sophisticated assessment and feedback of one's abilities or services. The use of simulated scenarios involving humans is rapidly expanding to meet the needs of many high-risk service fields outside of human health care.

(Gliva-McConvey, 2009),
Professional Skills Center,
Eastern Virginia Medical School, 2009;
http://www.aspeducators.org/sp_info.htm)

> The Simulated/Standardized Patient (SP) is a person who has been carefully coached to simulate an actual patient so accurately that the simulation cannot be detected by a skilled clinician. In performing the simulation, the SP presents the gestalt of the patient being simulated; not just the history, but the body language, the physical findings, and the emotional and personality characteristics as well.
>
> (Barrows, 1987)

What this shows is that there is not a simple, one-sentence definition of what an SP is or what one can do. This alone makes the idea of training one seem a daunting task. This chapter will hopefully show you that the task is not so daunting and that it is actually quite simple and can even be considered fun.

Now that we have tossed around a few definitions and explanations of what an SP is, let us now discuss who an appropriate candidate is to become an SP.

Contrary to popular belief, not all SPs are actors; neither do they need to be. In fact, many people within the SP training profession agree that actors are sometimes the least desirable people to use as SPs. There are a myriad of reasons for this belief; here are a few examples:

- Actors are not always very reliable. They often have agents or managers who call them at the last possible moment to send them on various auditions. Any actor worth his or her salt will choose to audition for a possible national commercial over playing someone with a pulmonary embolism for medical students to poke and prod all day. Hence, the SP program is left with the dilemma of last-minute coverage.
- Actors are trained to build an in-depth character. On the surface, this sounds beneficial to an SP trainer until he or she realizes that an "in-depth" character often involves a great deal of "character shading." "Character shading" tends to begin happening after the fourth or fifth encounter, when the actor is bored with the simple parameters of the case they are playing and they begin to embellish a bit. Suddenly, Mom did not just "die in a car accident," she "died in a car accident a year ago, in fact today is the anniversary of her death," and the encounter begins spiraling out of control from there.

This is not to say you should not hire actors to be SPs in your program. You should. This is just a cautionary example of why you should not hire *only* actors in your program.

A good rule of thumb for hiring SPs in a program is the diversity in your ranks. Your SPs should have a broad range of backgrounds and life experience. They should be of varying age ranges and demographics. They should especially be of varying racial and ethnic backgrounds. A well-diversified SP program is an SP program that can offer a broad spectrum of instructional practices, educational encounters, and valuable feedback sessions for clients.

Now we come to one of the most difficult areas of SP training: the interview process. How do we sift through hundreds of people and decide which ones to hire into our well-diversified SP pool? What is the correct process? What are the signs and signals of the perfect candidate? There is no easy answer to these questions as well as no correct method. A good amount of the time, the trainer (or whoever is in charge of hiring) simply has to go with their gut.

A good method of interviewing candidates is the group interview. The group should probably be no more than 10 candidates at one time. Ideally, there should be several key members of the SP program present at the interview, and their function is quite simple:

to quietly observe the candidates as they go through the interview process and to jot down their thoughts and observations of each individual candidate.

The interviewer's task is much more active. He or she defines what an SP is and describes the function of the SP's job—within their particular program, as it differs from one program to another—and the responsibilities it entails. The interviewer should cover all aspects of the benefits of the job, including pay and any perks there may be, and then get into the heart of what it really means to be an SP.

At this point, the interviewer can introduce a memory game of some kind. This kind of game serves several purposes: it gets the candidates' energy level up and their minds active, it gives the observers an activity to focus on that will give insight into the candidates' personalities and recall abilities, and it will show the individual candidate's willingness to participate in the unexpected.

This leads very nicely into introducing the sample case and checklist. The case and checklist should be given to each candidate for a five-minute review. Then the case should be read aloud with each prospective SP given an opportunity to read. This serves a dual purpose of having the interviewees both hearing and seeing the material. Some people are visual learners and others are audible learners, and this process helps both learn the materials in front of them. Then questions from the group should be fielded and answered so that everyone is on the same page with the case facts and checklist items.

After reading over the materials, a good practice is to do what is sometimes called a *lightning round* or *round robin*. This is a rapid-fire approach to checking the potential SP's case fact retention and recall. Even with only a few minutes' worth of coverage, it is amazing what the human mind can retain. This is another good source of information for the interview observers to jot down insights on particular candidates.

Once everyone has had an opportunity to respond to several round robin questions, it is a good idea for the interviewer to check in with his or her group to see how everyone is feeling and to get any feedback they may have. This is also a good point to take a five-minute break.

When the break is over, it is time for the interviewer to ask for a volunteer in the "hot seat." Using the same case the candidate has been working with, have the volunteer be the "patient" and the interviewer be the "student." It is a good practice to choose a very obvious student for the first volunteer: someone very nervous, or very obnoxious, or very empathetic. This gives the group something to chew on and fodder for checklist communication skills. A five-minute encounter without physical examination should be sufficient.

The group should be given the task to complete their checklists in real time, and the volunteer can complete his or hers after the encounter. When the encounter is over and all checklists are completed, then a group discussion invariably occurs over certain items on the checklist. This discussion gives the potential SPs their moment to ask questions, defend their checklist responses, and come to an agreement. Then another volunteer should be requested and given a different "student" to work with. The same postencounter process as above should occur.

After the discussion of the second encounter, the interview observers should have a fairly solid grasp of the candidates' potential. A big round of applause for the volunteers should be given and any questions the group may have should be answered.

Now you have your potential pool of diversified SPs. There could be a second, individual interview or not. At this point all you can do is give the newly hired SPs their shot and cast them in a case.

The interview scenario listed above is just one way of finding candidates. There are many different ways to conduct an SP interview and the example above has been proven to work quite well.

Another question that comes up from time to time regarding SPs is why they should be used over real patients with real findings. The answer is they should not. They should be used in conjunction with real patient experiences.

An SP encounter is the safest possible environment for a student because it provides them the opportunity to make mistakes without risk to the patient. No one is injured or dies if a mistake is made with an SP, and no one has irate patients or family members. An SP encounter gives the student a chance to make mistakes, to try again, and also to receive verbal feedback *from the patient* on how it felt to be in their care for however long the encounter might have been, which is a great way to improve students' bedside manners and expose them to the ways their actions or inactions affect a patient.

After being exposed to many SP encounters, a student can then meet real patients and interact with them with confidence in their ability and with professional empathy.

Training SPs on specific cases can and should be fun. It should be a collaborative process between the trainer and the SPs. If the SP feels involved in the material, they will stay involved with it when they perform it.

Case materials vary depending on the institution. Sometimes they are constructed by the faculty of individual departments; sometimes institutions would rather have a faculty member write a quick paragraph or "treatment" of a case, and then the SP program staff will flesh it out into a template form. Once the department faculty and the SP program staff are all in agreement, the case is ready for casting and training.

The amount of time to spend on training is always dependent on the complexity of the case. If it is a straightforward history with no physical examination, an hour or two should suffice. If it is a history that also has some kind of medical findings, it could take slightly longer. When a physical examination is added, then another hour is usually tacked on so the SPs get comfortable with maneuvers. If the case has not only a history and physical examination, but also some sort of physical findings (slurred speech, paralyzed legs, and so forth), an additional hour could be tacked on again.

In the earlier example of an interview, the process of training a history can be the same. The SPs should read over the materials for a few minutes, which should be followed with them reading it aloud. Then have them role-play it with you and then with another SP as a partner under your supervision. This gets the case facts ingrained in their minds, and they get to experience both sides of the encounter, which in turn gives them insight into the students' perspectives. Make sure the SPs are given ample opportunity to ask questions so there are fewer curveballs thrown at them the day of the encounters.

If the case has a physical examination attached to it, the training will take on a different tone. Train the history as discussed above and then take a break. Bring everyone back and go over the physical examination maneuvers they can expect to be practiced on them. It is an enormous help if a faculty member from the department to which the case is related could be present to really enhance the training process. In most cases, the faculty member is actually an MD, and this gives the SP confidence in the physical examination that is sometimes lacking when they are shown by a video or a trainer who is not an MD. Giving the SP a video of the maneuvers to take home with them to review after the training is also an enormous benefit.

If a given case also has physical findings, again it is a great boon to have a faculty member present to give physical examples for the SPs to mimic. Videos of actual people with the same findings are also very helpful. This part of the training, out of necessity, is much more one on one and can take time. However, the results of taking this time show very clearly when the students are given surveys on their SP experiences. Words like *real* and *believable* show up on those surveys, and you can be sure the encounter was a valuable experience for the student.

If the student catches a whiff of "ham acting" or overplaying a role from an SP, she is taken out of her "willing suspension of disbelief," and the encounter becomes a joke and is rendered useless. This is why it is so important the SP understands the person they are playing. They should be encouraged not to "act" the role but to infuse as much of their own personalities as possible. This makes the experience much more real and therefore much more believable.

Another aspect to consider while training is pain level. Many cases involve an SP being in pain. It is crucial in training that the pain level be agreed upon and shown in exactly the same way by each SP. One man's 5 out of 10 pain rating can be quite different than another man's rating, so it is recommended that the SP be shown examples of how to accurately portray their pain level so they do it consistently and in a standardized manner.

The same thing can be said for what is commonly known as the "communication challenge." A communication challenge is a phrase in a particular case that the SP is to speak, verbatim, at a specified point in the encounter. This phrase exists as a challenge to the student to field a question they may not have been expecting. For example: "Doc, am I gonna die?" or "This pain in my stomach, does it mean I have cancer?" This gives the examiner the opportunity to see how a student reacts to a surprise question. Do they answer directly and empathetically? Do they hedge? Do they ignore the question entirely? The question, although, must be delivered in the most realistic way possible or it stands out as being silly in a student's mind.

At this point, we have reached the subject that is really the bread and butter in the world of SP training: Verbal feedback from an SP to a student is the most important aspect of the job; thus, the delivery of verbal feedback is the most vital part of the training. If the case that is being trained requires verbal feedback at some point, it is very important that a good amount of training time is spent on making absolutely certain the SPs performing the case are comfortable in delivering vital, valuable, and, most importantly, specific feedback to their students.

Just like any aspect of the job, not every person is capable of delivering feedback effectively. Some programs have the luxury of grouping their SPs into categories:

- Group A contains SPs who are adept at all aspects of the job; History and Physical Examination performance and feedback delivery.
- Group B contains SPs who are adept at only History and Physical Examination performance. They should not be used for cases involving feedback.
- Group C contains SPs who should solely be used for encounters that require no case preparation: usually for Anatomy classes or Physical Examination practice sessions.

Of course, having a pool of SPs that are all in the Group A category would be fantastic and that group would be adept at delivering feedback.

Training feedback delivery requires giving the SPs tools to use and directives to follow. For example, give them a list of "feeling words" to draw from. Give them an outline or framework to follow. Give them ways to frame their sentences so that each SP is delivering feedback in the same way: a standardized way.

A good method for feedback delivery is as follows: having the SPs understand that feedback should be a conversation between themselves and their students. It should not feel as if they are delivering a sermon or giving a lecture. The SPs need to know that they are not professors or doctors and that it is vitally important that the students do see them that way. The students should see their SPs as friendly, helpful tools that are in the boat with them and not out to undermine or criticize them. A good way to achieve this is to train the SP to ask questions as a part of the feedback session, especially in the beginning: "How did you think our encounter went?" or "How are you feeling now that the encounter is over?" This allows the student to simply answer honestly and vent a little bit.

It is important to not let the questions stop there. Have the SP check in with the student and perhaps probe them a bit to see what the student felt they did well or needed to work on. If the student is the type of person who gives only one-word answers or is not one to dialogue easily, then the SP should be trained to be armed with two feedback points: one positive and one constructive. However, those two points both need to be delivered in a positive way. The constructive point should be delivered first and should not sound like criticism: "When you said, 'You drink *how* much on the weekends?' I felt a bit judged." This is quite different than an SP saying, "You judged me on how much I drink on the weekends" or "You were very judgmental."

Let us use a quick example of good, short feedback delivery. The encounter has just ended and the student is returning to the examination room after having left for a five-minute postencounter:

SP (with a big welcoming smile that shows the sick patient is gone and now we are just two people talking): "Hi. Come in! Please, sit down."

After the student sits, SP: "We only have a few moments to go over the encounter a little bit, so why don't we start with how you felt the encounter went?"

Student: Well, I was really nervous, but I thought it went okay.

SP: Being nervous is completely understandable. Tests are never easy. Let me ask you, you said you were nervous, how did you feel about your pacing throughout the encounter?

Student: I don't know. I guess it was okay. What did you think?

SP: Well, actually, there were times I felt a little bit rushed. For example, do you remember when you were asking me about my symptoms and when each one began?

Student: Yes, you said you started off feeling very tired and then a little later you felt like a fever, then you felt sick to your stomach and eventually vomited.

SP: That's really great. You just showed me you were really listening. The point I was trying to make was that when you asked me about my symptoms, you asked in a staccato kind of way where I could only answer in very short sentences. I felt very rushed.

Student: Oh, wow. I didn't realize that was how it came out. I'm sorry.

SP: There is no need to be sorry, this is what these encounters are for. How do you think you could have asked those same questions about my symptoms but in such a way that I wouldn't feel rushed?

Student: Well, I guess I could have asked about your symptoms kind of generally and then when you mention each one, I could maybe wait a moment or two before asking my next one to make sure you've said all you had to say.

SP: That sounds like an excellent way to do it. Did you feel like we made a connection at all?

Student: Actually, yes. During the part where you told me your wife died last year. I got the impression you were still very sad about it, and I wanted to make sure you were alright.

SP: I thought you handled that moment just beautifully. I was still sad and when you asked me, "How are holding up? Are you doing okay?" I felt nurtured. Like you understood me on a deeper level than what brought me into see you. Thank you for that. Did you have anything else about the encounter you wanted to discuss?

Student: Umm. No. Not right now. Thanks for the feedback.

The above example is a good feedback encounter because it is

- Conversational: The SP asked the student questions and when the student responded, commented on what the student expressed.
- Positive: Even the constructive point of rushed pacing was addressed gently and specifically. The student was able to remember the moment in question and was then asked to find *his own solution*. This is excellent feedback technique because it allows the student to be self-reflective. However, it is important that the SP be trained to have a solution of their own to a constructive feedback point in case the student doesn't arrive at one.
- Friendly: The SP smiled warmly at the student and invited them to sit down. It is so very important that feedback sessions be light and friendly. The students are much more receptive to feedback when the environment is warm.
- Supportive: The SP praised the student on his solution to the constructive point and then acknowledged the student's empathetic handling of the SP's wife's death.
- Feeling words were used: *rushed* and *nurtured*. This is why it is a good rule of thumb to provide a list of words that are both positive and constructive.

It is important that SPs be trained to look out for feedback points throughout the encounter and to refer back to their "feeling words" page as they are completing their checklists. This way, usually during the communication skills section of the checklist, the SP can jot down feedback points they may like to discuss and attach a feeling word to them.

A final word on the phrasing of feedback: it is suggested that SPs be trained to avoid negative sounding words like *shouldn't, don't, can't, wouldn't, wrong, inappropriate,* and so forth. Nothing turns a feedback session into an argument faster that putting a student into a defensive position.

We hope, after reading this chapter, you now feel more confident in bringing in people to join your SP pool and, more importantly, training them effectively. It is important to note that what was discussed in this chapter is just one person's way of screening, hiring, and training SPs. There are many other effective methods, and each program can and should develop its own take and put its own stamp on these methods.

REFERENCES

Barrows, H. S. (1987). *Simulated (standardized) patients and other human simulations.* Retrieved from http://www.aspeducators.org/sp_info.htm

Gliva-McConvey, G. (2009). Professional Skills Center, Eastern Virginia Medical School. Retrieved from http://www.aspeducators.org/sp_info.htm

CHAPTER 6

Incorporating Technology in Human Simulation

Fran Cornelius

OVERVIEW OF TECHNOLOGY TO SUPPORT HUMAN SIMULATION LEARNING EXPERIENCES

Technology, particularly mobile technology, can enhance the simulation learning experience. The value that technology brings to the simulation environment is the ability not only to provide a more realistic experience, but also to replicate the types of information-seeking and decision-support tools that the student is likely to encounter in the health care arena. Increasingly, technologies that can assist the health care practitioner, organize and deliver information, and improve patient safety are becoming integrated within the health care delivery system in all settings. Technological and informatics competencies among all health care providers have become a necessity. It is the responsibility of educators to provide opportunities for students to master the use of these technologies as they prepare to enter the workplace. What better place to provide these types of experiences than the simulation laboratory?

THE ROLE OF INFORMATICS COMPETENCIES

Since the Institute of Medicine's (IOM) landmark report in 1999, there has been heightened awareness of medication errors, patient safety, and the impact upon patient outcomes. As a result, there has been continued focus on health care delivery, patient safety, and the education of health professions. Recent reports call for the integration of evidence-based practice, quality improvement, and informatics within the education of all health professionals, emphasizing an interdisciplinary approach to patient-centered care (American Association of Colleges of Nursing [AACN], 2008; IOM, 2003, 2006). There is a growing belief within nursing, particularly in nursing education, that informatics and technical competencies among nurses are essential (Cornelius, Wilson, & Childs, 2010; Staggers, Gassert, & Curran, 2002; Westra & Delaney, 2008). The AACN has strongly recommended that education of students must be concurrent with current practice environments so that graduates are better prepared to enter the workforce (AACN, 2008).

TECHNOLOGICAL INNOVATIONS

The last decade has brought forth remarkable technological innovation, particularly in the area of mobile technology. The availability of smaller, progressively more powerful, portable computers and increasingly pervasive wireless technologies has lifted the restrictions of the past, allowing mobile access to information "anytime, anywhere." Many predict that improvements such as "high-bandwidth Internet access, high-definition video processing, and interactive video conferencing will be commonplace" and the eagerly anticipated fourth-generation wireless technology will offer increased "bandwidth to maximum data rates of 100 Mbps for high-mobility situations and 1 Gbps for stationary and low-mobility scenarios like Internet hot spots" (Woh, Mahlke, Mudge, & Chakrabarti, 2010, p. 81). This will bring forth capabilities to use stunning two- and three-dimensional images and flexible multiresolution image representations—all available in the mobile learning environment (Kristoffersen & Ljungberg, 1999; Kristoffersen, Nielsen, Blechar, & Hanseth, 2005). Imagine what this could do for extending the opportunities for simulation of collaborative practice.

The widespread use of cell phones with "smart technologies" such as Wi-Fi, cameras, Bluetooth, and built-in computing offers enormous potential for "opportunistic communications," particularly to support care at the bedside. Clearly, when one considers the recent explosion of cell phone use worldwide—more than 3.3 billion active cell phones currently, with an estimated annual growth of 22%—the potential for education and practice is enormous (Conti & Kumar, 2010; Woh et al., 2010).

In addition, the advances that have made larger capacity and faster laptops, netbooks, and tablet personal computers and introduced touch screen and pen-based interfaces while decreasing overall size have opened the door to an entirely new "mobile computing era that can be an integrated part of a distribute computing environment, one in which users change physical location frequently" described by Alonso and Korth as "nomadic computing" (Alonso & Korth, 1993, p. 388). This has shifted the learning environment dramatically by providing opportunities for richer in situ experiences for students.

TECHNOLOGIES TO SUPPORT HUMAN SIMULATION
LEARNING EXPERIENCES

All simulation scenarios can easily and appropriately incorporate technology. The key is to integrate the technology in a realistic manner using situations that the student is likely to encounter in practice. Providing students with opportunities to utilize "clinical automation tools that are proven to help deliver the most consistent, high-quality care to patients prepares them for success in real-world clinical practice" (Curran, Sheets, Kirkpatrick, & Bauldoff, 2007, p. 28). Technologies that can be easily integrated into the human simulation learning experience can be categorized into five groups: (a) mobile devices, (b) computers, (c) bar code scanners, (d) video and telecommunication, and (e) technologies that augment the simulation experience.

Mobile devices are generally small, pocket-sized devices such as personal digital assistants, iPod Touch, and smartphones. Since the mid-1990s, these devices have become more powerful, with increasing capacity and speed. Mobile devices can house a large library of references and connect the user to other resources through Wi-Fi,

Bluetooth, and in some instances cellular technology. Incorporating mobile devices within a simulation scenario can replicate realistically point-of-care information access to provide decision support.

The recently launched Apple iPad bridges the gap between mobile devices and computers by offering a larger screen. Its touch flow technology may offer value to the simulation learning environment by providing a very responsive, user-friendly interface with remarkable graphic and video presentation ideal for patient teaching. Current limitations include inability to multitask and nonswappable batteries—essential in health care, although it is anticipated that in the future, these limitations will be addressed and the iPad will become more widely used in health care (Dolan, 2010).

Computers that can be easily integrated into the simulation learning experience include net books, tablet PCs, and computers housed within mobile workstations, commonly referred to as *workstations on wheels* (WOW) or *computers on wheels* (COW). Computers can provide similar resources as the mobile device; in addition, computers can more realistically replicate the experience of working with electronic medical records (EMRs) and clinical information systems because computers tend to have more capacity, more power, and multitasking capability. Students can document patient assessment data and interventions and monitor patient status using imbedded trending tools. In addition, students can access decision-support resources and care protocols to ensure delivery of optimal care.

As such, these computers provide students with opportunities to build the technical and informatics competencies, including electronic data-management skills, long identified as priorities for nursing education programs by the AACN (2008) and IOM (2003). In addition, the expanded capacity and integrated sophisticated computer programs for academic environments permit longitudinal patient encounter experiences for students, following a patient through a series of simulated encounters and thereby creating a more realistic learning experience (EMR DailyNews, 2010).

"Bar-code point-of-care (BPOC) medication administration systems are designed to ensure that the right drug is being administered via the right route to the right patient in the right amount at the right time: the "five rights" of drug administration" (Sakowski et al., 2005, p. 2619). Although BPOC technology is not widely implemented, it has been documented that administration-related medication errors can be intercepted through electronic bar code scanning, reducing medication errors by more than 40% (Mahoney, Berard-Collins, Coleman, Amaral, & Cotter, 2007; Poon et al., 2010). Including bar code point-of-care technology in the simulation experience can model best practice care delivery while replicating medication administration experiences likely to be the norm within the health care industry of the future (Wideman, Whittler, & Anderson, 2005).

"Telehealth is the practice of health care delivery using telecommunications technology, including but not limited to diagnosis, consultation, treatment, transfer of medical data, education, dissemination of public health alerts and/or emergency updates" (Oregon Telecommunications Coordinating Council, 2002, p. 13). Telecommunication technologies can add another dimension to the simulation experience by providing students an opportunity to collaborate with other health care professionals using a technology that is being increasingly utilized to meet the challenges of access to health care. Scenarios that involve collaborative interaction with health care providers, specialists, and homecare patients can provide students with unique opportunities to practice remote monitoring and assessment skills and interdisciplinary communication. For disaster simulations, radio or cellular communication can be incorporated to manage triage and limited resources, and to arrange transport of priority victims among other things. Video consultation and family interviews can be prerecorded for viewing during the simulation activity to provide more depth to the simulation experience replicating the telecommunication experience. In addition, video recording of the actual simulation experience can be viewed postevent to provide even richer learning experiences via self-critique and debriefing.

There are many technologies that can augment the simulation experience, thereby providing a more realistic presentation of the scenario. Monitors can be programmed to provide specific vital signs or other symptoms that challenge assessment skills and warrant immediate response by the student. For example, fetal simulators can provide fetal and maternal ECG, fetal heart tones, and uterine activity for a realistic labor and delivery experience. In addition, fetal simulators can be programmed to "present various fetal parameters, including twins, as well as a wide range of clinical scenarios," providing students the opportunity to learn to distinguish normal and abnormal responses during labor (Fluke Biomedical, 2006). The more realistic these controlled experiences can be designed, the better the learning experience for the students. Often, it only takes a little imagination on the nurse educator's part to create a scenario that will help build student competencies. Creative use of technology can enrich the scenario by adding an element of reality to the experience by integrating technologies that are likely to be encountered in the real-world setting.

INCORPORATION OF TECHNOLOGY IN A SCENARIO RELATED TO PATIENT TEACHING AND MEDICATION ADMINISTRATION

Simulation Scenario: Patient Teaching and Medication Administration

SETTING: Medical surgical unit (inpatient hospital room)

SCENARIO: Mr./Mrs. Smith is a 58-year-old patient admitted to the unit 2 days ago, newly diagnosed with hypertension. Admission vital signs: blood pressure (BP), 200/134; AR, 92; R, 24; T, 98.6°F, exhibiting papillary edema and retinal hemorrhage. The patient must be closely monitored and is in need of considerable education regarding the new diagnosis of hypertension, newly prescribed medication, and lifestyle changes necessary to manage hypertension. This case can evolve over a period of days to allow opportunities for students to use trending and imbedded decision support tools to supplement patient care and teaching, as well as administration of recommended immunizations (i.e., flu or pneumonia vaccines).

INCORPORATED TECHNOLOGY:

1. Computer/laptop with
   a. EMR/electronic health record (EHR)
      - Review of patient history and laboratory results
      - Verification of medication orders
      - Documentation
   b. Patient education materials (customizable)
2. Bar code scanner for
   a. Medication administration and reconciliation
   b. Patient identification
   c. Allergy verification
3. Mobile device with e-books and Internet access for planned and ad hoc patient teaching in response to questions regarding diagnosis, disease process, medications, and lifestyle changes.

INCORPORATION OF TECHNOLOGY IN A SCENARIO
RELATED TO MEDICATION SAFETY

Simulation Scenario: In-House Consultation with Newly Ordered Medications

SETTING: Medical surgical unit (inpatient hospital room)

SCENARIO: The patient was admitted for elective surgery; total knee replacement—right knee; the patient has history of rheumatoid arthritis, chronic obstructive pulmonary disease. The patient has a long list of current medications and is complaining of a rash on his or her torso and upper extremities. A dermatology consult has been ordered by the admitting physician, and the patient was seen by the specialist. Medications for the rash (both oral and topical) were ordered. The new medication order was filled by the pharmacy and delivered to the unit. Nurse prepares to administer medications and begins initial teaching with regard to medications, asking the patient about any known allergies. The patient reports a history of allergies not previously documented on the EMR/EHR. Upon review of new medications, it is determined that the patient has an allergy that contraindicates one of the newly prescribed medications.

INCORPORATED TECHNOLOGY:

1. Computer/laptop with EMR/EHR
   a. Verification of drug allergies; updating patient allergies
   b. Check for drug interactions with current medications and newly prescribed medications
   c. Documentation
2. Telecommunications system for notifying physician of allergy and obtaining new orders, as well as notification of pharmacy

INCORPORATION OF TECHNOLOGY IN A SCENARIO
RELATED TO PATIENT SAFETY

Simulation Scenario: Failure to Rescue—Initiate Rapid Response Team

SETTING: Medical surgical unit (inpatient hospital room)

SCENARIO: The patient was admitted 2 days ago from the emergency department following a fall from a ladder at home while painting the exterior of their home. The patient sustained extensive bruising of the left side of their torso and a closed fracture of the left femur shaft with no loss of consciousness. The patient had surgery yesterday for insertion of an intramedullary rod; vital signs are as follows: BP, 140/88; AR, 126; R, 32; T, 98.2°F. The patient has an order of morphine IM q 4 to 6 hours as needed for pain and last received a shot 6 hours earlier. The patient is complaining of pain and is also complaining of lightheadedness and dizziness. It is observed that the patient has a cough.

INCORPORATED TECHNOLOGY:

1. Rapid response team activation system via a telecommunications system
2. Technologies to maintain and monitor airway, breathing, and circulation—monitors should be programmed to present expected findings for this scenario
   a. Oxygen
   b. Cardiac monitor
   c. Pulse oximeter
3. EMR/EHR
   a. Verification of allergies
   b. Documentation

INCORPORATION OF TECHNOLOGY IN A DISASTER SCENARIO

Simulation Scenario: Earthquake

SETTING: Medium-size city located close to the ocean in southern California

SCENARIO: The town of Sunshine Paradise, California, has just experienced an 8.4 earthquake resulting in significant building and infrastructure damage. Disaster response teams have been deployed, and several triage and treatment stations have been set up to care for victims of the earthquake.

INCORPORATED TECHNOLOGY:

1. Telecommunications technology/radio communications
   a. Coordinate efforts
   b. Allocate resources appropriately
2. Media—prerecorded media to build upon scenario and add compounding variables
3. Mobile bar code scanners for triage, tagging, and tracking victims before and after transport to health care facilities
4. Computer to coordinate information to facilitate and support family reunification and ensure that treatment is coordinated
5. Mobile devices/communications
   a. Emergency protocols and guidelines
   b. Wireless information system for emergency responders to identify potential hazardous materials and actions needed to protect responders and community at large

INCORPORATION OF TECHNOLOGY IN A RURAL SCHOOL HEALTH CLINIC SCENARIO

Simulation Scenario: Acute Otitis Media

SETTING: Rural school health clinic setting

SCENARIO: Pat is a 6-year-old child complaining of a severe earache. Vital signs are as follows: BP, 100/56; AR, 88; R, 18; T, 100.1°F. The school nurse examines the child and notes a bulging eardrum. Using the telehealth communications system connected to the urgent care clinic of a large regional health care system, the school nurse consults with the on-call physician, who is able to view the child's ear using a specially equipped otoscope held by the nurse. The physician is able to review the child's EHR, asking the nurse questions with regard to the child's history. The nurse reports that the child has a history of recurrent ear infections, has not been seen by an ear, nose, and throat (ENT) specialist, and has no known allergies. At the conclusion of the collaboration, the physician orders the following: observation, ibuprofen as needed, warm compress to the ear, head elevation, analgesic ear drops, and referral to an ENT specialist for evaluation of recurrent infections.

INCORPORATED TECHNOLOGY:

1. Live video conferencing or prerecorded video assets to mimic telecommunication interaction with hospital physician
2. Computer with EMR/EHR
   a. Review of patient health record
   b. Documentation
   c. Patient teaching materials (customizable)
   d. Physician's Orders
   e. Patient referral to an ENT specialist

INCORPORATION OF TECHNOLOGY IN A HOME CARE SCENARIO

Simulation Scenario: Medication Administration

SETTING: Home care setting

SCENARIO: Mr./Mrs. Jones is a 68-year-old home care patient with a history of congestive heart failure ×10 years and diabetes diagnosed 2 years ago. The patient was discharged from the hospital yesterday, where he or she was treated for gangrene of the toes on the right foot. Home care referral was ordered by the physician. Initial home visit vital signs: BP, 140/90; AR, 82; R, 16; T, 98.6°F; recent laboratory report of HbA_{1c} is 8.5%. Medications: Lanoxin, insulin, and hydrochlorothiazide. The patient is sitting in lazy boy chair with feet on the floor. Edema of lower extremities is present, and the patient is complaining of numbness and tingling of lower extremities. The dressing on the right foot is intact but appears to be too tight. On the table next to the patient is a large bag of licorice, half empty.

INCORPORATED TECHNOLOGY:

1. Computer
   a. EMR/EHR
      - Review of patient history and laboratory results
      - Verification of home care, diet, and medication orders
      - Documentation
   b. Blood sugar trending graph for enhanced patient teaching
2. Mobile device/computer with
   a. Drug guide to check for drug interactions (some forms of licorice may increase the risk for Lanoxin toxicity)
   b. Laboratory and diagnostic tests
   c. Camera to photograph wound for documentation

CONCLUSION

Nurse educators are charged with the responsibility of preparing students to be knowledgeable workers in a highly technological and information-infused health care environment. It is essential that all nursing students develop skills in the use of technology to manage information and to provide effective, safe, and high-quality patient care. It is through the integration of technologies described in this chapter in simulation learning activities and future technologies described in chapter 29 that students will have the opportunity to build competencies in a safe and secure learning environment that replicates "some or nearly all of the essential aspects of a clinical situation so that the situation may be more readily understood and managed when it occurs for real in clinical practice" (Hravnak, Beach, & Tuite, 2007, p. 3). It is in providing these opportunities for learning that we can adequately prepare our students to provide competent, high-quality care to patients under their care.

REFERENCES

Alonso, R., & Korth, H. F. (1993). *Database system issues in nomadic computing.* Proceedings of the 1993 ACM SIGMOD International Conference on Management of Data, 388–392.

American Association of Colleges of Nursing. (2008). *The essentials of baccalaureate education for professional nursing practice.* Washington, DC: Author.

Conti, M., & Kumar, M. (2010). Opportunities in opportunistic computing. *Computer, 43*(1), 42–50.

Cornelius, F., Wilson, L., & Childs, G. (2010). Leveraging technology to support doctoral advanced nursing practice. In H. M. Dreher & M. E. Smith Glasgow (Eds.), *Role development for doctoral advanced nursing practice.* New York: Springer Publishing.

Curran, C., Sheets, D., Kirkpatrick, B., & Bauldoff, G. S. (2007). Virtual patients support point-of-care nursing education. *Nursing Management, 38*(12), 27–28, 30, 33.

Dolan, B. (2010, January 28). 9 reasons the iPad falls short for acute care. *Mobihealth News.* Retrieved from http://mobihealthnews.com/6299/9-reasons-the-ipad-falls-short-for-acute-care/

EMR DailyNews. (2010, June 16). Education management solutions launches the first simulated EMR for nursing & medical student training.

Fluke Biomedical. (2006). *PS320 Fetal Simulator: Technical data.* Retrieved from http://www.maquet-dynamed.com/inside_sales/literature/fluke/ps_320_datasheet.pdf

Hravnak, M., Beach, M., & Tuite, P. (2007). Simulator technology as a tool for education in cardiac care. *Journal of Cardiovascular Nursing, 22*(1), 16–24.

Institute of Medicine. (2003). *Health professions education: A bridge to quality.* Washington, DC: National Academy of Sciences. Retrieved from http://www.acme-assn.org/valuable_resources/IOM-ABridgetoQuality.pdf

Institute of Medicine. (2006). Preventing medication errors: Quality chasm. In P. Aspden, J. Wolcott, J. L. Bootman, & L. R. Cronewett (Eds.), *Quality chasm series.* Washington, DC: National Academies Press.

Kristoffersen, S., & Ljungberg, F. (1999). Mobile informatics innovation of IT use in mobile settings: IRIS'21 Workshop Report. *Special Interest Group on Computer Human Interaction Bulletin, 31*(1), 29–34.

Kristoffersen, S., Nielsen, F., Blechar, J., & Hanseth, O. (2005). Ordinary innovation of mobile services. In *Designing ubiquitous information environments: Socio-technical issues and challenges.* IFIP International Federation for Information Processing (Vol. 185, pp. 305–319). IFIP TC8 WG 8.2 International Working Conference, August 1–3, 2005, Cleveland, Ohio.

Mahoney, C. D., Berard-Collins, C. M., Coleman, R., Amaral, J. F., & Cotter, C. M. (2007). Effects of an integrated clinical information system on medication safety in a multihospital setting. *American Journal of Health-System Pharmacy, 64*(18), 1969–1977.

Oregon Telecommunications Coordinating Council. (2002, December 5). *Report of the Oregon Telecommunications Coordinating Council.* Presented to the Joint Legislative Committee on Information Management and Technology, Seventy-Second Legislative Assembly.

Poon, E. M. M., Keohane, C. B. R., Yoon, C. M., Ditmore, M. B., Bane, A. R. M., Levtzion-Korach, O. M. M., et al. (2010). Effect of bar-code technology on the safety of medication administration. *New England Journal of Medicine, 362*(18), 1698.

Sakowski, J., Leonard, T., Colburn, S., Michaelsen, B., Schiro, T., Schneider, J., et al. (2005). Using a bar-coded medication administration system to prevent medication errors. *American Journal of Health-System Pharmacy, 62*(24), 2619–2625.

Staggers, N., Gassert, C. A., & Curran, C. (2002, November/December). Results of a Delphi Study to determine informatics competencies for nurses at four levels of practice. *Nursing Research, 51*(6), 383–390.

TIGER Informatics Competency Collaborative. (2009). *TIGER Informatics Competencies* [Data file]. Retrieved from http://tigercompetencies.pbworks.com

Westra, B., & Delaney, C. (2008). *Informatics Competencies for nursing and healthcare leaders.* Paper presented at the AMIA Annual Symposium, Washington, DC. Retrieved from http://www.ncbi.nlm.nih.gov/pmc/articles/PMC2655955/pdf/amia-0804-s2008.pdf

Wideman, M. V., Whittler, M. E., & Anderson, T. M. (Eds.). (2005). *Barcode medication administration: Lessons learned from an intensive care unit implementation* (Vol. 3, Implementation Issues). Rockville, MD: Agency for Healthcare Research and Quality.

Woh, M., Mahlke, S., Mudge, T., & Chakrabarti, C. (2010). Mobile supercomputers for the next-generation cell phone. *Computer, 43*(1), 81–85.

CHAPTER 7

Implementation of the Human Simulation Encounter

Carol Okupniak, John Cornele, and Robert Feenan

*T*his chapter will focus on the events and tasks necessary to implement a successful human simulation session. A simulation session usually consists of several timed face-to-face encounters with a standardized patient actor. There are distinct activities and management functions that must be addressed to maximize the effectiveness of the simulation and help to ensure that all of the teaching and learning objectives are met. The main components that will be reviewed include planning, scheduling, conducting the experience, and managing recordings.

PLANNING

Planning involves thinking about the overall operation of the simulation center as well as the needs of the individual session. The volume or number of programs or courses served by the center impacts how the cases are developed and the amount of time needed for an individual session. It is a good idea to determine the hours of operation early in the development of the center. As utilization increases, hours may be stretched and boundaries pushed. If care is not taken, the demand can easily outstrip the resources of the center.

The size of the suite impacts both the scheduling and the timing of the individual student encounter. Faculty must be aware of the limitations of the physical space of the simulation center. Primarily, this means how many rooms or stations you have. This number will determine how many students you will be able to accommodate per time increment. For example, if your center has 10 rooms available and a simulation encounter lasts 30 minutes per student, the center could accommodate 10 students every 30 minutes or 100 students in a 5-hour day with a lunch break. Hence, on the basis of the size of the class, the time of the actual session, and the number of rooms available, you can plan how many sessions over how many days will be needed to give all students in the given class or course the same simulation experience. Determine the timing for the encounter and session ahead of time, and doing a tabletop dry run to review timing and walk through the session can prevent issues the day of the actual session.

The type of encounter can also affect the planning and timing of the simulation session. Is the session designed to be formative or summative? The latter will more than likely be structured more rigidly with very specific timing on the basis of efficiently evaluating student performance and ensuring that all student encounters are standardized so the evaluation remains fair. A formative session may be structured with less rigidity to be more responsive to the learner's needs at the time of the encounter, and allow for learning in those unexpected directions that the learner brings to the encounter. Both designs need some constraint to make efficient use of the resources of time, space, equipment, and personnel. The degree of control can be adjusted but only within those limitations to ensure that the entire cohort involved in the session can complete the experience.

An integral part of the planning process is the construction and design of a standardized patient (SP) profile. Information about your patient that is not specific to the case should be generic. Information that is important must be carefully constructed and communicated to the SP during the training process. White (2007, p. 65) introduced the concept of the "backstory," which encompasses all of the information that serves to bring the "patient" to life for the student or trainee.

The design should take multiple factors about the patient's lifestyle into consideration. Not only is the patient's medical history important when designing your patient, their personal demographics as well as their name, age, and gender must also be considered. As the patient profile will be adapted by a variety of people of different genders, sizes, and ages, writing a profile for a very specific patient will limit your choices. As a rule, if not endemic to the case, leave it out of the profile or have the SP use personal information. The relevance of the information to the case is the factor that makes the exchange of information standardized.

Once you have determined all of the details of the case, organize the data in a format that will be used for training the SP. Include only information relevant to the case and organize it in a logical format. Clearly indicate words or phrases that you expect the SP to recite verbatim during the face-to-face encounter. Other data are given to the SP as information to recall in his or her own words should the student or trainee request the information.

If you are using multiple SPs for the same encounter, it is important to stress which words or phrases are required to be related to the student during the encounter. This will ensure standardization among all encounters. Once the script is written and the checklist items are formulated, it will be evident what necessary components will be required during the case. Catrell and DeLoney state, "Every presentation is standardized and a guide to every checklist restricts the SP's variation from the script." A well-trained SP will keep to the script and not introduce any information that deviates from that script.

When planning for a simulation session using SPs, it is important to schedule the training dates in association with the performance dates. Scheduling the SPs will be easier if these times are associated, as they are able to guarantee appearance at both events. This is crucial; SPs should not be scheduled for a case that they have not prepared and trained for. Using an ill-prepared SP in a test session seriously undermines and weakens the standardization of the case. This makes the scheduling a bit more difficult, but planning for it early and offering the performance opportunity to the SP coupled with the training helps the process.

SCHEDULING

Conflicts in scheduling will arise and require creative solutions. A procedure must be in place to deal fairly with requests for the same date and time of a simulation session by different courses or programs. Developing a master schedule on an academic year format is one solution that can deal with conflicts early and avoid problems when scheduling the individual session. This process can be complicated if the center serves multidisciplinary programs. Ensuring equity among groups of diverse needs can be challenging but is not impossible. Involving all in the planning and scheduling process early can help to avoid most conflicts. Choosing a single representative for the program and forming a steering committee to provide a forum for scheduling policy discussions will help to ensure that those policies are implemented on a daily basis.

Determining who uses the center and when will be governed in some respects by some of the previously mentioned limitations: the number of students, the number of rooms, and the length and type of encounter. There may be times when scheduling a session that the appropriateness of use may enter the equation. Having many requests for the same time and space may require a determination of the session based on who is using the center most appropriately. For example, quite a few centers have their simulation areas situated in the clinical skills laboratory and share the space. This can add another layer of complexity to the scheduling process. Having a matrix to determine usage by need may help. If the simulation center is the only place that video recording can be done, then the program who will be recording and using SPs has more of a need than a program who may only be using the space for a formative session that may only be using SPs, or even a program that is interested in the center for space only.

Planning for these situations in advance can avoid congestion and misuse of the center. Introducing the customers of the simulation center to the policies of operation and use will develop an informed customer base and thus more appropriate use of the resources.

CONDUCTING THE EXPERIENCE

Starting with a solid schedule and trialed timing helps to preserve the work flow on the day of the event by keeping everyone on track and the encounters standardized. The needs of the day can include the schedule, personnel assignments, room and equipment setup, and recording control. The schedule maintains the flow of the students through the center and determines the recording timing, if recordings are being done. The recording timing can in turn determine any announcements if they are being used to assist students and staff with timing.

EQUIPMENT

Make arrangements before the encounter for equipment that will be used. Will each SP need a cane? Do your SPs have any injuries, wounds, scars, and so forth, relevant to the encounter? Will a blood pressure cuff, stethoscope, thermometer, or watch with a second hand be needed? Careful attention to these details will help to add to the realism for the student or trainee.

As the student or trainee and patient encounter involves the assumption of the patient seeking medical care, there should be a vehicle for the student or trainee to retrieve necessary information about the patient. The student or trainee will be given information that is spoken, written, or digital. Deciding how that information is delivered is an often overlooked, but necessary, part of the planning process.

Undoubtedly, the easiest way to communicate information from the educator to the student or trainee is verbally. Having the current care provider read the report to the person who will assume the care of the patient and having that person write down necessary information is also a quick, easy, but limited way. A more efficient method of relaying information to the student or trainee is to have a written report outlining all necessary information about the patient that is easy for the student to refer to during the encounter.

An efficient and accurate method of relating information to the student or trainee is the use of an electronic medical record. This can aid in the realism of the simulation and make the student familiar with what is becoming a common form of documentation. This information can be made available to the student before the encounter for review. Having a well-constructed electronic medical record can serve not only to inform the student or trainee about the patient but also to help the student who is unfamiliar with electronic documentation experience in this form of communication, which exemplifies informatics technology in the medical field.

Personnel assignments are important to be sure all tasks are accomplished. Having one person assigned to prepare the students before the encounter and direct them to the encounter area is very valuable. It is also helpful if the person assigned to the students is associated with the program or course that is requiring the simulation, as they will be able to answer any program-or course-related questions from the students. This course representative is often best suited to deliver the prebriefing to the students. The personnel will need to be assigned to be responsible for the SPs as they will have last minute questions as well as procedural issues. Any case-related questions should be referred to the program or course representative, and the simulation center representative should handle logistical or technical questions. If the simulation is being video recorded, a camera and a video control person are essential. If recording is being handled manually, this person should not have any other responsibilities that could distract them from getting the best view of the student performance. Using all available personnel can help fill any gaps that may have been missed. For example, if extra SPs have been scheduled to ensure operation of the session in the event of an SP calling out for whatever reason, those "extra" backup SPs can be used to help with student flow or be assigned to perform quality assurance measures on recorded or live sessions.

Using computer software to aid in scheduling can simplify many of the operations both on the day of the encounter as well as during scheduling. Some programs use video capture software that automates some of the tasks associated with storing and indexing videos and associated student information and session information. This makes retrieval of the session information easier and more complete. The use of the software will require the collection of the information associated with the session before the day of the event to enter the data into the software. This can be incorporated into the scheduling process and as the information is received about the session.

Having a staging area for the students can help to maintain the flow of the students through the session. This will allow an area to brief the students before their encounter and an area to wait for the beginning of their session. An additional area may be needed if students have activities after the SP encounter.

Unscheduled interruptions, although not welcome, must be prepared for as much as practical. These may include fire drills, sick students, sick SPs, or sick faculty. Absent students will disrupt the schedule at the least, and if the session is a summative test, they may necessitate the creation of a makeup session.

The final action of a session day is to clean up and restore the center or prepare for the next session. It can help if much of the materials needed for encounters are stored in the center. SPs can assist with the process by restoring the room that they have been scheduled in and properly dealing with their linen and trash.

MANAGING RECORDINGS

Recording the simulation session and associating the supporting documentation and files require some degree of organization and management. If a manual system is used, the simulation specialist involved will have to enter the information from the session, including student name or ID number, video file name, SP responsible for presenting the case, faculty involved in evaluation of the student, and any other information needed by the case. The schedule of the recordings will have to be developed as well as any announcements needed to direct the students and faculty to keep the session running smoothly. Many of the video capturing software systems available today are capable of automating most, if not all, of these functions. However, some of the data will still need to be entered into the system, but in most cases it can be done ahead of the session date. The use of a computer-based system will also allow for easier retrieval of the session information for distribution and review. Camera control during the session is still best handled by personnel.

When choosing recording capabilities, choose a file format that supports your distribution system, if possible; the recordings need to be easily distributed to your intended audience, students, or faculty or outside reviewers. If you have access to informational technology support, it can be helpful with these decisions as well as in troubleshooting during an actual session. Many centers find it helpful to include information technology personnel on their staff.

The personnel assigned to manage the daily recordings will need to know the distribution and storage requirements for the recordings. Recorded video files of any length of time can tend to be large files, so if they are being saved locally on the center's servers, storage capacity may become an issue. Will the students be viewing the recordings, and how long will they have access to them? This needs to be set after the session. How will the students access the recordings? Will they have to return to the simulation center to view them or will the recordings be posted on the web for remote access. In either case, the recorded information will need to be secured and filed so the student will only have access to their own material. The center will need to have a policy on data retention and destruction. Information used for evaluation of students is sensitive and confidential, and the policy needs to address the length of time the videos will be stored as well as who will have access to them and how access is granted. Some centers will house the data on secure servers at their location, whereas others will prefer to outsource this function.

Frequent review and analysis of the center procedure will keep the process up to date. All of these procedures will collectively provide a smooth, secure, and standardized session.

CONCLUSION

Simulation is a powerful tool to enhance learning and to provide the student with opportunity to reflect on their performance in a nearly real-life setting. The better the simulation environment is constructed and the more efficiently it is run, the more disbelief is suspended. A well-organized session also makes retrieval of data for review and reflection easier.

REFERENCES

Canrell, M. J., & Deoney, L. A. (2007). Integration of standardized patients into simulation. *Anesthesiology Clinics, 25,* 377–383.

White, P. (2007). *Coaching standardized patients for use in the assessment of clinical competence.* New York: Springer Publishing.

CHAPTER 8

Debriefing After Simulated Patient Experiences

Catherine Jean Morse

This chapter explores different models and approaches of debriefing after student participation in simulated patient experiences. Debriefing can be defined as a learning experience in which reflective thinking on past actions is linked to theoretical frameworks and didactic knowledge and then integrated into a new perspective for managing similar situations in the future (Morse, 2009). In simulated experiential learning, debriefing exercises are essential not only to enhance student learning and clarify concepts, but also to acknowledge and support the student. However, how to debrief, when to debrief, and what the critical elements are in an effective debriefing have not been clearly established (Fanning & Gaba, 2007).

Experiential learning is not a new pedagogy in the education of prelicensure or advanced practice nursing students. Types of experiential learning have included clinical rotations, cooperative experiences, service learning, skills laboratories, and internships. However, the focus of this discussion is on the debriefing of students after participation in standardized patient laboratory (SPL) or hybrid scenarios that include student interaction with the standardized patient(s) and high-fidelity mannequin(s) in one scenario. Despite different approaches, such as SPL and hybrid scenarios, all experiential learning modalities have the potential to simultaneously engage students in the cognitive, affective, and behavioral domains of learning. One key difference between experiential learning and traditional didactic lecturing is that it is not teacher focused; rather, it is student focused. Another underlying assumption of experiential learning with simulation is that it is particularly well suited for the adult learner: that is, most students, albeit with varying backgrounds, in undergraduate and graduate nursing programs. Although the graduate nursing student may have a greater repertoire of prior experience, second degree programs at the undergraduate level involve students who also bring a greater depth of prior experience to the learning environment.

Therefore, effective design, implementation, and evaluation of simulated experiences require an understanding of the pedagogy of experiential learning. Although the literature is replete with theories of experiential learning, Kolb's (1984) experiential learning theory, which describes learning as an active experience in which the learner interacts with the environment and engages in reflective processes, is well-suited to learning in the simulated patient environment. The experiential learning cycle is described as a cyclical or spherical pattern of learning from experience that has four elements: concrete experience, observation and reflection, forming abstract concepts, and testing in new situations (Kolb, 1984). The typical learning experience in the simulated environment encompasses a prebriefing that includes describing the scenario objectives (orientation to the environment and provision of time to answer student questions), the simulated scenario, and lastly, the debriefing. Experiential learning with simulated patients has been described using the experiential learning theory as a framework: concrete experience (simulation experience), observation and reflection (debriefing and reflective thought), forming abstract concepts (stimulates new ideas, debriefing, lectures, reading, or PDA use), and testing in new situations (new simulation exercises, clinical experiences, or life experience; Overstreet, 2008). The typical experiential learning experience in SPL also includes a prebriefing that can be written or verbal, patient interaction, and feedback from the standardized patient, after which debriefing can be conducted individually (faculty–student) or in small groups of students and faculty. Although it is a different experiential learning experience, the principles of debriefing remain the same and will be discussed later in the chapter. Student engagement in reflective practices is an essential element in the experiential learning cycle.

Reflection during debriefing allows participants to consider their decisions and actions during the simulated scenario, integrate the experience into established theories or evidence-based protocols, and then, if needed, create a new framework or perspective for working through a similar situation in the future. The faculty member serves as the students' guide in the reflective process and ensures that the integration of correct patient care principles is achieved.

Teaching and learning in simulation provides safety for the practitioner and patient and an opportunity for repeated deliberate practice with the intent to improve patient safety and patient outcomes. Critical self-reflection in debriefing may be one mechanism to translate student learning from simulation to authentic patient experiences (Issenberg, McGaghie, Petrusa, Lee, & Scalese, 2005; McGaghie, Issenberg, Petrusa, & Scalese, 2010; Rudolph, Simon, Raemer, & Eppich, 2008). Conducting simulation experiences and not engaging students in debriefing, and thereby not fostering reflection, could result in erroneous or negative learning or, at best, represent a squandered learning experience. Reflection is an active process for the participant and debriefing leader. It requires the debriefing leader to facilitate students' self-analysis in a productive, nonpunitive fashion. Engaging students in reflective exercises is a complex but worthwhile endeavor.

The concept of a reflective practitioner is based on more than three decades of work, not just in the health care professions, but in law, engineering, and business (Schon, 1983). This body of work describes the intuitive processes that some practitioners bring to uncertain situations as "knowing in practice," meaning that there are certain actions, recognitions, and judgments that are completed without thinking consciously. *Reflection in action* refers to the ability to combine and recombine the incoming stimuli, being willing to reconsider decisions or actions based on new information while immersed in the situation (Schon, 1983). The professional is not only thinking while they are doing, but also evolving their way of doing. The reflective practitioner is able to revise their understanding of a situation in the thick of it and is able to reflect on their understanding of the rules governing the situation, the feelings associated with it, or how the problem is framed. Conversely, *reflection on action* is the active process that can be facilitated in the debriefing after participation in simulated experiences or any experiential learning opportunity. Clearly, developing these skills in nurses, advanced practice nurses, and other health care professionals will hopefully translate to thoughtful, safe, and creative care of patients. One model of debriefing that is described in the medical literature, which has rigorous reflection as a core element, is debriefing with good judgment (Rudolph, Simon, Rivard, Dufresne, & Raemer, 2007). These authors describe rigorous reflection as a process that "brings to the surface and helps resolve the clinical and behavioral dilemmas and areas of confusion raised by the simulation experience" (Rudolph et al., 2007, p. 362).

Assumptions and beliefs about reflection in nursing include (a) reflection can be an intuitive practice used in everyday life, but transferring those skills to the professional arena may require further development; (b) reflection is always good and develops a thinking practitioner; (c) increased reflection will result in improved learning; and (d) student reflective journaling will translate into a reflective practitioner (Scanlan & Chernomas, 1997). Faculty members need to examine their own assumptions about reflection and, in particular, the role of reflection in debriefing. It is also critical to differentiate reflection and debriefing from evaluation and feedback.

Because evaluation can be summative or formative, faculty members need to have clearly identified if an experiential learning experience entails an evaluative process. A formative evaluation provides learners with feedback from the educator, encouraging self-reflection to improve future performance (Jeffries & Rogers, 2007). A summative evaluation is conducted at the end of a learning period, and although there is feedback, there is no opportunity for improvement (Jeffries & Rogers, 2007). Nurses and advanced practice nurses will face many new, uncertain, and stressful situations in their careers. Developing skills in reflection will better equip them to provide safe and effective patient care. The use of simulation and appropriate debriefing techniques may be one approach to achieve that goal.

Facilitating the development of a reflective practitioner is paramount for nursing students at all levels. The experiential learning offered by simulation and debriefing can emulate the authentic, complex patient environment and allow the student to practice reflection in action (during the scenario) and reflection on action (debriefing). Remember, debriefing without reflection could result in a missed learning opportunity or negative learning if clinical errors are not discussed and corrected.

DEBRIEFING IN NURSING

Although there are an increasing number of studies on simulation in the nursing literature, few address the process of debriefing (Nehring, 2009; Solnick & Weiss, 2007). A summary of the current nursing literature on debriefing follows.

The effect of a structured debriefing session on prelicensure student learning was evaluated in 11 senior level nursing students after participation in three pediatric simulations (Cantrell, 2008). A verbal debriefing was performed immediately postsimulation and a structured, investigator-led debriefing, including an audiotape review, was conducted 2 weeks later. Content analysis of the students' comments revealed three critical components that influenced students' learning: adequate student preparation, demeanor of the faculty involved in the simulation, and debriefing at the end of the simulation experience. The students reported that the format of the debriefing was less important than the timing, and debriefing immediately after the experience was judged to be critical to the discussion of the experience and integration of the knowledge gained.

Debriefing with the outcome present state test (OPT) model of clinical reasoning was described in a study with 44 undergraduate nursing students in a medical and surgical clinical course (Kuiper, Heinrich, Matthias, Graham, & Bell-Kotwall, 2008). The

OPT model of clinical reasoning requires creative thinking, emphasizes framing clinical situations with the patient's story, and focuses on patient outcomes. The process of student completion of the OPT worksheets was defined as structured debriefing in this study. In a 14-week clinical course, the study participants engaged in authentic clinical experiences and rotated through the simulation laboratory for simulated patient experiences. OPT worksheets were completed after both types of clinical experiences, and the highest scoring worksheets from the authentic clinical experience were compared with the highest scoring worksheets completed after participation in simulated experiences. The OPT worksheets were scored and reflected student level of clinical reasoning. No significant differences were reported between the mean scores of the OPT worksheets of the two groups ($t = -1.34$, $p = .194$; Kuiper et al., 2008). The students' written reflections revealed that the simulation experience prompted them to think on their feet, quickly, and for themselves; challenged clinical decision-making skills; and provided an opportunity to practice without being in a real situation. The format of debriefing in this study was written and structured with the OPT model, making it difficult to generalize the results beyond this study.

A qualitative study was conducted in a small sample of experienced Australian psychiatric mental health nurse educators to describe and clarify the structure used by faculty members when teaching with experiential exercises (Brackenreg, 2004). In particular, the author was interested in the phases of reflection and debriefing. Nine nurse educators, 8 of whom had at least 3 years of teaching experience and reported using experiential methods, and 1 participant without experiential teaching experience, participated in structured telephone interviews. Data analysis revealed that 8 faculty members took explicit steps, including a planned time frame for introducing the experience and an explanation of the conduct and design of the action phase of the process; 5 allocated the greatest percentage of time during the overall experience for the action phase; only 3 faculty members preplanned the debriefing or reflection phase and allowed at least half the total time of the experience to be spent in this phase. Most educators did not have a plan for the debriefing phase and only allotted 10% to 25% of the total time to debriefing. The one participant who reported never having used experimental teaching methods expressed concern that if the experiences were not conducted correctly, the experience could harm students. The findings highlighted the variability in faculty practice and the importance of further empiric study of the contribution of different debriefing models to participant learning.

A descriptive correlational study was conducted with 68 baccalaureate nursing students to clarify the relationship between the 5 elements of the nursing simulation design framework (Jeffries, 2007), student satisfaction, and self-efficacy (Smith, 2008). The 5 elements, as described by Jeffries (2007), include objectives, support, problem solving, guided reflection, and fidelity. Students were enrolled in the first medical and surgical nursing course and simulated experience was part of the curriculum. The students participated in a simulated scenario, including debriefing, and then were invited to participate in the study. If they agreed, the simulation design scale and student satisfaction and self-confidence in learning scale were completed.

The debriefing was described as a guided reflection and included a discussion of the following elements: student feelings, simulation activity, and patient's condition and student responses. The author also used the advocacy-inquiry approach described in the model "debriefing with good judgment" (Rudolph, Simon, Dufresne, & Raemer, 2006). The clinical scenario and debriefing were each approximately 20 minutes long. The results revealed that whereas all 5 design characteristics were rated favorably, guided reflection was rated the highest on the simulation design scale (mean = 4.8, *SD* = 0.41). The correlational analysis demonstrated a moderately strong correlation between all 5 design characteristics and student satisfaction and self-efficacy. The author concluded that consideration of the design characteristics, including guided reflection or debriefing, is an important step in creating an effective teaching–learning experience. The study was limited by the small sample size and lack of a control group.

Thirteen primary themes were identified in a qualitative, focus group study of eight undergraduate nursing students after participation in a patient simulator experience (Lasater, 2007). Themes related to debriefing included the following: "Debriefing was the most important phase for determining clinical judgment, but not enough time was spent on it"; "More honest, forthright feedback from the facilitator was needed" (Lasater, 2007, p. 272). The student feedback supports the notion of critical self-reflection and the potential value of the teaching–learning experience of debriefing. Also, it suggests that simply focusing on the good or correct actions that a student performs in simulation does not necessarily aid in their learning.

A concept analysis of debriefing in simulation learning in nursing identified the defining attributes of reflection, emotion, reception, and integration and assimilation (Dreifuerst, 2009). The author elaborates on the attributes as follows: reflection is the reexamination of the simulation experience; emotion and emotional release is an important part of affective learning and that emotional release can facilitate reflection; reception or openness to feedback has a primary role for the participant; and lastly, integration and assimilation of the experience into a conceptual framework as one of the most difficult attributes of debriefing.

The review of the literature on debriefing and simulation in nursing education reveals that there is much work to be done. Despite this fact, it is clear that the inclusion of debriefing in the planning of experiential learning exercises is critical. It also seems clear that critical self-reflection is a key component of debriefing. The development of faculty expertise in debriefing is required and should not be felt to be intuitive.

DEBRIEFING IN MEDICAL EDUCATION

The effect of timing of debriefing was investigated in a study of 161 third-year medical students who were randomly assigned to one of two groups: debriefing after participation in simulated experience or debriefing during simulation (Van Heukelom, Begaz, & Treat, 2010). The postsimulation debriefing was described as a three-step structured process that incorporated (1) decompression and reflection, (2) clarification of proper case management and review of errors, and (3) generalization and application. In contrast, debriefing during simulation was provided only if the participants appeared stuck or unable to make treatment decisions. Significant differences between the two groups were found in the responses to the following statements: debriefing helped me learn effectively ($p = .0001$), debriefing helped me to understand the correct and incorrect actions ($p = .001$), and debriefing style was effective ($p = .001$), with the postsimulation debriefing group scoring significantly higher on all the aforementioned categories (Van Heukelom et al., 2010).

A randomized controlled trial was conducted to evaluate the efficacy of debriefing on the performance of 58 practicing anesthetists (Morgan et al., 2009). The experimental group received the debriefing intervention led by an experienced facilitator, whereas the other 2 groups either received a home study program or no educational intervention.

Significant ($p = .03$) improvements were noted in the debriefed group on the scenario-specific checklist, which supported the efficacy of debriefing.

The outcome of different approaches to debriefing was evaluated in anesthesia residents (Savoldelli et al., 2006; Welke et al., 2009). Savoldelli et al. (2006) compared three randomly assigned groups of anesthesia residents ($n = 42$). Group 1 received no feedback, Group 2 was exposed to verbal feedback only, and Group 3 received verbal and video feedback. There were significant differences among the three groups, $F(2, 39)$, $p < .005$, and a post hoc analysis revealed that improvement was greatest in the group that received verbal feedback only (+15%), followed by those receiving video-assisted verbal feedback (+11%). A decrement was observed in the control group (–1%). Furthermore, the study findings suggested that exposure to the patient simulator without debriefing was of little educational value (Savoldelli et al., 2006).

In contrast, Welke et al. (2009) compared personalized, video-assisted, verbal debriefing to a standardized, computer-based, multimedia debriefing. The standardized computer-based multimedia debriefing was an author-designed computer program that included text, voice-over, and standardized videos. The scores on the anesthesia nontechnical scoring system improved for both groups in the posttest and retention scenarios; however, there were no significant differences between the groups. The study demonstrated a very small effect size of .02 for this type of instruction modality, and the results suggested that multimedia standardized debriefing was as effective as a personalized verbal and videotaped debriefing (Welke et al., 2009). However, there was no detailed description of the approach or duration of the personalized verbal debriefing or of the expertise of the facilitator in debriefing.

This review of the medical education literature evaluating debriefing after simulated experiences reveals one major conclusion: trends toward the positive benefit of the inclusion of debriefing exist, but clear empirical evidence does not. However, there is convergence in the literature that one of the essential elements of experiential learning in simulation is debriefing (Issenberg et al., 2005; Jeffries, 2005; McGaghie et al., 2010; Nehring, 2009). Despite this agreement, a review of the literature does not reflect agreement on the essential elements of debriefing or empiric evidence supporting one approach over another.

MODELS OF DEBRIEFING

There are various models of debriefing described outside the health care education literature (Lederman-Costigan, 1992; Petranek, Corey, & Black, 1992). The four E's of debriefing have been described in the simulation and gaming literature as events, emotions, empathy, and explanations (Petranek et al., 1992). Lederman-Costigan (1992) identified the seven elements of debriefing in higher education as the facilitator, the participants, the experience, the impact of the simulation, the recollection of the simulation, the process of discussing the experience, and the time to process it. Similar to previously presented approaches, Lederman described the three phases of debriefing as "the introduction to systematic reflection and analysis, the intensification and personalization of the analysis of the experience, and the generalization and application of the experience" (Lederman-Costigan, 1992, p. 151)

Although not considered a model of debriefing, but rather a checklist for use in medical simulation, the GREAT debriefing checklist includes the following: G, guidelines;

R, recommendations; E, events; A, analysis; and T, transfer of knowledge (Owen & Follows, 2006).

Hertel and Mills (2002) did not describe a specific model of debriefing but instead discuss the following as essential elements of an effective debriefing within a higher education setting:

- acknowledgment of participant emotions
- a discussion of the roles that the participants held during the simulation
- a summary reviewing the simulation in terms of learning objectives and an exploration of how the knowledge or skills derived from the simulation exercise can be applied to future situations

These authors also emphasized the importance of illuminating the thinking process of the participants and facilitating the discovery of faulty thinking that can be corrected in the debriefing. This is very similar to the approach taken in debriefing with good judgment (Rudolph et al., 2006), which recommends ascertaining the participants' internal frames that drove their actions observed in the simulation experience and engagement in rigorous self-reflection.

A three-step approach to the debriefing phase of experiential learning—defined as a systematic evaluation—entails returning in thought to the experience to highlight significant events and a closer examination of details, focusing on the feelings generated by the experience, and a cognitive reappraisal of the experience and associated principles toward developing a new cognitive map (a result of participation in the experiential learning process; Boud, Keogh, & Walker, 1985).

Although a single approach or model of debriefing may not be appropriate for all simulation experiences, the inclusion of critical self-reflection is supported as a crucial element in the experiential learning process (Brackenreg, 2004; Hertel & Mills, 2002; Issenberg et al., 2005; Jeffries & Rizzolo, 2006; Kolb, 1984; Lederman-Costigan, 1992; Owen & Follows, 2006; Petranek et al., 1992; Schon, 1983). Faculty members' knowledge of different models and theoretical frameworks supporting debriefing is essential to provide students with the most effective learning experience. As previously noted, it is important to differentiate the type of teaching–learning experience as a formative or summative assessment. Although debriefing and formative assessment are not interchangeable concepts, there can be significant overlap. When a formative assessment is conducted in a debriefing, it can lead to new insights during the dialogue between student and instructor (Rudolph et al., 2008).

An approach to debriefing that includes critical self-reflection as an essential element is the debriefing with good judgment model, as described by Rudolph et al. (2006). This is a structured model of debriefing with roots in the experiential learning model, cognitive science, and reflective practice (Rudolph et al., 2006, 2007, 2008). The authors, with more than 3,000 debriefings, sought to create a learning environment in which the participants felt "simultaneously challenged and psychologically safe enough to engage in rigorous reflection" (Rudolph et al., 2006, p. 49). Engaging in rigorous reflection during debriefing will hopefully lead to the development of a reflective practitioner when engaged in the complexities of patient care. This is potentially important to clinical practice, as nonreflective practitioners have been found to ignore inconsistent data and maintain ineffective practice patterns, whereas reflective practitioners are able to self-correct when competing data with new solutions to improve practice become available (Argyris & Schon, 1974, 1978; Schon, 1987). Rigorous self-reflection is incorporated in the steps of the debriefing with good judgment model.

The underlying assumptions of the debriefing with good judgment model include (1) participants' observable actions are driven by their internal frames or mental models; (2) these frames are invisible but can be inferred from the observed actions, which can include speech, nonverbal communication, and psychomotor clinical skills; (3) internal frames or mental models are the frameworks that participants use to make sense of the external world and are influenced by the participants' knowledge, assumptions, and feelings; (4) understanding the participants' internal frames is integral to changing future behavior; and (5) transparency of the faculty or instructor's internal frames is equally important to the process (Rudolph et al., 2006, 2007).

In this model, the faculty members' internal frames have shifted from the judgmental style of debriefing to a good judgment stance, a subtle shift that is critical to the success of the approach. Judging what went wrong and supplying the correct answer, assuming that their view is the only correct view, and shaming or blaming the participants to change their internal frames do not conclude the debriefing (Rudolph, 2010). Rather, the faculty member, well knowing the correct answer to the clinical dilemma, does not want to place the participant on the defensive. It is better for the participant to find the answer. In addition, the faculty member does not hide his or her frames in the debriefing with a good judgment model but openly shares them with participants. This means that a student does not have to guess what the instructor is thinking.

Debriefing with this model has three primary steps: (1) reactions to the scenario—includes facts and feelings and sets the stage for discussion; (2) understanding—review of what happened and exploration of the deeper meaning; and (3) summary—the faculty member reviews the lessons learned and the application to future practice (Rudolph, 2010). The understanding phase is where the real work of debriefing with good judgment occurs. Actions and clinical outcomes observed in the simulation are approached as intellectual puzzles to be solved, rather than inherently "bad" decisions. This is achieved by identifying the participants' "internal frames" or mental models using the advocacy-inquiry approach, in which the faculty member maintains a stance of genuine curiosity to discover through inquiry each student's internal frames. Actions are not viewed as erroneous, but as the inevitable result of the student's internal frame (Rudolph et al., 2006, 2007, 2008).

A conversational technique is used in a joint exercise to allow the judgment of the faculty member to be integrated with the frames of the student. The hallmarks of the conversational technique are advocacy and inquiry. This combination allows faculty members to counterbalance the natural tension that arises when making critical evaluative judgments with a trusting relationship that is established with each student being critiqued. The faculty members' perspective is clearly stated and invites the participants to share their perspective. The faculty member pairs their observations of the simulation (advocacy) with a question to discover the student frames that produced the clinical behaviors observed in the simulation (Rudolph et al., 2006, 2007, 2010).

For example, "I noticed that the patient's oxygen saturation was in the 70s and you were really focused on placing a peripheral intravenous line and did not initiate treatment. I was concerned, as hypoxemia can be a precursor to respiratory arrest—what were your thoughts at the time?" Uncovering the student's internal frames shift the learning from single-loop to double-loop learning. That is to say that the focus is not just on actions that create a result, but understanding and potentially changing the frames that drive the actions (Argyris & Schon, 1974; Rudolph et al., 2006).

This model of debriefing allows for critical constructive feedback to be provided to students in an atmosphere of mutual trust and avoids the historical "shame and blame" or "guess what you did wrong" approach that has been present in some health care training. However, this approach requires faculty investment and training to become proficient. It may not be appropriate in all situations, such as when patient safety and time is of paramount concern, discipline or counseling is needed, or criminal or negligent behavior occurred (Rudolph, 2010).

CONCLUSIONS

As a practice discipline, experiential learning is the core of the nursing educational foundation. Historically, those experiences all occurred in clinical sites. However, with the advances in technology, simulation can provide another venue for practice. Although simulation will never be a replacement for authentic clinical practice, it is an important adjunct. Designing clinical scenarios using a patient simulator and SPL is time-consuming, and sometimes the bulk of the work is expended in planning the active simulation experience and little thought is given to the debriefing.

However, the importance of debriefing and developing reflective thinking cannot be underestimated. To conduct effective debriefing sessions, faculty members are required to be versed in experiential learning theories and trained to facilitate a structured debriefing. Much uncertainty still exists in nursing about debriefing, and many confuse the process with feedback. Further research to explicate the core elements of debriefing will help to build an evidence-based approach to teaching and learning with simulation.

Simulation is labor-intensive and financially costly; therefore, it is critically important to demonstrate the most time- and cost-effective method to conduct experiential learning for our students with optimized outcomes in learning.

Finally, it is important that faculty members who lead simulation experiential teaching–learning experiences examine their own assumptions about reflection, and in particular, the role of reflection in debriefing. It is extremely important to differentiate reflection and debriefing from evaluation and feedback. Facilitating the development of a reflective practitioner is of paramount importance in nursing students of all levels, as it contributes to a lifelong approach to learning and professional practice.

REFERENCES

Argyris, C., & Schon, D. A. (1974). *Theory in practice: Increasing professional effectiveness* London: Jossey-Bass.

Argyris, C., & Schon, D. A. (1978). *Organizational learning: A theory of action perspective.* Reading, MA: Addison-Wesley.

Boud, D., Keogh, R., & Walker, D. (1985). *Turning experience into learning.* London: Kogan Page.

Brackenreg, J. (2004). Issues in reflection and debriefing: How nurse educators structure experiential activities. *Nurse Education in Practice, 4*(4), 264–270.

Cantrell, M. A. (2008). The importance of debriefing in clinical simulation. *Clinical Simulation in Nursing, 4*, e19–e23. doi:10.1016/j.ecns.2008.06.006

Dreifuerst, T. K. (2009). The essentials of debriefing in simulation learning: A concept analysis. *Nursing Education Perspectives, 30*(2), 109–114.

Fanning, R. M., & Gaba, D. M. (2007, Summer). The role of debriefing in simulation-based learning. *Simulation in Healthcare, 2*, 115–125. doi:10.1097/SIH.0b013e3180315539

Hertel, J., & Mills, B. J. (2002). *Using simulations to promote learning in higher education.* Sterling, VA: Stylus.

Issenberg, B. S., McGaghie, W. C., Petrusa, E. R., Lee, G. D., & Scalese, R. J. (2005). Features and uses of high-fidelity medical simulations that lead to effective learning: A BEME systematic review. *Medical Teacher, 27*(1), 10–28.

Jeffries, P. (2005, March/April). A framework for designing, implementing and evaluating simulations used as teaching strategies in nursing. *Nursing Education Perspectives, 26*(2), 96–103.

Jeffries, P. (Ed.). (2007). *Simulation in nursing education.* New York: National League for Nursing.

Jeffries, P., & Rizzolo, M. A. (2006). Designing and implementing models for innovative use of simulation to teach nursing care of ill adults and children: A national multi-site, multi-method study. Retrieved from https://www.nln.org/research/LaerdalReport.pdf

Jeffries, P., & Roger, K. (2007). Evaluating simulations. In P. Jeffries (Ed.), *Simulation in nursing education* (pp. 87–103). New York: National League for Nursing.

Kolb, D. (1984). *Experiential learning: Experience as the source of learning and development.* Englewood Cliffs, NJ: Prentice-Hall.

Kuiper, R., Heinrich, C., Matthias, A., Graham, M., & Bell-Kotwall, L. (2008). Debriefing with the OPT model of clinical reasoning during high fidelity patient simulation. *International Journal of Nursing Education Scholarship, 5*(1), 1–24.

Lasater, K. (2007). High-fidelity simulation and development of clinical judgment: Students' experience. *Journal of Nursing Education, 46*(6), 269–277.

Lederman-Costigan, L. (1992). Debriefing: Toward a systematic assessment of theory and practice. *Simulation and Gaming, 23*(2), 145–160.

McGaghie, W. C., Issenberg, B. S., Petrusa, E. R., & Scalese, R. J. (2010). A critical review of simulation-based medical education research: 2003–2009. *Medical Education, 44*, 50–63.

Morgan, P. J., Tarhis, J., LeBlanc, V., Cleave-Hogg, D., DeSousa, S., & Haley, M. F. (2009). Efficacy of high-fidelity simulation debriefing on the performance of practicing anaesthetist in simulated scenarios. *British Journal of Anesthesia, 103*(4), 531–537. doi:10.1093/bja/aep222.

Morse, K. (2009). *Concept analysis: Debriefing in high fidelity simulation.* Unpublished manuscript, College of Nursing, Villanova University, Villanova, PA.

Nehring, W. M. (2009). Nursing simulation: A review of the past 40 years. *Simulation and Gaming, 40*(4), 528–552. doi:10.1177/1046878109332282.

Overstreet, M. (2008). The use of simulation technology in the education of nursing students. *Nursing Clinics of North America, 43*(4), 593–603.

Owen, H., & Follow, V. (2006). GREAT simulation debriefing. *Medical Education, 40*(5), 488–487.

Petranek, C., Corey, S., & Black, R. (1992). Three levels of learning in simulation: Participating, debriefing and journal writing. *Simulation and Gaming, 23*(2), 174–185.

Rudolph, J. (2010). *Debriefing in a simulation environment: An introduction and immersion.* Paper presented at the Comprehensive Instructor Workshop, Institute for Medical Simulation, Harvard Medical Simulation Center.

Rudolph, J., Simon, R., Dufresne, R., & Raemer, D. (2006, Spring). There's no such thing as "non-judgmental" debriefing: A theory and method for debriefing with good judgment. *Simulation in Healthcare, 1*(1), 49–55.

Rudolph, J., Simon, R., Raemer, D., & Eppich, W. (2008). Debriefing as formative assessment: Closing performance gaps in medical education. *Academic Emergency Medicine, 15*(11), 1010–1016.

Rudolph, J., Simon, R., Rivard, P., Dufresne, R., & Raemer, D. (2007). Debriefing with good judgment: Combining rigorous feedback with genuine inquiry. *Anesthesiology Clinics, 25*, 361–376. doi:10.1016/j.anclin.2007.03.007.

Savoldelli, G. L., Naik, V. N., Park, J., Joo, H. S., Chow, R., & Hamstra, S. J. (2006). Value of debriefing during simulated crisis management: Oral versus video-assisted oral feedback. *Anesthesiology, 105*(2), 279–285.

Scanlan, J., & Chemomas, W. (1997). Developing the reflective teacher. *Journal of Advanced Nursing, 25*, 1138–1143.

Schon, D. A. (1983). *The reflective practitioner: How professionals think in action.* New York: Basic Books Inc.

Schon, D. A. (1987). *Educating the reflective practitioner: Toward a new design for teaching and learning in the professions.* San Francisco, CA: Jossey-Bass.

Smith, S. (2008). *High-fidelity simulation in nursing education: Design characteristics and their effect on student satisfaction and self-efficacy.* PhD dissertation, University of Northern Colorado.

Retrieved from http://proquest.umi.com/pqdweb?did=1545632991&Fmt=7&clientId=3260&R QT=309&VName=PQD.

Solnick, A., & Weiss, S. (2007). High fidelity simulation in nursing education: A review of the literature. *Clinical Simulation in Nursing, 3*, e341–e345. doi:10.1016/j.ecns.20090.5.039.

Van Heukelom, J. N., Begaz, T., & Treat, R. (2010). Comparison of postsimulation debriefing versus in-simulation debriefing in medical simulation. *Simulation in Healthcare, 5*(2), 91–97.

Welke, T., LeBlanc, V., Savoldlli, G., Joo, H., Chandra, D., & Crabtree, N. (2009). Personalized oral debriefing versus standardized multimedia instruction after patient crisis simulation. *Anesthesia and Analgesia, 109*(1), 183–189. doi:10.1213/ane.0b13e318a323ab.

CHAPTER 9

Reports and Analysis

Laurie L. Kerns and Sukhtej S. Dhingra

INTRODUCTION

Well-planned simulation experiences promote state-dependent learning—that is, practicing a skill in the environment and emotional state wherein the skill will be used. The trainee is provided an opportunity to exercise his or her clinical judgment and the resultant behaviors can be observed. Events from the simulation may be recorded for feedback, evaluation, or learner self-reflection, and measures of performance may be obtained. Other chapters in this publication discuss the benefits of simulation and the development of evaluation instruments. This chapter describes the basic styles of performance measurement and the methods by which to collect, interpret, and publish the data.

For the purposes of this manuscript, we will describe reports and measurements in broad terms that may be suitable for individual or team-based performance within health professionals' education, as well as simulation-based exercises with clinicians within integrated delivery systems.

DOCUMENTING CLINICAL PERFORMANCE

Medical education has traditionally used a "see one, do one, teach one" apprenticeship model (Rodriguez-Paz et al., 2009). The learner was expected to practice on real patients and evaluation was based on faculty observation, oral examination, multiple-choice examination, and treatment consequence. Clinician performance tended to be measured by volume and profitability (Lee, 2010). The focus on patient safety requires a new practice approach and has paved the way toward the adoption of simulated skills exercises. The movement toward learner-led experiences, problem-based learning, and competency-based training has helped to create a paradigm shift and the opportunity for performance-based education and assessment has been introduced.

The use of clinical performance–based education and assessments has been growing in medical and nursing education. Simulation using standardized patients (laypeople trained to portray a medical condition) was introduced by Dr. Howard Barrows in the 1960s to provide the medical student with an exercise that could be repeated and controlled (Wallace,

1997). Nursing education has long used basic simulation: CPR on a mannequin, subcutaneous and intramuscular injection skills practice using oranges, and role-play (Sanford, 2010). The advancement of technology has provided additional opportunities to simulate clinical conditions using task trainers and low- and high-fidelity electromechanical mannequin simulators. These technologies have been embraced and have driven new learning and assessment strategies within the curriculum of nursing, medical, and health professionals' education. Simulation participants are provided an opportunity to practice technical and communication skills, experience role expectations, and review the behaviors and communication patterns of the individual and the team within a controlled environment. The adoption and use of standardized patient examinations for licensure and certification has elevated the credibility of the examination and driven the use of simulation into the educational and continuing medical education arenas (Boulet, 2009).

WHY COLLECT DATA?

Once simulation with participants begins, the next logical questions are: "Did it make a difference?" "Did the training do what it was intended to do?" "Are we changing behavior?" "Are we getting our money's worth?" Interviews with simulation center directors from 2005 to 2009 revealed that early adopters were more interested in the simulation experience than in tracking outcomes, but that the trend is beginning to shift (Kerns, 2009). Although the goal of simulation is to provide a safe place to learn complex skills (Prion, 2008), it may be necessary to collect data to record utilization, feedback, and performance data. Simulation is expensive, and nursing programs are spending money on simulators, laboratory space, administration, maintenance, and training (Adamson, 2010). Utilization information may be necessary to satisfy stakeholders, whereas feedback may be collected to record participants' experience and confidence levels, and performance data provide information relative to training and skills improvement. The act of documentation may increase learner motivation and identify deficiencies within curricula and organizational systems. As certification requirements and licensure boards require documentation of competencies to make inferences about proficiency (Boulet, Gimpel, & Errichetti, 2003) and liability insurance companies record team training experiences, simulation learning becomes the vehicle to collect that data.

Prion (2008, p. e76) states, "Careful attention to input variables such as prerequisite knowledge and skills, environmental variables such as the educational practices of the simulation, and direct measurement of learner outcomes will provide the most comprehensive and credible feedback about student learning from the simulation experience."

Thus, it is important to collect these data right from the beginning and include all types of simulation to provide the basis for review and analysis of simulation laboratory utilization, learner feedback, and performance evaluation.

WHAT DATA DO WE WANT TO COLLECT?

Evaluating the effectiveness of the simulation might be done via a simple satisfaction self-report. This could be captured via paper form (bubble sheet) or computer-based online survey software. Measuring the participant buy-in and success within the exercise may provide helpful feedback for the simulation operator. Surveys conducted before and after the simulation exercise may provide insight into trainee confidence levels, as well as information about opportunities to practice the learned skills. Pre- and postexercise evaluation examinations can be conducted to check for increased content knowledge. This cycle of feedback and performance evaluation between simulation exercises provides an opportunity for the trainee to demonstrate the improvement and behavior changes with this practice-based learning. Global (holistic) performance ratings are effective measurements to record communication skills and professionalism (Boulet, 2009). Documentation may be obtained to reflect outcomes (the simulated patient status), processes (how well a task was performed), or volume (how many tasks were completed).

ASSESSMENT AND EXAMINATION STYLES

Formative Assessments

Often referred to as *learning exercises*, formative assessments establish baseline data and are considered low stakes. Rarely are important decisions, such as competency, connected with a formative exercise. The goal is to provide feedback to the examinee about his or her performance.

Summative Assessments

Summative assessments usually occur at the end point of the training or learning curriculum. Decisions may be made as to the success and readiness of the examinee to continue onto the next phase of training or for the training to be considered complete. Summative exercises are frequently considered high stakes in that the examinee, if failing the exercise, may be denied a required status (Boulet, 2008).

Norm-Referenced Examination

In a norm-referenced examination, achievement or pass-fail decisions tend to be based on a sample of examinee scores. An examinee's performance is measured on the basis of how well she or he performs relative to other examinees in the sample. Often, pass-fail decisions are made on the basis of a cut point of 1 or 2 standard deviations (SDs) below the mean. This information may be useful in determining percentile scores, student rank, or required remediation, but may not define what the examinee can do. However, it may be implied that examinees obtaining the same or similar scores demonstrate similar levels of performance. The norm reference may change as the ability of the group changes over time.

Criterion Reference Examination

A criterion-referenced examination is designed to measure an examinee's performance as compared with an acceptable standard. In the case of simulation, it is the measure of the examinee's mastery of a particular skill or ability to match their performance to what the test author considered important.

ASSESSMENT APPROACHES

Feedback from the participants and instructors in the form of evaluation instruments or surveys at the time of the exercise provides valuable insight into the learning experience. Assessment data will document the degree to which the learning outcomes are met and will offer feedback to instructors regarding the course or curricula. Survey data from participants and instructors will provide information regarding the process including, but not limited to, learner preparedness for the exercise, realism of the scenario, and attitudes toward the event.

Explicit Process

A case-specific performance checklist, used to identify the knowledge and skills the candidate is expected to perform correctly, would be considered an explicit process.

Implicit Process

An implicit process is the global judgment by an evaluator as to the performance of the examinee. Often used as a humanistic domain rating scale to evaluate communication or professional skills or to evaluate the timing or sequence of events.

Explicit Outcome

The consequence or gain at the completion of the exercise, such as the patient status, would be considered an explicit outcome. (Boulet & Swanson, 2004). This would include "value sensitive" assessments that consider not only the learning outcomes but also the personal value and choices made by the trainee.

HOW DO WE COLLECT THE DATA?

As mentioned previously, additional chapters in this publication address the creation of measurement instruments. We believe that instruments, when properly designed and used, can produce meaningful outcome measurements. "If skills are to be tested and pursuant performance criterion are well-defined, the focus should simply rest on modeling performance scenarios that are in line with practice patterns" (Boulet, Gimpel, et al., 2003, p. 225). The scenario may seek to replicate the entire environment or may elicit a particular skill to be observed. Recorded video provides powerful evidence that may be used for self-reflection or debriefing. Associating the video with simulation events or behavior provides a structure to review performance. Written records collect opinions and performance data. Introducing realism and complexity may provide a valid assessment of the examinee's skills and abilities and may provide inferences about their behavior outside the simulated exercise. Conducting the evaluation in an "unobtrusive" manner, such as from a remote location or via video recording, is important if aspects of behavior are to be assessed (Boulet & Swanson, 2004).

The type of information we collect (feedback or examination) as well as the style of collection (in person, on paper, via a web-based learning management system, anonymously, or by name) will have some impact on the data collected.

Types of Data/Assessment Instruments

Assessment instruments may be designed to collect qualitative (anecdotal) information or quantitative (score) data.

Surveys

Instruments of opinion tend to provide qualitative information. Information relative to perceptions, attitudes, opinions, and attributes may be collected. Participant feedback may be collected in the form of surveys or polls. Satisfaction surveys may be collected anonymously and may provide feedback about the experience. In addition, the opinions may be correlated to performance scores to study the verisimilitude of the simulation and its impact on performance.

A confidence survey may be administered as a pretest or posttest, or the participant may be surveyed minutes, days, or weeks after a simulation exercise. This is intended to record the trainee's confidence after having practiced a particular skill or to measure a change in attitudes after a training exercise (Figure 9.1).

A postsimulation self-reflection instrument via debriefing or independent video review may assist the learner in internalizing a learned skill, attitude, or behavior.

Performance Rating Checklist

Documenting performance through the use of a checklist can link the scenario events to observable behaviors. The instrument may capture competency assessment as well as performance processes (teamwork, leadership, communication, and professionalism) in addition to outcomes.

Global ratings rely on judgment by trained evaluators to recognize and evaluate within defined parameters or anchors.

It may be instructive to categorize checklist items by domain or skill/competency. These performance-based categories allow for the review of the information in more detail. This may expose a deficiency the learner has within a particular domain area

ANONYMOUS SURVEY STATISTICS

Scenario Survey

All Responses — Total Sample Size: 6

The scenario experience was realistic	Sample Size:	6
Option Text	**No of Responses**	**Percentage**
Yes	4	66.67
No	2	33.33

Have you had an opportunity to apply the communication skills practiced in the Infant Transport Scenario?	Sample Size:	6
Option Text	**No of Responses**	**Percentage**
Yes	4	66.67
No	2	33.33

Have you had an opportunity to apply the technical skills practiced in the Infant Transport Scenario?	Sample Size:	6
Option Text	**No of Responses**	**Percentage**
Yes	1	16.67
No	5	83.33

I have increased confidence in my ability to perform the skill practiced in the scenario	Sample Size:	6
Option Text	**No of Responses**	**Percentage**
Yes	3	50
No	3	50

Figure 9.1 *Example of a Participant Survey.*
Source: Adapted from Education Management Solutions. © 2008

CHECKLIST SCORE

INSTITUTE NAME : EMS Institute 4.6

STUDENT NAME   : Learner, One   STUDENT ID : learner1

SESSION NUMBER: 2   DATE   : 08/04/2009

	SCORE	RESULT
FORM: Z Form	SCORE: 82.11%	RESULT:PASS
CASE: Sarah W.	SCORE: 82.11%	RESULT:PASS
CATEGORY: History	SCORE: 92.86%	RESULT:PASS
Q1 : Location of the pain: "Where does it hurt?" (Yes)	SCORE: 100.00%	
Q2 : What makes this problem better? (Yes)	SCORE: 100.00%	
Q3 : What makes this problem worse? (Yes)	SCORE: 100.00%	
Q4 : Has it changed since it started (N)	SCORE: 50.00%	
Q5 : Associated Symptoms: "Anything else going on?" (Yes)	SCORE: 100.00%	
Q6 : How much alcohol do you consume" (Yes)	SCORE: 100.00%	
Q7 : Have you tried to treat this? (N)	SCORE: 50.00%	
Q8 : Are you currently taking any medication? (Yes)	SCORE: 100.00%	
CATEGORY: Physical Exam	SCORE: 81.25%	RESULT:PASS
Q9 : Auscultated Heart (Incomplete)	SCORE: 50.00%	
Q10 : Auscultated Lungs (Listened 2 location)	SCORE: 100.00%	
Q11 : Auscultated abdomen (Done)	SCORE: 100.00%	
Q12 : The student lightly palpated my abdomen (Done)	SCORE: 100.00%	
Q13 : The student percussed my abdomen (Done)	SCORE: 50.00%	
Q14 : The student deeply palpated my abdomen (Done)	SCORE: 100.00%	
Q15 : The student examined for rebound tenderness (Done)	SCORE: 100.00%	
CATEGORY: Interpersonal Comm SCORE:	72.22%	RESULT:PASS
Q17 : Communication Skills: The student adequately addressed my concerns, offered adequate information, did not lecture me. (6Superior-7)	SCORE: 72.22%	
Q18 : Empathy: The student demonstrated concern for me/my condition.	SCORE: 72.22%	

Figure 9.2 *Performance Checklist.*
Source: Adapted from Education Management Solutions. © 2008

that may not be observable from the overall case score. The learner may compensate in his or her overall scores by performing exceptionally well within another domain area. For accurate scoring, it may be important to keep the categories equal or to weight the items in such as a way as to equalize the categories; however, raw data may also be important to obtain. Several of the reports presented on the following pages demonstrate the use of categories to display the results.

The checklist example (Figure 9.2) records the events of an encounter between a standardized patient and a trainee. The patient records the events (questions asked, physical examinations performed) as well as a global rating (a Likert rating scale—in this case, a scale from 1 to 9) documenting the subjective judgment of the patient in response to the trainee's treatment of the patient. The standardized patient is carefully trained to recognize the correct maneuvers as well as the anchors of the global rating scale. The checklist, when completed via a computer-based software-management system, may use predefined scoring criteria to efficiently score the exercise and disseminate the information.

At the basic level, the result of the checklist or assessment instrument may be produced. In the simplest form, a raw score may be obtained, or in this example, a weighted mean score is used to produce a percentage score for each item, for the category, and finally for the case, encounter, or event.

Item banking or maintaining a library of checklist items will help to maintain the integrity of the data over time. This will reduce or eliminate the potential of similar but different items or misinterpretation of items.

The following checklist (Figure 9.3) provides information about actions completed by the trainee to document the event without scores.

CHECKLIST RESPONSE

INSTITUTE NAME	: Institute	SESSION NAME	: Asthma
PARTICIPANT NAME	: Student, Mary (3456789)	DATE	: 08/14/2010-1(09:00)
SCENARIO NAME	: Asthma, Acute		

Category Name   Nursing scenarios

Q.No	Question Text	Admin, TSC (FAC)
1	Wash hands	1-Done
2	Introduce self	1-Done
3	Identify the patient (name, ID band, DOB, MR#)	1-Done
4	Obtain BP, pulse, respiratory rate, temperature, SpO2	1-Done
5	Perform respiratory assessment	2-Done incorrectly or incompletely
6	Attach ECG monitor leads	1-Done
7	Give oxygen	1-Done
8	Monitor level of consciousness	1-Done
9	Recognize severe respiratory distress	2-Done incorrectly or incompletely
10	Call for help	1-Done
11	Administer emergency medications per order	1-Done
12	Maintain cardiovascular and respiratory stability	1-Done

Figure 9.3 *Checklist Report Without Scores.*
Source: Adapted from Education Management Solutions. © 2008

SOAP Scoring Template

Review or edit the scores below. Click on the submit button to save your changes.

Institute	EMS Institute 4.6	Test Date	12/22/2010
Student Name	B. Steve	Session Number	1
User Name	laurie.kerns	Case Name	Greg R.

Patient input regarding the problem(s)

Well-nourished 68 year old male presents complaining of a cough and SOB. Patient reports he had a cold three weeks ago. The cold has apparently subsided but the cough has persisted and he has experienced SOB x2 days. Patient reports he has to sit upright, limit activity, and has to use two pillows to sleep.

	UNACCEPTABLE	ADEQUATE	SUPERIOR
Subjective	Omits many key elements of history	Provides enough correct detail for adequate assessment and plan May be missing some elements of HPI, PMH, Family or Social Hx	Accurate and complete information as with standard; identifies patient's concern(s) Key elements listed (CC, HPI with OPQRST, etc)
Medical History CC HPI	○1 ○2 ○3	○4 ⦿5 ○6	○7 ○8 ○9
Pertinent ROS Includes relevant PMH, FamHx, SocHx	○1 ○2 ⦿3	○4 ○5 ○6	○7 ○8 ○9

Figure 9.4 *Patient Note With Scoring Rubric.*
Source: Adapted from Education Management Solutions. © 2008

Medical Knowledge Examination

Examinees may be assessed on their medical knowledge either via their critical thinking within a simulated examination or exercise, or through a patient note, electronic health record, or content questionnaire delivered after the exercise. The postsimulation exercise, as with the checklist, when completed via a computer-based software management system may utilize predefined scoring criteria to efficiently score the exercise and disseminate the information. Figure 9.4 is an example of a trainee patient note with a scoring rubric for the instructor. In the example, the examinee is asked to document the subjective and objective findings for the patient. The instructor is given a web-based scoring rubric to evaluate the examinee documentation.

HOW DO WE INTERPRET THE DATA?

Mean, Median, and Mode

Once scores are obtained, they must be interpreted. Common measures of central tendency (mean, median, and mode) are used to interpret the results. The mean is the average score obtained by the group. It is the sum of all scores divided by the number of scores.

The median is the midpoint of scores or the center of the data set. This is the point at which there is an equal number of scores above and below. This may not be a student score, but it is the point at which 50% of the examinees scored above and 50% scored below. The mode is the score attained by the greatest number of examinees.

These scores by themselves may not provide much detail as to the performance of the examinee or group. The score distribution may be positively or negatively skewed depending on item difficulty and performance by the group. In a negatively skewed distribution, most scores fall above the mean. In a positively skewed distribution, most scores fall below the mean. Figure 9.5 illustrates how knowing only the mean will not tell us much about the performance of the group.

Because the mean alone is not enough, we need more information as to the measures of variability. One of these measures is the range of scores. The range is measured by subtracting the lowest score from the highest score. The standard deviation (SD) is another measure of variance and measures how far the score is from the mean. It is, in basic terms, the average distance from the mean. A larger SD indicates more variance in the scores. Figure 9.6 demonstrates how SD affects the score distribution. Larger SDs produce flattened curves, whereas a smaller SD produces more elongated curves.

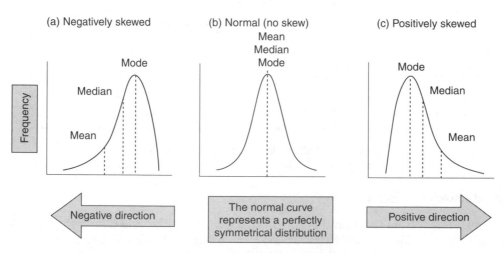

Figure 9.5 *Score Distributions.*

PROBABILITY DENSITY FUNCTION

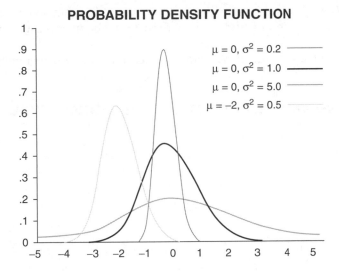

Figure 9.6 *Score Distributions. The **black** line is the standard normal distribution*

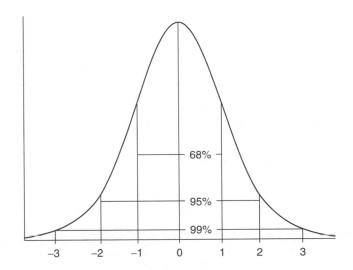

Figure 9.7 *Normal Score Distribution.*

A normal score distribution is commonly referred to as a *bell curve*. In a bell-shaped curve, most of the scores will appear near the center, and the outliers (scores to the extreme lowest and highest point) will appear at either end. Figure 9.7 demonstrates where most scores will fall within a normal distribution. The numbers within the graphic illustrate the percentage of scores and where they will fall in the distribution. The numbers on the *x* axis of the plot indicate the number of SDs. In other words, 68% of the scores will fall between 1 *SD* above and 1 *SD* below the mean. Ninety-five percent of the scores will fall between 2 *SD* above and 2 *SD* below the mean.

The reported sample (Figure 9.8) displays the examinee's score for the case (represented by the circle). The line represents the mean score for the case and each bar represents 1 *SD* above and below the mean. The graphic offers a visual representation of the information. The scores are available on the x axis; however, they are not the single piece of information provided. This report may be useful for reviewing case or category scores.

Figure 9.9a provides score information per case for an entire cohort (examination group).

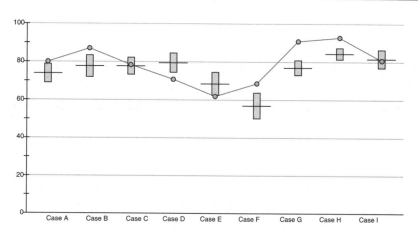

INDIVIDUAL PERFORMANCE - FORM LEVEL

Institute Name :
Test Session   :
Student   :
Form   :

Figure 9.8 *Examinee Performance Report.*
Source: Adapted from Education Management Solutions. © 2008

CLASS SUMMARY

Institute Name   :
Session   :
Class   :

Case	Total	Mean	Variance	SD	Minimum	Maximum	Range	Pass%
A	140	73.77	99.76	9.99	42.25	95.63	53.38	0.00
B	140	77.74	141.80	11.91	46.51	100.00	53.49	0.00
C	140	77.72	81.30	9.02	51.77	95.94	44.17	0.00
E	140	79.51	99.95	10.00	51.50	98.56	47.06	0.00
G	140	68.36	146.20	12.09	33.00	100.00	67.00	0.00
J	140	57.03	187.62	13.70	15.42	84.75	69.33	0.00
L	140	77.01	62.65	7.92	50.87	92.21	41.34	0.00
S	140	84.23	37.24	6.10	58.84	96.19	37.35	0.00
T	140	81.55	96.23	9.81	56.69	97.50	40.81	0.00

Figure 9.9 *Class Performance Report.*
Source: Adapted from Education Management Solutions. © 2008

A histogram (bar graph) report is essentially a frequency count. It offers details as to the number of examinees gaining credit for a correct checklist item. This information may be helpful in determining those checklist items that may be too easy (every examinee receives credit) or those items that may be too difficult or misinterpreted (no examinee receives credit). If all examinees fail to receive credit, the item may not be appropriate for the level of training or interpretation of the scoring criteria may be incorrect (Boulet, McKinley, Whelan, & Hambleton, 2003). This report also provides a shape for the data and how the scores are distributed (Figure 9.10).

Percentage Score Versus Percentile Rank

A percentage score is the total number of points accumulated divided by the total number of points available. A percentile rank score is the number at which a percentage of scores falls below the examinee's score. Thus, an examinee at the 85th percentile is described as performing better than 85% of the examinees taking the examination. Figure 9.11 shows an example of a percentile report.

ITEM SURVEY HISTOGRAM

Institute Name:
Case   :
Date Range   :

Category Name: Physical Exam

5 AB: Palpate abdomen in 4 quadrants   Sample Size: 140

Performed   140(100%)
Performed Incorrectly   0(0%)
Not Performed   0(0%)

Category Name: Physical Exam

6 AB: Palpated the liver   Sample Size: 140

Performed   82(58.57%)
Performed Incorrectly   18(12.86%)
Not Performed   40(28.57%)

Category Name: Physical Exam

7 AB: Palpated the spleen   Sample Size: 140

Performed   57(40.71%)
Performed Incorrectly   37(26.43%)
Not Performed   46(32.86%)

Figure 9.10 *Histogram Report.*
Source: Adapted from Education Management Solutions. © 2008

PERCENTILE SCORE

Institute Name:
Test Session :
Student :

Legend
SS : Student Score
PR : Percentile

Case Name	Case Score (%)		POST ENCOUNTER (%)		Physical Exam (%)		Professional Comm (%)		PPQ (%)		History Questions (%)	
	SS	PR	SS	PR	SS	PR	SS	PR	SS	PR	SS	PR
Tom	66.38	7.86	77.50	14.29	70.00	43.57	100.00	100.00	100.00	100.00	50.00	24.29
Steve	69.06	2.86	76.75	42.86	78.21	62.86	100.00	100.00	88.33	22.14	50.00	2.86
Leslie	88.72	96.43	100.00	100.00	90.00	98.57	100.00	100.00	95.00	45.00	77.78	57.86
Joseph	73.42	88.57	94.00	72.14	70.00	82.14	100.00	100.00	100.00	100.00	58.33	87.86
Gregory	77.92	80.71	95.67	72.86	---	---	100.00	100.00	100.00	100.00	70.00	86.43
Coma	83.56	61.43	80.25	39.29	80.00	38.85	80.00	28.06	66.67	4.32	90.00	93.53
Carlos	80.56	62.14	87.50	67.86	56.25	43.57	80.00	32.14	91.67	47.14	100.00	100.00
Bealrice	65.46	15.71	---	---	63.64	15.71	100.00	100.00	---	---	---	---
OVERALL	75.07	46.43	88.55	69.29	70.66	56.43	94.44	53.57	92.71	58.57	69.83	28.57

Figure 9.11 *Percentile Rank Report.*
Source: Adapted from Education Management Solutions. © 2008

HOW DO WE PROVE THE DATA?

"Quantitative data...is useless by itself. You've got to ask the data the right questions" (Lehrer, 2009, p. 104). The purpose of a clinical skills assessment is to provide a sample set of data from which to make a determination about the examinee's competency and to infer that the behavior will be repeated in practice. For an examination to be considered effective, it must be both reliable and valid (Boulet, 2009). "Fortunately, assessments do not need to be perfect to give worthwhile information about student abilities. If however the assessment lacks sufficient evidence to support reliable and valid interpretations, it should be used very carefully if at all" (Howley, 2004, p. 289).

Data Reliability

Reliability refers to the precision and consistency of assessment outcomes and the reproducibility of scores over time (Downing, 2004). Low reliability would be reflected in large variations of scores in retesting. High score reliability indicates that if a test were to be repeated, the examinee would receive approximately the same score each time. Examinations are considered more reliable when the scores are spread across the entire range.

The test/retest method for measuring reliability is rarely used as it is difficult to administer and may be expensive. For this reason, statisticians developed a formula to determine internal consistency: for example, Cronbach's α coefficient or Kuder–Richardson formula KR-20. The formula compares alternating items as if the single test was administered at two different times (see Figure 9.12). The coefficients may be most effective with dichotomous items (yes/no or performed/did not perform) and when

RELIABILITY COEFFICIENT

Institute Name:

Test Session: **Case :** (All)

Case	Category Name	Alpha Value	Questions	Students
A	All	0.7624	36	140
B	All	0.9583	37	140
C	All	0.6000	35	140
E	All	0.8349	36	140
G	All	0.6724	30	140
J	All	0.7965	41	140
L	All	0.6024	40	140
S	All	0.6369	38	140
T	All	0.5943	36	140

Figure 9.12 *Cronbach's α Correlation Formula Report.*
Source: Adapted from Education Management Solutions. © 2008

the examination is measuring the same construct. Each formula measurement range is between .00 and 1.00. A value of 1.00 indicates perfect reliability or that that the test is free of error variance. A value of .70 or better is commonly considered reliable. Recommendations for moderate stakes summative examinations are in the .80 to .89 range and high stakes examinations as high as .90 (Downing, 2004).

The report in Figure 9.13 is an example of a point-biserial correlation, also known as discrimination analysis. Best used with dichotomous items (yes/no, done/not done), it measures the correlation between a right and wrong score for a checklist item and the total test score when summing up the remaining items (Graham-Frees, 2010). Therefore, we would expect the top-performing examinees to receive credit for a particular item. The point-biserial calculates the correlation value for the item with the examinee's performance. The higher the point-biserial value, the more likely the top performing examinees gained credit for the item. The lower the point-biserial value, the more likely the bottom performing examinees gained credit for the item. Removal of an item with a negative point-biserial correlation will increase the reliability of the examination.

Rater Reliability

Assessments utilizing human raters depend on consistent ratings. One form of inter-rater reliability measures the percentage of agreement, or how often two or more independent raters agree in their interpretations. However, simple agreement does not account for chance or guarantee accuracy. The kappa (κ) statistic formula corrects for chance agreement. This report is most meaningful when the sample size (pairs of data) is relatively large (Figure 9.14). The value range for κ statistics is –1.0 (total disagreement) and +1.0, which is in considered complete agreement.

The designation "NA" refers to no disagreement whatsoever. Therefore, if there was an item in which every evaluator and every observer gave the same answer for every examinee, then it is out of range and returns as an NA. For example, an item such as

DISCRIMINATION ANALYSIS REPORT - TEST

Institute Name :   Session Name :   Session
Case Name: Mean Score: Median Score: Sample size:
Max Score: 100.00   Highest Score: Lowest Score: SD:

| | Correct Group Responses | | | | | Responses Frequencies | | | | | | | | | |
Item No.	Overall	Upper 27%	Lower 27%	Point Biserial	Correct Answer	1	2	3	4	5	6	7	8	9	Non Distractor
1	66.67%	75.00%	50.00%	0.34	Y	8	4								
2	41.67%	50.00%	25.00%	0.17	Y	5	7								
3	50.00%	75.00%	50.00%	0.51	Y	6	6								
4	66.67%	75.00%	75.00%	0.05	Y	8	4								
5	83.33%	100.00%	100.00%	0.11	Y	10	2								
6	50.00%	50.00%	50.00%	-0.08	Y	6	6								
7	58.33%	100.00%	25.00%	0.56	Y	7	5								
8	75.00%	50.00%	75.00%	-0.14	Y	9	3								
9	75.00%	100.00%	75.00%	0.46	Y	9	3								
10	75.00%	100.00%	75.00%	0.42	Y	9	3								
11	50.00%	50.00%	50.00%	0.25	Y	6	6								
12	75.00%	75.00%	50.00%	0.05	Y	9	3								

Figure 9.13 *Discrimination Analysis Report.*
Source: Adapted from Education Management Solutions. © 2008

"examinee performed skill x." If every examinee was marked with a "yes" by every evaluator and every observer, then there is no disagreement and no distinguishers, so the value is NA (rather than 1).

If, using the same example, 5 examinees were given a "yes" to "examinee performed skill x" and all 5 observers agreed, and 5 examinees were given a "no" for this item and all observers agreed, then it would be a score of 1.

A value of 0 refers to equal numbers of agreement and disagreement. For example, of 10 evaluators and 10 observers, if 5 observers agreed on the item and 5 observers disagreed, then the disagreement would be equal. Therefore, the result would be "no better than what could be expected by chance." A κ value between 1.0 and .7 is desired. Again, recommendations for moderate-stakes summative examinations are in the .80 to .89 range, and high-stakes examinations as high as .9 (Downing, 2004).

For increased reliability, if possible, items should be clearly written and evaluated by content experts. Downing (2004) recommends pretesting and item banking to increase reliability.

Figure 9.15 identifies the average case and category score provided by each rater (in this case a standardized patient). The information provides insight into the potential leniency or stringency of raters or discrepancy between raters. Here, if one assumes that the examinees seen by the various raters are "randomly equivalent," the mean values should be close.

Threats to reliability include ambiguous test items, items that attempt to measure more than one construct, and nested or sequenced items. Evaluator fatigue, training, and consistency or inconsistency in ratings will negatively affect the reliability of the examination (Swanson & Norcini, 1989).

QUALITY ASSURANCE (KAPPA STATISTICS)

Institute Name :   **Case :**   A

Statistics :

Question	Sample Size	Kappa Value
1. The learner allowed me enough time and space to tell my story (open ender approach)	6	-0.0345
2. I understood the words and explanations this learner used.	6	-0.0714
3. This learner was empathetic in his/her communication with me.	6	-0.3333
4. I was respected as a person	6	0.0000
5. This learner demonstrated compassion for me.	6	0.3333
6. This learner used reflective listening techniques with me (summarizing periodically).	6	-0.0435
7. This learner elicited my feelings and thoughts about my concerns.	6	0.1818
8. This learner elicited and answered my questions.	6	-0.3333
9. This learner demonstrated sensitivity and responsiveness to my needs.	6	0.5000
10. This learner made consistent eye contact with me.	6	0.0000
11. I could trust this learner to be my advocate.	6	0.5000
12. This learner understood my health beliefs and concerns.	6	0.0000
13. This learner demonstrated patience and did not rush me into making decisions that I was not yet prepared to make.	6	0.5714
14. Overall, how satisfied were you with this interaction?	6	-NA-

Figure 9.14 *Kappa Statistics Report.*
Source: Adapted from Education Management Solutions. © 2008

SP AVERAGE SCORE

Institute Name:

Test Session:

SP Name	N	Case Name	Case Score (%)	Physical Exam (%)	Professional Comm (%)	PPQ(%)	History Questions (%)
Angie	33	A	73.45	68.83	95.45	91.62	65.53
Sara	26	A	74.28	70.86	96.00	97.13	68.00
Allison	36	A	74.42	75.59	89.72	96.25	63.89
Pam	18	A	68.39	60.71	91.67	88.98	63.89
Nicole	9	A	70.58	65.87	100.00	93.33	56.94
Leslie	18	A	78.49	72.22	98.89	89.91	70.14

Figure 9.15 *Comparing Raters.*
Source: Adapted from Education Management Solutions. © 2008

Validity

Validity is the degree to which a test measures what it intends to measure (Graham-Frees, 2010). Validity refers to the score interpretation rather than the examination. "Assessments are not valid or invalid, rather assessments have more (or less) validity evidence to support or refute meaningful score interpretation" (Downing, 2003, p. 831). Measurement of validity is the impartial collection of data from multiple sources. It asks the question "are the inferences based on the scores correct?" (Boulet, 2009).

Sources of validity evidence include:

- Content validity—do the experts agree that the content and desired learning outcomes match the curriculum?
- Response process—is the data entry accurate?
- Internal structure—is there data and rater reliability?
- Relationships to other variables—were there other measures that could be correlated to this examination?
- Consequences—did the examination produce curricular change, examinee pass-fail decisions?
- Feasibility—was the exercise operationally and fiscally acceptable?
- Acceptability—did the participants agree that the exercise was realistic? Did the evaluators agree that assessments could be made (Varkey, Natt, Lesnick, Downing, & Yudkowsky, 2008)?

HOW DO WE PUBLISH THE DATA?

Once the data are gathered, measured, and validated, there will be additional feedback to be shared with trainees, instructors, stakeholders, and operators. In addition to the examples provided within this essay, there are more styles of reporting to be considered.

Reports for Trainees

Consider the kind of feedback required and whether the information provided will threaten the integrity of the examination. Within formative assessments, it is instructive for the learner to be provided information regarding the skills that were performed correctly as well as those that are in need of improvement. It may also be important for the learner to know how they performed relative to their peers. Checklist ratings and evaluator comments may be appropriate to distribute to provide the learner with as much information as possible.

Within summative assessments, it may be important to provide score or pass-fail information but not provide the level of detail that could change the performance of future learners. Consider how the information will be distributed. Will this be via a debriefing session, supervision session, or published to a learning management system?

Reports to consider:

- *Skills summary*—a snapshot report that displays an overall score, all case and scenario scores, categories and skill areas, and class and cohort means and range.
- *Performance history*—statistical information for performance over time including comparison with class means and comments by evaluators.
- *Performance chart*—a graph representation of a student's performance as compared with the class for the selected session or date range.
- *Checklist ratings*—with or without scores and comments.

Reports for Instructors

Providing volume reports, such as the item histogram, to instructors gives a picture of the performance of an entire examination cohort. This can clearly identify training deficiencies or problem examination items.

Reports to consider:

- *Course summary scores*—scores for an exercise, course, or group of trainees or over time.
- *Percentile rank*—ranking of learners.
- *Students in need of remediation*—immediate information for those trainees falling a percentage or number of SDs below the rest of the examinees.
- *Item analysis*—analysis of the examination items.
- *Reliability*—data and rater reliability and quality assurance.
- *Accreditation and course information*—coursework and accreditation accomplishment and center usage.

Reports for Stakeholders

Return on investment as well as proper utilization may be of particular interest to the administration and fiscal agents of the institution.

Reports to consider:

- *Utilization reports—track the use of the center by department, the number of learners served or create invoices for billable time.*
- *Equipment and maintenance*—capital and disposable equipment and supplies, usage, and maintenance costs.

REPORTS FOR OPERATORS

When the operator is responsible for the administration of the simulation, feedback in the form of satisfaction surveys will provide tips for improvement in setting design and realism. Although the focus of this essay is on performance reports, the operators will also benefit from a management system that will provide data for inventory, maintenance, scheduling, and utilization.

Reports to consider:

- *Survey statistics*—feedback from the trainees and instructors.
- *Inventory list and inventory status*—capital equipment and supplies in stock, order information, maintenance, repair, loan, and availability.
- *Inventory utilization*—usage of capital and disposable supplies.
- *User reports*—to manage users of a simulation center or learning management system.

CONCLUSIONS

The use of simulation seeks to construct or recreate a scenario wherein trainees' competence, problem-solving skills, and behavior may be observed and measured. Using a learning management system with video recording provides a convenient tool to capture and generate the data described in this chapter. It also allows online feedback regarding these skills and behaviors. Data collection adds credibility to the simulation exercise and ultimately to the laboratory. The trainees' focus will be the sense of achievement (or survival!). The instructor will be interested in knowing if the learning objectives match the performance outcomes, and the operators' focus will be on the operational and administrative components of the exercise and of the laboratory. Feedback in the form of surveys, skills ratings, data integrity, and operational information will serve to validate the efforts of the simulation facilitators and improve the experience of the participants over time.

REFERENCES

Adamson, K. (2010). Integrating human patient simulation into associate degree nursing curricula: Faculty experiences, barriers, and facilitators. *Clinical Simulation in Nursing, 6*, e75–e81. doi: 10.1016/j.ecsns.2009.06.002

Boulet, J. R. (2008). Summative assessment in medicine: The promise of simulation for high-stakes evaluation. *Academic Emergency Medicine, 15*(11), 1017–1124.

Boulet, J. R. (2009). *Pretzel logic.* Conference Proceedings of the Arcadia Summit. Philadelphia, PA, August 13, 2009.

Boulet, J. R., Gimpel, J., & Errichetti, A. (2003). Evaluating the clinical skills of osteopathic medical students. *Journal of the American Osteopathic Association, 103*(6), 267–279.

Boulet, J. R., McKinley D. W., Whelan G. P., & Hambleton, R. K. (2003). Quality assurance methods for performance-based assessments. *Advances in Health Sciences Education: Theory and Practice, 8*(1), 27–47.

Boulet, J. R., & Swanson, D. B. (2004). Psychometric challenges of using simulations for high-stakes assessment. In W. Dunn (Ed.), *Simulations in critical care education and beyond* (pp. 119–130). Des Plains, IL: Society of Critical Care Medicine.

Downing, S. M. (2003, September). Validity: On the meaningful interpretation of assessment data. *Medical Education, 37*(9), 830–837.

Downing, S. M. (2004, September). Reliability: On the reproducibility of assessment data. *Medical Education, 38*(9), 1006–1012.

Graham-Frees, L. (2010). *Data: What does it mean?* Conference Proceedings of the Arcadia Summit, Oakland, CA, August 20, 2010.

Howley, L. D. (2004, September). Performance assessment in medical education: Where we've been and where we're going. *Evaluation and the Health Professions, 27*(3), 285–303.

Lee, T. H. (2010). Turning doctors into leaders. *Harvard Business Review, 88*(4), 50–58.

Lehrer, J. (2009). *How we decide* (1st ed.). Houghton Mifflin.

Kerns, L. (2009). *Are medical education centers addressing what users need or want?* Modsim World Conference, Virginia Beach. October 14, 2009.

Prion, S. (2008). A practical framework for evaluating the affect of clinical simulation experiences in prelicensure nursing education. *Clinical Simulation in Nursing, 4*(3). doi:10.1016/j.ecns.2008.08.002

Report sample graphics: Arcadia—Simulation Learning Management System from Education Management Solutions Inc., Exton, PA.

Rodriguez-Paz, J. M., Kennedy, M., Salas, E., et al. (2009). Beyond "see one, do one, teach one": Toward a different training paradigm. *Quality and Safety in Health Care, 18,* 63–68. Retrieved August 12, 2010, from qshc.bmj.com

Sanford, P. (2010, July). Simulation in nursing education: A review of the research. *Qualitative Report, 15*(4), 1006–1011.

Swanson, D., & Norcini, J. (1989). Factors influencing reproducibility of tests using standardized patients. *Teaching and Learning in Medicine, 1*(3), 158–166.

Varkey, P., Natt, N., Lesnick, T., Downing, S., & Yudkowsky, R. (2008). Validity evidence for an OSCE to assess competency in systems-based practice and practice-based learning and improvement: A preliminary investigation. *Academic Medicine, 83*(3), 775–780.

Wallace, P. (1997). Following the threads of an innovation: The history of standardized patients in medical education. Originally published in *Caduceus, A Humanities Journal for Medicine and Health Sciences, 13*(2), 5–28. Retrieved from http://www.aspeducators.org

SUGGESTED READING

Boulet, J. R. (2005). Generalizability theory: Basics. In B. S. Everitt & D. C. Howell (Eds.), *Encyclopedia of statistics in behavioral science* (pp. 704–711). Chichester: John Wiley & Sons, Ltd.

Boulet, J. R., Gimpel, J., Errichetti, A., & Meoli, F. (2004). Using national medical care survey data to validate examination content on a performance-based clinical skills assessment for osteopathic physicians. *Journal of the American Osteopathic Association, 103*(5), 225–231.

Boulet, J. R., Smee, S. M., Dillon, G. F., & Gimpel, J. R. (2009). The use of standardized patient assessments for certification and licensure decisions. *Simulation in Healthcare, 4*(1), 35–42.

Burns, H. K., O'Donnell, J., & Artman, J. (2010). High-fidelity simulation in teaching problem solving to 1st-year nursing students: A novel use of the nursing process. *Clinical Simulation in Nursing, 6,* e87–e95. doi:10.1016/j.ecns.2009.07.005

Downing, S. M., Tekian, A., & Yudkowsky, R. (2006). Procedures for establishing defensible absolute passing scores on performance examinations in health professions education. *Teaching and Learning in Medicine, 18*(1), 50–57.

Grant, J. S., Moss, J., Epps, C., & Watts, P. (2009). Using video-facilitated feedback to improve student performance following high-fidelity simulation. *Clinical Simulation in Nursing.* doi:10.1016/j.ecns.2009.09.001

Harvill, L. M. (1991). Standard error of measurement. *Educational Measurement: Issues and Practice, 10,* 33–41.

Johnson. (n.d.). *Descriptive statistics lecture 15.* Retrieved from http://www.southalabama.edu/coe/bset/johnson/lectures/lec15.htm

Koslosky, B. *Digital lifestyle gadgets.* Retrieved from http://billkosloskymd.typepad.com/lexicillin_qd/2007/09/mean-vs-median-.html

Newble, D. (2004, February). Techniques for measuring clinical competence: Objective structured clinical examinations. *Medical Education, 38*(2), 199–203.

Norcini, J. J., & Boulet, J. R. (2003). Methodological issues in the use of standardized patients for assessment. *Teaching and Learning in Medicine, 15*(4), 293–297.

Petrusa, E. R. (2004). Taking standardized patient-based examinations to the next level. *Teaching and Learning in Medicine, 16*(1), 98–110.

Roberts, C., Newble, D., Jolly, B., Reed, M., & Hampton, K. (2006, September). Assuring the quality of high-stakes undergraduate assessments of clinical competence. *Medical Teacher, 28*(6), 535–543.

Traub, R. E., & Rowley, G. L. (1991). Understanding reliability. Educational measurement. *Issues and Practice, 10*(1), 37–45.

Whelan, G. P., Boulet, J. R., McKinley, D. W., Norcini, J. J., van Zanten, M., Hambleton, R. K., et al. (2005). Scoring standardized patient examinations: Lessons learned from the development and administration of the ECFMG Clinical Skills Assessment (CSA). *Medical Teacher, 27*(3), 200–206.

Wilkinson, T., & Frampton, C. (2004). Comprehensive undergraduate medical assessments improve prediction of clinical performance. *Medical Education, 38*, 1111–1116.

CHAPTER 10

Patient Safety in Human Simulation

Susan E. Will and Joanne Weinschreider

INTRODUCTION

*T*his chapter provides an overview of the patient safety movement in the United States, including tools that can be used to promote safe change and the role of simulation in building a culture of safety in medicine. Teams must achieve true interprofessional collaboration and function in high-reliability organizations to ensure the delivery of quality health care. Teams that are able to achieve both collaboration and a high-functioning work environment are able to provide quality care. Unfortunately, although the consumers and technologies of health care have changed dramatically over the years, the systems, the culture, and the means for training in health care have lagged behind considerably. Only recently has simulation been used as a learning tool for both students and professionals to improve skill-based competencies along with team-based competencies. Understanding the history of the patient safety movement, the tools for assessing current health care culture, the methods to incite culture change, and the role simulation can play in building a stronger and safer health care market for tomorrow is vital to every educator, manager, leader, and health care professional who seeks to ensure a culture of safety in medicine.

PATIENT SAFETY OVERVIEW

The patient safety movement is not a new movement. It is, however, a rather young movement and has only recently begun to attract the attention it deserves in the United States. In 1999, the Institute of Medicine (IOM) released the report, *To Err Is Human: Building a Safer Health System.* This pivotal work uncovered, identified, and highlighted evident risks within the U.S. health care system. Included in the report was this disturbing fact: 44,000 to 98,000 Americans die each year from hospital-related medical errors. Until this report, the extent of health care–related harm was medicine's hidden secret. Of course, we can also understand this loss of life another way: It equals 3 fully loaded jumbo jets crashing every other day for a 5-year period (Health Grades, 2004)—with congruent restitution costs to hospitals averaging between $17 and $29 billion each year. In addition, those dollars flowing out of the health care system cannot be used for other essential items, such as system, staffing, and infrastructure upgrades and support. We do not mention here the undue harm, pain, and suffering that occurs to family and friends in the wake of these preventable events.

In 2001, the IOM's second report, *Crossing the Quality Chasm: A new health system for the 21st century*, built upon its predecessor, provided a strategic safety plan for the years ahead, with steps to satisfy that plan. The committee outlined 6 aims for improvement, 10 rules for system redesign, and 4 main areas for change. The committee then asked health care leaders to forge ahead and change systems, behaviors, and ultimately the culture of health care. What the committee had not taken into account, however, was medicine's well-established, strongly rooted culture, which makes cultural change difficult to enact and slow to implement.

Today, medical error remains the third leading cause of death in the United States after heart disease and cancer (Starfield, 2000). Years after uncovering the harm that exists within our health care system and a path toward quality improvement, little advancement has been made. Health care has taken small steps forward but, as a whole, the system remains unsafe and unreliable (Health Grades, 2004).

To truly comprehend patient safety and medical error, one needs to understand how they are defined:

> Patient safety is the "freedom from accidental injury due to medical care, or medical errors."
>
> Medical error is defined as "the failure of a planned action to be completed as intended or the use of a wrong plan to achieve an aim...[including] problems in practice, products, procedures, and systems." (Health Grades, 2004, p. 2)

Health care continues to struggle with the basic concepts of safety science. The industry has looked repeatedly to other high-risk industries (e.g., aviation and nuclear power) for safety-related toolkits and strategies with little success. As previously noted, it is health care's unwillingness to move away from its historic and strongly rooted cultural standards that has been blamed for the lack of progress. Quite simply, to become safe, medicine must abandon hierarchical medical traditions, autonomy, and the practice of silo medicine (Amalberti, Auroy, Berwick, & Barach, 2005).

Therefore, many of our health care organizations can be identified as suffering from what James Reason (2000) has called "sick system syndrome." It is a health care system that lacks transparency and mutual respect and where hierarchy runs rampant and true collaboration is rare, is "sick," and in need of repair. Historically, physicians have had difficulty in being team players, which hampers collaboration and true interdisciplinary learning. For their part, nurses are constantly "nursing" their paperwork and computer systems, leaving the concept of patient-centered care just out of reach. Nonetheless, a hospital that suffers from sick system syndrome can be transformed by making safety a standard, not a priority in a list of other priorities that need to be accomplished. The second step in truly transforming medicine is to adopt or to develop a culture that is transparent, integrated, consumer driven, has meaning and joy, and refocuses medical education (for all professionals) on safety (Leape et al., 2009).

TRANSFORMING THE HEALTH CARE SYSTEM

Transformation is a powerful word. Medicine must become a high-reliability organization to truly transform health care. From top-down and bottom-up, everyone who plays either a direct or an indirect role in patient care must be focused on patient safety. This type of adherence to safety can fundamentally change the ways in which health care is delivered. As we abandon our medical roots and historical behaviors, we can transform health care into a safer place for our patients. Nursing and medicine have long looked at their professional roles in patient care as individual performers. If they complete their role-related tasks, then they have done their part and provided quality care. What has been uncovered and commonly cited is that to provide safe quality care, nurses and medical providers must be taught to work together and to collaborate to ensure that the team is providing safe care (Leape & Berwick, 2005).

FIRST, DO NO HARM

Errors and a lack of quality in health care are the leading causes of mortality and morbidity in the U.S. health care system. Patients are harmed in a variety of ways, and it can happen anytime—from a patient's first encounter through a patient's last encounter within a health care system. Harm can be as small as a missed dose of a medication that then has a domino effect on a patient's hospital course or as large as wrong-sided surgery.

In an effort to identify and share lessons learned from adverse events, the Joint Commission (JC) tracks certain "sentinel events"—defined by the JC as "an unexpected occurrence involving death or serious physiological or psychological injury, or the risk thereof" (Agency for Healthcare Research and Quality [AHRQ], 2010, p. 3). The most frequently reported sentinel events include wrong-sided surgery hospital suicide, operative and postoperative complications, delay in treatment, medication error, and patient falls (AHRQ, 2010). Sentinel events have trended up significantly in the last 5 years in the United States. In 2005, there were approximately 575 sentinel events reported. In 2008, there were more than 800 sentinel events reported (JC, 2010a, 2010b). It is unclear if this increase is a result of an increase in the occurrence of events or if the upward trend is related to the fact that the JC now requires reporting of these events.

The JC and the State Department of Health also track "never events"—events that should never happen and typically result in death or severe disability. Over the last 12 years, 71% of such events occurring in the United States resulted in death. Despite the fact that never events are very rare and a hospital can go for years without having one, they do occur. Never events can be classified in six main domains, with related criteria (AHRQ, 2010). The six domains include surgical (e.g., wrong-sided surgery), product or device (e.g., death related to contaminated equipment), patient protection (e.g., infant discharged to wrong legal guardian), care management (e.g., death or serious disability related to a medication error), environmental (e.g., death or serious burn from any hospital source), and criminal events (e.g., abduction).

From 2007 to 2008, the Minnesota Department of Health captured 312 never events. Their never events included pressure ulcers (39%), falls (30%), retained objects (12%), wrong-sided surgery (7%), wrong procedure (5%), medication errors resulting in patient death (2%), suicide (1%), and other (4%) (AHRQ, 2010).

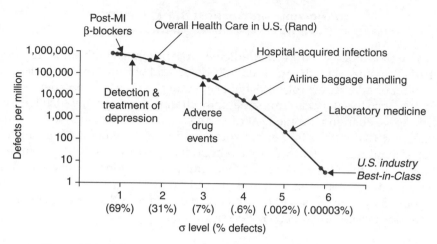

Figure 10.1 *Defect Rates in Medicine Compared With Other Sectors.*
Source: From Leape, L. (2009). Errors in medicine.

Never events continue to happen at alarming rates in health care. Although the need to make health care safer is evident, the path to satisfy that need remains long and winding.

Harm exists not only in the form of sentinel and never events. A recent study tracking adverse drug events (ADEs) in adult intensive care units reported that 50% of such patients will suffer from at least 1 ADE during their hospital stay. Twenty percent of these patients will suffer either death or disability related to the ADE. Medication errors remain the most common type of medical error in health care. The same holds true for even our tiniest health care consumers. There is strong evidence that patients in neonatal intensive care units are also at risk of experiencing a medical error (Leonard, 2010; Usprung & Gray, 2010).

Another way to look at the harm within health care is to use the six sigma process. Six sigma seeks to improve processes by identifying and removing causes of defect toward this goal: having 99.9997% of the outcome defect free. A six sigma rate equals 3.4 defects per million opportunities. A rate of 6 identifies best industries. Overall, health care in the United States functions at a six sigma rate of slightly less than 2. This is an error rate of roughly 31% defects per 1 million exposures. In comparison, let us return to the airline industry for a moment, where baggage handling is at a six sigma rate of 4, with 0.6% defects per million exposures (see Figure 10.1; Leape, 2009, p. 5). Unfortunately, a checked bag in an airport is safer than a patient in a U.S. hospital.

IDENTIFYING AND LEARNING FROM FACTORS THAT CONTRIBUTE TO ERRORS

There are a variety of factors that contribute to or weaken the ability to ensure consistent quality in health care. The biggest contributor to errors in health care are the systems in which that care is provided, not the individuals that provide the care, who are rarely to blame. This acknowledgement of system accountability represents a change in thinking in health care. Historically, errors have been viewed as a single person's fault, with that person being exclusively blamed for adverse events that occur related to human error. This approach of blame is neither correct nor productive when looking toward changing culture. Nurses and physicians provide care in systems that allow for and contribute to errors that result in harming patients. Moving toward a just culture, a culture not of blame and train but a culture where systems, educational factors, and environment factors are scrutinized and improved, can bring about the transformation that health care needs (Leape, 2009).

Of course, there are a variety of factors that should be considered when analyzing an event that results or could have resulted in patient harm (a near miss). Addressing all the factors outlined in Table 10.1 when reviewing an adverse event or near miss is vital to identifying system-based weaknesses. The JC has a tool available to assist in the comprehensive and systematic review of adverse events. This tool, *A Form for a Root Cause Analysis and Action Plan in Response to a Sentinel Event,* can be accessed at the JC web site. Objectively, reviewing events for causative factors enables one to identify new system, infrastructure, and educational processes that should be adopted to decrease the risk of the adverse event reoccurring in the future or the near miss being repeated and actually reaching the patient. Following through on the process of discovery, implementation, and evaluation of the factors that contribute to errors in medicine is vital to taking the first steps toward cultural change.

In health care, the risk for errors and harm lurk at every turn during a patient's health care encounter. A model repeatedly used to identify types of errors and to drill down and explore why accidents occur in health care is James Reason's (2000) "Swiss cheese" model. Reason's model of accident causation compares health care to layers of Swiss cheese. The layers of Swiss cheese are the institution's defenses, safeguards, and systems, and the holes in the Swiss cheese represent weaknesses in these systems. When the usual defenses, safeguards, and systems are weak or worked around, an injury or accident can occur and the adverse consequences may reach the patient. Visually, this can be seen as all the holes in the Swiss cheese, analogous to weaknesses in the health care system, lining up so that the error reaches the patient. Reason refers to this as the "sharp end," or the point when the holes align and the patient is harmed (see Figure 10.2). The sharp end is where the bedside care providers practice whereas the blunt end represents the health care system. Too frequently, accountability for the error and resulting patient harm is assigned to the bedside care provider at the sharp end of the process, although responsibility actually rests at the blunt end or the health care organizations poorly designed system of care (Reason, 2000).

Reason's (2000) model provides a framework for studying accidents, errors, and injuries and for identifying opportunities for improvement so vital changes can be made. This can be accomplished as each layer is pealed back after an adverse event to identify the root cause. By identifying the failures in each layer related to systems, policies, and

Table 10.1 *Factors to Consider When Reviewing an Event*

Work environment	Staffing numbers, acuity, lack of working equipment, and high census coupled with a lack of leadership and administrative support can contribute to a patient being harmed.
Work-related factors	Understanding one's role and institutions policies and having a clear understanding of the task required is vital to ensuring patient safety.
Professional factors	Knowledge, skills, and competence as well as motivation and ability to work in a high-stress environment is needed to provide safe care.
Present cultural factors	Maintaining a strong focus on safety, transparency, and teamwork will decrease adverse events.
Teamwork factors	Communication (verbal and written), teamwork, and collaboration are vital to building and maintaining a culture of safety.

Source: Adapted from Handyside and Suresh (2010).

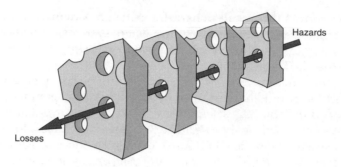

Figure 10.2 *James Reason's Swiss Cheese Model. From Reason, 2009.*
Source: Reproduced from Human error: Models and management, James Reason, *BMJ*, 320, 768–770.
Copyright © 2000 with permission from BMJ Publishing Group, Ltd.

team members, one can identify the root cause(s) that contributed to the patient harm or near miss. Scrutiny of adverse events should include more than the typical JC and state-mandated and catastrophic events. It should include all events, both near misses and those causing patient harm. These events should be studied to identify opportunities for improvement (Veltman, 2007).

COMMUNICATION, COLLABORATION, AND TEAMWORK

In reviewing reported sentinel events to identify causation, the JC discovered that in health care, 70% of patient adverse events are related to ineffective communication and collaboration among team members. Perhaps one member of the team had critical information but did not share this information with all the members of the care team because of a lack of respect or intimidation. Respect, nonhierarchical, open communication, and collaboration are vital to ensure safety in patient care. Unfortunately, this is rarely realized in the present health care environment (Leape et al., 2009).

> The American Nurses Association includes four major elements in their definition of collaboration. These are "1) a partnership with mutual valuing, 2) recognition of separate and combined spheres of responsibility, 3) mutual safeguarding of legitimate interests of each party and 4) recognized shared goals."
>
> Healthcare has its own definition of collaboration which is "a complex phenomenon that brings together two or more individuals, often from different professional disciplines, who work to achieve shared aims and objectives." (Fewster-Thuente & Velsor-Friedrich, 2008, p. 41)

Collaboration and teamwork are commonly thought to be interchangeable. However, teamwork is actually one characteristic of true team collaboration. True collaboration within a team is seen when hierarchical behaviors are decreased, communication is increased, and a high level of cooperation is reached. In this type of environment, information flows easily to and from all members of the care team (Fewster-Thuente & Velsor-Friedrich, 2008).

Barriers commonly cited as impeding true collaboration in health care are related to the patriarchal relationship between nurses and physicians, lack of time, lack of role clarification, gender, and medical culture. Historically, the nurse–physician relationship has been a power struggle in which the physician has more power and authority than the nurse. This creates a hierarchy or power distance that can negatively impact a person's willingness to speak up against the power gradient (Leonard, Graham, & Bonacum, 2004). Lack of time has also been cited as a barrier in achieving team collaboration. Nursing and medicine are constantly under time pressure to do more with less, and this is true now more than ever with the increased acuity of hospitalized patients. Nursing is also a profession where one can flex in and out of service working both full- and part-time. Flexing in and out of the profession and varying schedules impede the ability of teams to achieve true collaboration (Fewster-Thuente & Velsor-Friedrich, 2008).

Another factor that can negatively impact collaborative communication has its roots in the silos of nursing and medical education. Physicians are taught to be diagnosticians and to quickly evaluate a situation and determine the best medical management. They learn to be concise and to quickly get the "headlines" and make decisions. Nurses are taught to be "broad and narrative in their descriptions of the clinical situation" and often reminded that it is not within their scope of practice to diagnose (Leonard et al., 2004, p. 86). This can result in what has been labeled the *doctor–nurse game*, where the nurse has important patient care data or observations to contribute but does not communicate this in a direct and assertive manner, rather uses a *hint and hope* approach. Unfortunately, the patient and the family are caught in the middle of this game. Assertiveness training and structured communication, such as the use of situation–background–assessment–recommendations (SBAR), are recommendations to address this concern.

A lack of individual role clarification can negatively impact a team's ability to function effectively. Not understanding one's role on the team can be detrimental to the team's ability to provide safe care. Another barrier to open communication is gender. Historically in health care, nurses are females and physicians are males, and this has resulted in a relationship where the nurse is viewed as subordinate and the physician is viewed as dominant. Although this is beginning to change, physician dominance is often still present in current medical cultures (Fewster-Thuente & Velsor-Friedrich, 2008).

A study that looked at male and female interactions in health care found that female teams of nurses and physicians had a higher rate of collaboration than the blended teams of males and females. The impact of culture on team collaboration is not limited to the roles in the hospital. It includes each person's unique cultural background as well as the culture of the country and the organization. In the United States, individuals are encouraged to be innovative and maintain a certain level of autonomy. This has always and still does carry over to medical culture. When physicians and nurses achieve true collaboration, patient safety increases, resulting in fewer adverse events (Fewster-Thuente & Velsor-Friedrich, 2008).

True collaboration in health care is not easy to attain. Health care is a very hierarchical system, where staff may recognize the need to speak up to prevent harm but do not speak up because of the authority gradient or intimidation. Intimidation affects patient safety. In a survey by the Institute for Safe Medication Practices, almost half of the respondents reported that their past experiences with an intimidating provider impacted future interactions, with that provider often resulting in work-arounds to avoid speaking with that provider (Smetzer & Cohen, 2005). Intimidation erodes trust and "trust is essential for teamwork"... it "influences communication and communication is the lubricant for collaboration" (Reina, Reina, & Rushton, 2007, pp. 103 and 105). Trust and open communication are critical to achieve true collaboration and improve the flow of information among all care providers. According to Hunt, Shilkofski, Stavroudis, and Nelson (2007), flattening the hierarchy will allow for better communication to and from the team leader. Reducing hierarchical behaviors will result in safer care for patients.

In 2008, the JC released Sentinel Event Alert No. 40, titled *Behaviors that Undermine a Culture of Safety*. In this alert, the JC acknowledges that intimidating and disruptive behaviors exit in most health care facilities. They recommend that all hospitals adopt a policy of *zero tolerance* for these unprofessional and unsafe behaviors. One of the action items in this event alert recommends that all leaders and managers receive education in the areas of relationship building and collaborative practice. This includes conflict resolution skills to address unprofessional behavior. Best practice would be for all staff to receive this type of training.

Research by Maxfield, Grenny, McMillian, Patterson, and Switzler (2005) reinforces the need for training all staff in conversation and conflict resolution skills. These research-ers have identified seven safety concerns that most staff are unwilling to address with their peers, even when they perceive that a patient is at risk of harm. The concerns are as follows: broken rules, mistakes, lack of support, incompetence, poor teamwork, dis-respect, and micromanagement. Maxfield et al. view these conversations as crucial con-versations. They have also outlined approaches for staff in how to address and not avoid these types of conversations. Staff who are skilled and willing to speak up to have these crucial conversations with other care providers are "the most effective, satisfied, and committed in the organization. Crucial conversation skills are beneficial to patient safety as the staff are not only empowered but also skilled in how to speak up for safe care."

BUILDING A CULTURE OF SAFETY IN HEALTH CARE

Building a culture of safety requires that one first recognize the opportunities that exist in health care across all levels. Cultural change is not easy. It takes engagement and commitment from all members of the team to make progress. The lack of safety in health care has been studied from many angles, and as previously stated, the prog-ress in truly transforming health care has been very slow. This slow progress has been linked to a variety of factors. Researchers conclude that the current state of health care is related to a lack of leadership involvement, poor teamwork and communication among frontline staff, a lack of transparency, and failure in building a just culture (Sammer, Lykens, Singh, Mains, & Lackan, 2010).

One must first understand the characteristics of a culture of safety and what is needed to construct this culture of safety to effectively transform health care to a safer system of care. "A safety culture is expressed in the beliefs, attitudes and values of an organization's employees regarding the pursuit of safety" (JC, 2009, p. 1). The required building blocks of a culture of safety include strong and supportive leadership, true collaborative teamwork, practiced standardization, effective communication, transpar-ency, and a just and patient-centered culture.

Assessing Current Safety Climate

The next step is to understand the processes that can be used to achieve cultural change. Changing culture is a slow but amazing and rewarding process that requires many tiny steps forward to achieve even the smallest amount of change. It takes time to change culture, and it is often best to attempt culture change slowly and locally.

Sexton et al. (2007) viewed and recommended the culture of safety as unique to each unit and recommended obtaining a baseline measurement of each unit's safety climate before attempting to make changes. There are several valid instruments available to measure the unit's culture (Colla, Bracken, Kinney, & Wells, 2005; Sexton et al., 2006). These safety culture surveys evaluate staff perceptions of a variety of domains, including safety climate, teamwork climate, perception of management, stress recognition, job satisfaction, and working condition (Pronovost & Sexton, 2005). When administering a safety culture survey, the participant response rate is very important. Sixty percent of the unit staff must complete and return the questionnaire for the results to be reflective of the culture of the unit rather than the attitudes of the individuals who completed the survey. Once a baseline measurement is obtained, leadership should review the domain scores and determine which scores are at goal (>80% agreement) and which scores are in the danger zone (<60% agreement). Leadership and staff can then focus on the problematic scores, work together to identify specific areas of concern, and provide insights and ideas for addressing these concerns. Because safety culture is local and identified interventions will be specific to the unit, it is best to have a local safety champion lead these discussions, and ideally, all unit roles should be engaged in this process. Sexton et al. (2007) developed a safety culture checkup tool to facilitate this process. The discussion should start with a quick review of the unit scores and then staff selecting one culture item, which is meaningful to those present, for a more detailed discussion. With this item in mind, staff focus on the following:

1. What does this item mean to you?
2. How accurately does the unit score reflect your experience on this unit?
3. How would it look on this unit if 100% of staff strongly agreed with this item?
4. Identify at least one actionable item to improve unit results in this area (Sexton et al., 2007, p. 701).

After several of these focused discussions, the safety champion can consolidate the feedback and organize it by theme. Then unit leadership and staff can work together to develop an action list and timeline for addressing the safety items. The practice of evaluating a unit's culture of safety and teamwork is more than an academic exercise. Researchers have linked higher safety scores to better clinical outcomes. These include lower rates of nurse turnover, decubitus ulcers, catheter-related bloodstream infections (CRBSI), and in-hospital mortality (Pronovost et al., 2006). In 2009, researchers studying organizational culture concluded that there is a direct link between safety climate and organizational culture. Higher team culture scores correlated with a higher level of safety, whereas a more hierarchical culture was correlated with a lower level of safety (Singer et al., 2009).

Staff empowerment and engagement are critical to the development of a culture of safety and teamwork. Patient safety leadership walk rounds can help achieve these goals (Woodward et al., 2010). During administrative safety walk rounds, unit leadership meet informally with staff in the clinical area to discuss potential sources of harm for patients. Questions that are asked on the rounds often include the following:

1. How might the next patient be harmed?
2. What are the system weaknesses that need to be addressed?
3. What thoughts about work keep you up at night?

Staff concerns and recommendations for increasing patient safety become action items for follow-up, and communication of the outcomes is shared with all staff members. This open rounding process reinforces for staff the critical role that they have in identifying and decreasing areas of risk for patients. The discussion also fosters a more open relationship between management and staff (Woodward et al., 2009).

Some units will formalize this process and develop a comprehensive, unit-based safety program (Johns Hopkins Hospital, 2010) on the unit—when a hospital administrator adopts a unit and partners with staff to identify and address risks to patient safety. These 2 programs recognize and empower the bedside care provider to advocate for safe care for patients and be vigilant, constantly evaluating the clinical area for risks to patient safety.

The Cultural Change Process

John Kotter and Holger Rathgeber (2005) outlined eight steps to implement successful cultural change. When the eight steps are used appropriately in health care, they can set the stage for a cultural transformation. There are 4 phases and eight steps in Kotter's cultural change process. These steps can be nicely adapted to the health care industry (see Table 10.2).

Leadership is another key component in designing, building, fostering, and promoting a culture of safety in health care. Without leadership commitment, there is little movement, and the few changes that are made will not last. It is vital to the survival of all patient safety initiatives that senior leadership be verbally and physically supportive.

Table 10.2 *Kotter's Eight Steps for Cultural Change*

Set the stage	
1. Create a sense of urgency	Assist others in seeing the true need and value in moving toward change.
2. Build a guiding team	Pull together a team that has strong leadership, credibility, authority, and ability to communicate and articulate the problem.
Choose a direction	
3. Develop the vision and the steps to accomplish it	Clearly identify how things will change, the steps needed to accomplish it, and what types of resources will be needed to get there.
Make it happen	
4. Gain buy-in and communicate the plan	Communicating out the plan and gaining buy-in from all levels for the vision is vital to the success of any patient safety movement.
5. Remove barriers to change	Encourage, support, and assist all that try to adopt and support the new vision. Break down and remove all barriers that exist within the current system that will impede change.
6. Celebrate short-term wins	Share with all levels of your institution the smallest successes.
7. Keep pushing	Do not give up.
Make it stick	
8. Create a new culture	When systems, behaviors, and perceptions change, hold the type to them, celebrate them, and share the successes with others.

Source: Agency for Healthcare Research and Quality (2010b). As adapted from Kotter & Rathgebar (2005).

Some people relate this as *walking the walk and talking the talk*. Setting the groundwork for an organizational culture of safety starts with the most senior leader in the organization and permeates out to all care providers from there. An engaged leader will continually work to promote a culture of safety where staff are empowered to speak up in all venues to support safe care. An engaged leader is vested in the process and is able to truly identify opportunities for improvement that exist within the organization. Once leadership with the team has created a safety vision and a sense of urgency, they can start to work on changing and transforming the culture. A lack of leadership, on the other hand, is detrimental and will destroy the best efforts. When there is a lack of leadership and support, typically people are less willing to speak up and address the real issues that lead to adverse outcomes out of fear for retribution (JC, 2009).

INTERPROFESSIONAL TEAM TRAINING—ADDRESSING THE HIERARCHY OF HEALTH CARE

Building a culture of safety can only be accomplished with a well-constructed plan targeting the underlying causes of unsafe practices. Promoting true team collaboration is vital to the success of every patient safety initiative.

One program commonly cited in the literature that will promote collaboration and communication is team training. The aviation industry introduced cockpit resource management in the early 1970s as aviation accident reviews determined that the primary causes of loss of life and equipment were failures of crew communication, decision making, leadership, workload management, and task prioritization. Cockpit resource management soon transitioned to crew resource management (CRM) as aviation leadership realized that all crew members, not just those in the cockpit, impacted safety. CRM emphasizes the importance of all team members in promoting safety and empowers all members to speak up if they have concerns about safety. Crew members who identify and communicate sources of potential error are celebrated, and all crew members are empowered to stop a flight if any potential for harm is identified. In aviation, commitment to a culture of teamwork and safety has resulted in a decrease in the loss of life and an increase in consumer trust and confidence in the safety of commercial aviation (Kosnik, Brown, & Maund, 2007; Marshall & Manus, 2007; McConaughey, 2008; Thomas, Silverwood, & Helmreich, 2003).

Realizing the positive impact of team training on aviation safety and the continued risks in the existing health care system, individuals started to see team training as an opportunity to decrease harm in health care. This new focus on team performance also made sense as health care becomes ever more complex, eliminating each team member's ability to practice effectively as a solitary provider (Carroll & Messenger, 2008). In addition, research supports that the collective decisions made from the diverse input of all members of a team are better than those decisions made by an individual. Nurses and doctors and other members of the interprofessional team must depend on each other to realize the best patient outcomes.

Hunt et al. (2007, p. 302) state that "a team represents a synergy, in that a well functioning team should be able to do things more effectively, efficiently, reliably or safely than an individual or a group of individuals working separately could do had they been alone."

Implementation of team training in health care started in an operating room (OR) in a hospital in Basel, Switzerland, in 1997. Since then, the CRM concepts have been applied in the emergency departments, ORs, anesthesia departments, labor and delivery units, and intensive care units. All these clinical areas are very fast paced with rapidly fluctuating censuses and patient acuity. The application of the CRM concepts of crew communication, workload management, and task prioritization to the clinical arena certainly seemed to make sense (McConaughey, 2008).

There are several available programs to teach team training, some that are copyrighted (e.g., MedTeams®; Locke, 2002) and some that are available in the public domain (e.g., TeamSTEPPS; Department of Defense & AHRQ, n.d.). Often an organization creates their own program using the key principles of CRM. Whichever program is selected, successful implementation requires commitment and buy-in from all levels of staff, especially physicians. It also requires careful program planning. A team training champion who can constantly reinforce the use of the team skills and tools in the clinical area will serve as a role model and promote success of the program. Physician support and willingness to participate in the interprofessional education process are vital to the team training concept and the program's success (Kosnik et al., 2007; Marshall & Manus, 2007). An effective team training program must be built on a solid foundation of safety science concepts and adult learning principles. According to the Department of Defense and AHRQ (n.d.), a team training program should focus on 4 main competencies. These include leadership, communication (briefings, debriefing, SBAR), situational awareness (cross monitoring, chain of command), and mutual support (two challenge rule). In the MedTeams® program, these concepts are also addressed within the dimensions of team structure and climate, problem-solving strategies, team communication, management of workload, and team skill improvement (McConaughey, 2008; Weaver et al., 2010).

Recognizing the impact of teamwork on patient safety, the Department of Veterans Administration (VA), National Center for Patient Safety, developed a comprehensive CRM team training program that has been or is being implemented in about one-third of the VA Medical Centers (Dunn et al., 2007). Table 10.3 provides a summary of CRM communication principles, tools, and techniques of the VA's curriculum. Although these elements are specific to the VA National Center for Patient Safety Medical Team Training, they are representative of concepts and behaviors included in most CRM team training programs and provide a nice summary of the key aspects of team training.

Whichever CRM program is selected, one must recognize that team training is an ongoing process and requires constant attention and nurturing to affect the current hierarchical health care system. Team training education is best provided in an active learning environment including role-playing and simulation to maximize learning and retention of knowledge and skills. Incorporation of real stories from adverse events on the clinical unit can be helpful in personalizing the team training for the staff. Simulation is an excellent modality to use to reinforce expected teamwork and communication behaviors. Simulating the most stressful team failures in a safe learning environment allows the staff the opportunity to openly discuss the clinical aspects of the situation and their feelings about the situation, and to identify opportunities for better practice. This approach can help teams personalize the team concepts and better transition the use of the learned concepts and tools into their clinical practice. Teams that practice team training as active learners are more likely to demonstrate those behaviors in actual practice (Salas, Weaver, DiazGranados, Lyons, & King, 2009). Team training research conducted by Salas, DiazGranados, et al. (2008) concluded that in team training, both task work and teamwork have a positive impact on a team's ability to function. This type of interprofessional training can impact cognitive, affective, process, and

Table 10.3 *CRM Communication Principles, Tools, and Techniques*

CRM Tool	Communication Principle/Method
Rules of conduct	Ground rules for communication that focus on mutual respect and shared responsibility
SBAR	Situation–Background–Assessment–Recommendations: a structured framework for reporting patient information for hand-off in care responsibility (holistic approach with bottom line recommendations)
Graded assertiveness	Methods for increasing levels of assertiveness in the normal course of work to optimize patient care; especially relevant for an individual facing an authority gradient (e.g., nurse addressing a physician)
Two-attempt rule	Method for escalating assertiveness before ascending the chain of command
Feel the pinch	Intuitive sense that something is wrong
Call out	"Speaking up" to team members when completing a task, making an important observation, or when something appears to be wrong
Step back	Method for stopping a process or a procedure to reflect on the course of events, reassess prior assumptions, and question the efficacy of the action plan (e.g., "Stop what you are doing and listen to my concern.")
Repeat back	Method of repeating a verbal order or information to confirm mutual understanding (e.g., nurse repeating an order by a physician in the OR, emergency room, or Med-Surg unit)
Read back	Method of transcribing a verbal order or information and reading it back to confirm mutual understanding (e.g., nurse reading back telephone order from a physician)
Dynamic skepticism	Attitude of questioning the validity of previous assumptions by constantly evaluating incoming data—accept only what you see and know
Situational awareness	Understanding of the current status with impact on activity goals in a dynamic and changing environment
Work load distribution	Balanced distribution of work among all team members to achieve optimal outcome
Fatigue management	Acknowledging the effect of fatigue on human performance by developing strategies for fatigue management to optimize the safety of patients and staff

Source: From Dunn et al. (2007). Used with permission

performance outcomes in health care. In medicine, this can mean more efficient teams, better communication, and less adverse events. CRM or team training fills a void in the educational curriculum, as little has been done to date to teach nurses, physicians, and other members of the care team human interaction skills (McConaughey, 2008).

One tool that has successfully been adopted into many areas of medicine and is commonly viewed as a safety tool is the aviation preflight and in-flight checklist. An aviation style checklist both pre- and in-flight is being used to increase team communication and awareness during health care procedures that have high potential for error (e.g., before starting a surgical case or placing a central line). A checklist should include 3 parts: a team sign-in, a universal time-out, and a team sign-out. When the checklist is related to perioperative services or preprocedure, it should include the names of team members (first and last), 2 patient identifiers, patient position (when required), allergies, and all health care–related error "traps" (e.g., deep vein thrombosis prophylaxis and antibiotics). Checklists should be posted to allow all team members to visualize, to participate, and to speak up if things are not checked off or the standard of care is not met before or during the procedure (Sax et al., 2009).

Sax et al. (2009) discussed the use of a preoperative checklist that was developed and implemented in the OR suites in an academic medical center in the Northeast. The group tracked the progress of compliance over a 5-year period. During this period, the group reports a compliance rate change from 75% (2003) to 100% (2007). More important, the use of the checklist was helpful in assuring compliance with specific surgical criteria (e.g., antibiotic timing and deep venous thrombosis prophylaxis) (2009). The goal of a checklist is to limit or hopefully reduce the amount of errors and harm associated with procedures and health care encounters that contain a large amount of risk.

Although the use of the checklist for procedures has been associated with a decrease in errors, patient harm, and even deaths, some health care providers are still very reluctant to make the checklist a standard part of their everyday practice. In the book *The Checklist Manifesto: How to get Things Right*, Atul Gawande (2009) discussed his somewhat frustrating experience in getting hospitals in the United States to consistently use the OR checklist. Perioperative staff when interviewed conveyed that they did not think the checklist was necessary, and yet many of these same staff said that they would want the checklist used if they were having surgery themselves. Peter Pronovost, an international expert on patient safety, recently coauthored a book titled *Safe Patients, Smart Hospitals: How One Doctor's Checklist Can Help Us Change Health Care From the Inside Out* (Pronovost & Vohr, 2010). Part of the book focuses on the implementation of a safety checklist for use during the insertion of a central line. Implementation and adoption of this type of procedure checklist required that the physician and the nurse partner together to ensure that the procedure is carried out safely. This was accomplished by giving the nurse the responsibility and the right to stop the procedure if the physician breaks sterile technique or misses a critical step on the checklist. Despite the fact that the use of this checklist is credited with saving lives, some hospitals are still not using it. One reason cited for not using the checklist focused on current medical culture on one of the units. The unit had a culture that did not support the nurse speaking up, when indicated, to stop the procedure. Pronovost also reinforces the need for health care providers to remember the *science* in science of safety and seek opportunities to research and measure the impact of safety initiatives so that health care is providing patients with both safe and evidence-based care.

PATIENT SAFETY AND SIMULATION

The positive relationship between simulation and patient safety is commonly referenced in both the patient safety and the health care simulation literature. The IOM (2001) refers to simulation as a method to prevent and to mitigate harm. Health care simulation is a mechanism to practice clinical interventions and teamwork skills in a safe environment without any danger of harming a patient. The simulated health care setting offers a risk-free, nonjudgmental, and safe environment in which one can practice, make mistakes, and learn from experience without risk of exposing patients or providers to actual harm (Cato & Murray, 2010; Hunt et al., 2007). Dunn and Murphy (2008) propose the use of simulation as a health care safety and quality learning laboratory.

Simulation provides a mechanism to decrease patient harm and to improve patient outcomes. Although there are recommendations for additional research studies to be completed, there are data that link both high- and low-fidelity simulation-based training with improved performance with patients (Issenberg & Scalese, 2008; Salas, Wilson, Burke, & Priest, 2005). Salas, Wilson, et al. (2008) and Weaver et al. (2010) stated that the health care community can gain significantly from using simulation-based training to reduce errors and to improve patient safety as long as the process is designed and delivered appropriately. It is important for educators to view simulation as a tool to enhance the learning process and to promote patient safety, rather than thinking that it is the simulation that leads to the actual learning of the related concepts. For simulation to be successful, attention to all aspects of the program is critical. This includes clearly identifying the goals and objectives for each simulation experience.

OVERVIEW OF THE HISTORY OF PATIENT SAFETY SIMULATIONS

Health care simulation, which started as a skill-focused educational modality in the 1960s, is now used "to promote and improve team communication and construction, procedural skill training, educational evaluations and technologic innovations, such as the usability of devices" (Hunt et al., 2007, p. 306). Simulation has become part of the culture of health care education and performance improvement programs. One of the primary driving forces for this has been the public and institutional demand to improve the quality and safety of patient care. Carroll and Messenger (2008) support the above factor as a rationale for the continued growth of simulation. The decreasing resources and the ever-increasing expectations for medical education, coupled with the continued accelerations of innovations in care with new knowledge, diagnostics, devices, and drugs, clearly support the need for the ongoing use of simulation for health care education. This is both at the preclinical and the clinical levels. It is expected that the use of simulation will continue to grow rapidly in the next 5 to 10 years. Carroll and Messenger stated that the "next five to 10 years may be known as the golden age of medical simulation" (p. 47).

The approaches to simulation are varied but often include a presimulation briefing, a simulated clinical scenario, and a postsimulation debriefing. Some simulation exercises also include didactic content relative to the simulation. Ideally, the simulation is videotaped so that the participants can view the tape and observe both the clinical and relational aspects of the scenario. The debriefing process is where many say the true learning occurs. It should be 2 to 3 times the length of the simulated clinical event. Debriefing provides the interprofessional team the opportunity to honestly discuss what went well, what could have been done better, lessons learned, and how to perform better the next time, as well as system opportunities for improvement. All team members, regardless of their position in the hierarchy, have an equal voice in the debriefing process. Sometimes, this is the first time individuals from the separate disciplines have had this experience, and it can be very enlightening and empowering. The use of debriefing during the simulation process can set the stage for more open and honest communication in the clinical setting and more frequent in situ clinical debriefings as the team becomes more experienced and comfortable with each other and the debriefing process. Debriefing is one of the most important aspects of the simulation (Weinschreider & Dadiz, 2009).

As previously stated, poor communication among the care providers has been identified by the JC as a root cause in up to 70% of reported sentinel events. Simulation provides an excellent avenue to focus on improvement of critical aspects of the communication process. Marshall, Harrison, and Flanagan (2008) reported that the use of structured communication tools with medical students improved the content and clarity of telephone referrals in a simulated clinical environment. The researchers used the identify, situation, background, assessment, and recommendation (ISBAR) tool during the study. It is a modification of the well-known SBAR communication tool. Although limitations of this study preclude generalization of these findings to other areas, it does reinforce the use of simulation to test communication opportunities.

Nursing education has a long history with the use of task trainers and simulation to help prepare students for their clinical placement and to ensure the provision of safe care. Research supports the use of human patient simulation in helping patients learn key patient safety principles (Henneman, Cunningham, Roche, & Curnin, 2007). Simulation can also successfully support the transition of new graduates through their orientation process and their transition to the clinical area (Beyea, Von Reyn, & Slattery, 2007).

Simulation has also been used to study the impact of hand-off communication from the anesthesia provider to the PACU nurse. The 3 aims of the project were (1) to develop a simulation-based training intervention directed toward hand-off in the PACU, (2) to determine if the implemented hand-off simulation program impacts quality of hand-off in the PACU, and (3) to evaluate the impact of the hand-off initiative on overall team-work in the PACU. The author reports that the preliminary outcomes of this research are promising (Clancy, 2008).

On the interprofessional team level, simulation provides an excellent forum for CRM education and addressing individual behaviors that undermine a culture of safety. The JC (2008, p. 1) includes the following in the category of disruptive behaviors: "verbal out bursts and physical threats, passive activities such as refusing to perform an assigned task or quietly exhibiting uncooperative attitudes during routine activities." Often the overt disruptive behaviors are associated with a position that has more power within the organization, but the covert behaviors can be just as damaging. They also undermine the team effectiveness and compromise patient safety. Interprofessional team simulation should never be designed to focus solely on skill attainment, but rather always highlight the importance of team interaction and communication and how it relates to patient outcomes and quality care. Simulation is an excellent modality to use to reinforce expected teamwork and communication. One reason for this is that the simulation process allows for interprofessional team members to slow down the usual "time-constrained processes" and step back and reflect on the clinical scenario as well as their perceptions of their own roles and the roles of others during the simulation (Forsythe, 2009, p. 148).

For more advanced teams, simulations can be designed with confederates (simulation facilitators, faculty, actors) who demonstrate difficult or disruptive behaviors. This requires that the participating team members maintain their focus on the clinical aspects of the simulation and the interprofessional communication skills, as well as support the patient and family. With this approach, the postevent debriefing not only should focus on the identification and discussion of the observed patient and family behaviors but also must address the impact of these behaviors on the team and any increased risk of harm to the patient. Participants can debrief the patient and family behaviors to determine the best way to access the reason behind these behaviors and the best approach to safely manage these behaviors without alienating the patient or negatively impacting care.

Simulation can also be used to test the safety of new clinical equipment in a simulated clinical environment without risk of patient harm. It can also test the functionality of new clinical areas, buildings, or processes. Trbovich, Pinkney, Cafazzo, and Easty (2009) looked at the use of smart pump technology in a simulated clinical environment and based on their finding reinforced the need for setting hard override settings, focusing adequate attention on the training and implementation processes, and evaluating the impact of other systems related to the new technology.

Another use of simulation is to promote safe patient care using clinical rehearsals, also called *just-in-time* or *just-in-place* education. This can be helpful with high-risk, low-occurrence clinical procedures such as central line placement and dressing changes. An example of the just-in-time simulation education is when a simulation cart is prepared and made available for staff use immediately before completing the required clinical procedure. This allows the staff member to practice until competent with the procedure through the use of the simulator, limiting the risk of harm to the patient (Weinstock et al., 2005).

As the focus on patient safety and improved clinical outcomes continues, a key stakeholder and driver in the simulation movement is the medical malpractice insurer. With the ultimate goal of reducing financial exposure, some insurers have provided financial support and coordinated focused training for simulation in those clinical areas that are considered most at risk for adverse outcomes (obstetrics, anesthesia, and perioperative). Insurers are starting to transition from a reactive position of paying claims to a proactive approach of partnering with health care organizations and clinicians to decrease risks and promote patient safety. The Controlled Risk Insurance Company (CRICO) was one of the first insurers to assess their areas of risk and become active in the concept of "applied learning—taking new concepts and applying them in practice environments for both the intake of new knowledge and for the development of new skills" (Hanscom, 2008, p. 985). CRICO views simulation as an excellent partnership opportunity between the malpractice insurer and the health care organization. As such, CRICO has implemented simulation-based training in 3 high-risk specialty areas: anesthesia, obstetrics, and laparoscopic surgery. Outcomes in the anesthesia initiative have enabled CRICO to decrease insurance premiums for some care providers.

Another example of an insurer partnering with health care to decrease risk is in the funding of obstetrical patient safety nurses who are charged with the development, implementation, and evaluation of simulation programs and in situ drills with the focus on decreasing claims (Will et al., 2006). The foci of these activities include team interaction and clinical management of high-risk, low-occurrence events. Within health care organizations, risk-management departments are using simulation as an opportunity to reenact and learn from sentinel events. Lessons learned from the root cause analysis process can be incorporated into simulation experiences and shared with participating front line clinical staff. Disruptive patient behavior, communication errors, lack of teamwork, and failure to activate the chain of command can be scripted into a simulation experience and then become a focus in the postsimulation debriefing process.

Understandably, there are some limitations to the use of simulation. Hunt et al. (2007) talked about the approach of "practice with plastics first" and many technical skills that can and should be learned on task trainer simulators. The approach of *see one, do one, teach one* using patients in the learning process is being replaced by the safer approach of *simulate, simulate, simulate* before ever touching a real patient. Still, it is important to avoid the concept of mannequin think. Mannequin think is seen when learners have difficulty transferring skills learned in isolation during simulation to the complex clinical setting with its many distractions. This reinforces the need to incorporate interactions with patient, family, and other members of the patient care team into simulated learning events. Incorporating the use of interactive exercises and role-play simulations with acquisition of even the most basic technical skills will help the learner transition the skill successfully to the clinical setting (Kneebone, 2009).

Table 10.4 *Seven Key Elements of JC Speak Up™ Initiative.*

Seven Key Elements of JC Speak Up™ Initiative
1. Speak up if you have questions or concerns. If you still do not understand, ask again. It's your body and you have a right to know.
2. Pay attention to the care you get. Always make sure that you are getting the right treatments and the right medicines by the right health care professionals. Do not assume anything.
3. Educate yourself about your illness. Learn about the medical tests that you get and your treatment plan.
4. Ask a trusted family member or friend to be your advocate (advisor or supporter).
5. Know what medicines you take and why you take them. Medicine errors are the most common health care mistakes.
6. Use a hospital, clinic, surgery center, or other types of health care organization that has been carefully checked out. For example, The JC visits hospitals to see if they are meeting the JC's quality standards.
7. Participate in all decisions about your treatment. You are the center of the health care team.

Source: From Joint Commission (2010a). Used with Permission.

Another concern with task simulation training is introducing or reinforcing the concept of doing to the patient instead of with the patient. Dissociation with the human patient reinforces the outdated and unsafe concept that the role of the provider is to provide care and the role of the patient is to consume care (Spath, 2003). With this approach, providers lose an additional set of eyes—those of the patient—in the work of detecting error and in preventing error from reaching the patient and causing harm. The use of actors—adding the human aspect to simulation—reinforces the critical role of patient and family involvement in care. Actors in roles of patients and family members will serve as a constant reminder to the health care team that the patient must always have a voice in their care and thus a voice in the efforts to reduce harm (Spath, 2003). This also supports the JC's emphasis on partnering with the patient to promote patient safety and encourage patients and their families to speak up for safety. The seven key elements of the JC "Speak Up™" initiative should be incorporated into simulation activities (see Table 10.4).

BUILDING SIMULATIONS TO PROMOTE PATIENT SAFETY

Building patient and family roles into simulation provides for increased interaction and continued adjustment of the clinical scenario. Simulation facilitators can adjust scenarios and objectives based on each staff member's actions and interactions with the patient and the patient's reactions and questions. Kneebone et al. (2006, p. 922) argued for the inclusion of real people within all simulations.

> From our experience, we believe that the presence of a real person within a simulated scenario adds enormously to the perceived authenticity of the experience. Involving a human 'patient' creates an anchor to each clinician's actual practice, which in turn taps into a complex Web of conscious and unconscious professional responses. These include empathy, communication and decision making. Accessing such responses through mannequins and computer simulators alone is not feasible, given the current state of technology. Indeed, there seems to be a danger that the

practitioner may learn to play the simulator. Yet the ultimate focus of any health care training must be the patient.

The use of real patients presents an opportunity for the participants to use patient-appropriate jargon during the simulation and for the patient and family to ask questions and validate their understanding or lack of understanding throughout the simulation. For advanced interprofessional simulations, patient and family profiles can be built from real clinical situations in which disruptive or combative patient or family behavior impacted the quality of care provided. For these more complex simulations, it is advantageous to include additional members of the interprofessional team, such as social work and security in the scenarios. When additional teams are added to a simulation, it is especially important to include them in the debriefing process. Teams that simulate together should always debrief together.

Patients and their families can also be utilized in designing simulations to promote patient safety. This is an excellent way to engage patients and their families in the health care transformation process toward building a culture of safety. According to Balik and Dopkiss (2010, p. 2), "Patients and families are the only source of information about complex healthcare systems across all settings and are best equipped, if carefully listened to, to identify the unknowable aspects of unsafe systems." This outside view of the health care system can benefit the simulation process and the learners. The true and often heartbreaking stories from real patients and families who have experienced harm can serve as powerful lessons for staff. This type of partnering is also helpful for the involved consumers who want to ensure that their experience is not repeated again. There are several patient safety advocacy groups (e.g., Consumers Advocating for Patient Safety) that are currently partnering with health care institutions to decrease medical errors. Members of these groups are available as expert resources in planning patient- and family-centered simulations. These groups also work to enact legislation to improve the health care system and to help prevent harm. Patient- and family-activated emergency response teams are an example of a system change enacted as a result of patient and family involvement in the patient safety movement.

Simulation also allows for health care providers to practice the process of disclosure of an adverse event with patients and their families. According to Woodward et al. (2010, p. 486), "Disclosure of errors is perhaps the most direct way to engage the patient in safety issues." The current standard of medical ethics and care supports transparency with disclosure of adverse events that impact the patient. The Leapfrog Group, which represents the nation's largest purchasers of health care benefits, has recommended that hospitals, by policy, respond to never events with 4 principles: apologize, report the event, complete a root cause analysis of the event, and waive all associated fees (Binder, 2010). Thoughtful disclosure helps to mitigate the emotional distress associated with unanticipated outcomes for both the patient and the provider. Although this is recognized as the best approach, certainly, it is not always the easiest approach. The limited available evidence suggests that "a full and frank disclosure offers potential benefits for improved patient experience and provider–patient relationships" (O'Connor, Coates, Yardley, & Wu, 2010, p. 6). Simulation provides an opportunity for staff to role-play all aspects of the disclosure conversation with immediate feedback from the simulated patient and family. In addition, the debriefing discussion provides an opportunity for all the team members to consider and to share their thoughts about the disclosure process.

During the postsimulation debriefing, individual and team errors can be discussed in addition to system errors. Emphasis can be placed on the team's feelings related to the errors or harm that may have been caused. This provides an opportunity to review resources that are available to support staff that err and become the second victim.

THOUGHTS ON THE FUTURE OF SIMULATION AND PATIENT SAFETY: A CALL TO ACTION

Now, there is much passion and creativity being expressed in the use of simulation to promote patient safety. Although some research supports the impact of simulation for staff competency and perceptions of competency, questions remain as to whether the lessons and skills learned in a simulated learning environment will translate to improved patient outcomes, higher quality care, and a decrease of adverse events. More research is needed to evaluate the impact on patient outcomes and overall patient safety. Although this evaluation of simulation effectiveness and impact on decreasing patient harm is not easy, it is very important work.

Support is available. Regulatory agencies are verbally and financially supporting the use of simulation to promote patient safety. AHRQ has provided funding for projects that evaluate the role of medical simulation in promoting patient safety (Clancy, 2008). There are currently bills in both the U.S. House of Representatives and the U.S. Senate requesting increased federal funding for health care simulation.

Even with the limited number of outcome studies that link simulation to improved patient outcomes, it just makes sense to provide the opportunities for staff to practice. Don Berwick, MD, past president and chief executive officer of the Institute for Health Care Improvement, a member of the original committee that produced *To Err is Human*, and current Administrator of the Centers for Medicare and Medicaid Services, describes medical simulation as "one of the most exciting areas of healthcare improvement especially in patient safety and liability" (Voelker, 2009, p. 2191).

According to Dunn and Murphy (2008, p. 8), "We cannot afford not to implement medical simulation and the associated evolving safety education techniques."

SUMMARY POINTS

1. The patient safety movement is 20 years in the making. All health care consumers and providers must recognize, acknowledge, and address the potential for harm within the health care system and the required course for change.
2. The transformation of health care to a safe and harm-free system is a twofold process. Organizations must become high-reliability organizations, and the teams within those organizations must practice true interdisciplinary collaboration.
3. Harm exists within health care at an alarming rate. A number of regulatory agencies (e.g., JC and State Departments) mandate hospital reporting of sentinel and never events, along with the action plans of the completed root cause analysis. The JC then tracks and disseminates sentinel alerts that summarize incidence, causation, lessons learned, and recommended actions to allow other organizations the opportunity to improve processes and systems without having to live through yet another tragic event.

4. Learning from the health care errors of today is vital to shaping a safer tomorrow. To accomplish this, one must evaluate the true multidimensional factors that contribute to error. Most of the time adverse events result from weaknesses within organizational systems and infrastructure, and the fault does not rest with the bedside care providers.

5. A just culture shifts the blame from the health care provider and allows for true transparency and review of systems, infrastructures, and educational processes for all health care providers. It abandons the historic methods of blame and train. It is only by peeling back and assessing all the layers of the system that one is able to identify the true opportunities for improvement and decrease the potential for future harm.

6. Communication errors play a major role in team and system failures. The use of CRM behaviors and skills in team training programs provides frontline staff with the necessary tools to improve communication, to increase collaboration, to decrease hierarchical behaviors, and ultimately to provide safer care.

7. Changing culture takes time and requires interprofessional commitment, planning, and, most importantly, consistent and visible leadership support throughout the process.

8. Culture is local to each clinical unit, and measuring the unit culture should be the first step in determining the safety opportunities within that unit.

9. Simulation is an excellent modality for teaching both clinical and interpersonal skills. The active learning process embedded in simulation training ensures retention and future use of learning objectives. Although the true value of simulation is yet to be clearly defined, it has been proven as a vital educational tool with the ability to enhance teamwork-related skills.

10. There are a variety of approaches to simulation. These include the use of high and low fidelity and the use of actors and standardized patients. Careful planning is necessary to match the learning goals with the appropriate educational modality.

11. Medical malpractice companies are visibly and financially supportive of using simulation as a means to decrease patient harm and the resulting claims. Nurses, especially patient safety nurses, are well-positioned to develop, to implement, and to evaluate patient safety–focused simulation programs.

12. Simulation facilitators or faculty should partner with patients and their families to develop simulation curriculum from actual adverse events. This approach will increase the realism of the simulation for the staff, while supporting the patient's goal of limiting future exposure and risk to ensure that another family does not suffer from the same event.

13. Simulation is a valuable tool in the toolkit for health care transformation. Its use can assist in building a culture of safety in medicine and hopefully a safer future for patients. Simulation has the potential to reshape the U.S. health care industry.

14. There is a need for additional research to determine the best interventions to improve patient outcomes and the role of simulation in translating best practices from the simulation center to the clinical unit.

REFERENCES

Agency for Healthcare Research and Quality. (2010a). *Patient safety primer: Never events*. Retrieved August 24, 2010, from http://www.psnet.ahrq.gov/primer.aspx?primerID=3

Agency for Healthcare Research and Quality. (2010b). TeamSTEPPS® Fundamentals Course. Retrieved from http://www.ahrq.gov/teamsteppstools/instructor/fundamentals/module1/igintro.htm#actions

Amalberti, R., Auroy, Y., Berwick, D., & Barach, P. (2005). Five system barriers to achieving ultra safe health care. *Annals of Internal Medicine, 142*(9), 756–764.

Balik, B., & Dopkiss, F. (2010) 10 years after *To Err Is Human*: Are we listening to patients and families yet? *Focus on Patient Safety, 13*(1), 1–3.

Beyea, S. C., von Reyn, L. K., & Slattery, M. J. (2007). A nurse residency program for competency development using human patient simulation. *Journal for Nurses in Staff Development, 23*(2), 77–82.

Binder, L. (2010). The importance of dealing with never events, focus on the harm to patients, not the blame game. *Modern Healthcare, 40*(18), 23.

Buerhaus, P. I. (2007). Is hospital patient care becoming safer? A conversation with Lucian Leape. *Health Affairs, 26*(6), 687–696.

Carroll, J. D., & Messenger, J. C. (2008). Medical simulation: The new tool for training and skill assessment. *Perspectives in Biology and Medicine, 52*(1), 47–60.

Cato, D. L., & Murray, M. (2010). Use of simulation training in the intensive care unit. *Critical Care Nursing Quarterly, 33*(1) 44–51.

Clancy, C. M. (2008). The importance of simulation: Preventing handoff mistakes. *AORN Journal, 88*(4), 625–627.

Colla, J. B., Bracken, A. C., Kinney, L. M., & Weeks, W. B. (2005). Measuring patient safety climate: A review of surveys. *Quality and Safety in Health Care, 15*, 364–266.

Department of Defense & Agency for Healthcare Research and Quality. (n.d.). *Team STEPPS instructor guide.* Washington, DC: U.S. Government Printing Office.

Dunn, E. J., Mills, P. D., Neily, J., Crittenden, M. D., Carmack, A. L., & Gagian, J. P. (2007). Teamwork and communication Medical team training: Applying crew resource management in the veterans health administration. *Joint Commission Journal on Quality and Safety, 33*(6), 317–352.

Dunn, W., & Murphy, J. G. (2008). Simulation about safety, not fantasy. *Chest, 133*, 7–9.

Fewster-Thuente, L., & Velsor-Friedrich, B. (2008). Interdisciplinary collaboration for healthcare professionals. *Nursing Administration Quarterly, 32*(1), 40–48.

Forsythe, L. (2009). Action research, simulation, team communication, and bringing the tacit into voice society for simulation in healthcare. *Simulation in Healthcare, 4*(3), 143–148.

Gawande, A. (2009). *The checklist manifesto: How to get things right.* New York: Metropolitan Books.

Handyside, J. & Suresh, G. (2010). Human factors and quality improvement. *Clinics in Perinatology,* (37), 123–140.

Hanscom, R. (2008). Medical simulation from an insurer's perspective. *Academic Emergency Medicine, 15*(11), 984–987.

Health Grades. (2004). *Health grades quality study: Patient safety in American hospitals* [Report]. Denver, CO: Health Grades Inc.

Henneman, E. A., Cunningham, H., Roche, J. P., & Curnin, M. E. (2007). Human patient simulation teaching students to provide safe care. *Nurse Educator, 32*(5), 212–217.

Hunt, E. A., Shilkofski, N. A., Stavroudis, T. A., & Nelson, K. L. (2007). Simulation: Translation to improved team performance. *Anesthesiology Clinics, 25*, 301–219.

Institute of Medicine. (1999). *To err is human: Building a safer health system* [Report brief]. Retrieved January 9, 2009, from http://www.iom.edu/CMS/8089/5575/4117.aspx

Institute of Medicine. (2001). *Crossing the quality chasm: A new health system for the 21st century* [Report brief]. Retrieved January 9, 2009, from http://www.iom.edu/CMS/8089/5432/27184.aspx

Issenberg, S. B., & Scalese, R. J. (2008). Simulation in health care education. *Perspectives in Biology and Medicine, 51*(1), 31–46.

Johns Hopkins Hospital. (2010). *Comprehensive unit based safety program, CUSP.* Retrieved August 30, 2010, from http://www.inovationas.ahrq.gov/content.aspx?id=1769

Joint Commission. (2008). *Behaviors that undermine a culture of safety* (Sentinel Event No. 40). Retrieved August 25, 2010, from http://www.jointcommission.org/SentinelEvents/SentinelEventAlert/

Joint Commission. (2009). *Leadership committed to safety* (Sentinel Event Alert No. 43). Retrieved August 25, 2010, from http://www.jointcommission.org/SentinelEvents/ SentinelEventAlert/

Joint Commission. (2010a). *Facts about the Speak Up™ initiatives.* Retrieved August 25, 2010, from http://www.jointcommission.org/GeneralPublic/Speak+Up/about_speakup.htm

Joint Commission. (2010b). *Sentinel event statistics.* Retrieved August 26, 2010, from http://www.jointcommission.org/SentinelEvents/Statistics/

Kneebone, R. (2009). Simulation and transformational change: The paradox of expertise. *Academic Medicine, 84*(7), 954–957.

Kneebone, R., Nestel, D., Wetzel, C., Black, S., Jacklin, R., Aggarwal, R. …Darzi A. (2006). The human face of simulation: Patient-focused simulation training. *Academic Medicine, 81*(10), 919–924.

Kosnik, L. K., Brown, J., & Maund, T. (2007). Patient safety: Learning from the aviation industry. *Nursing Management, 38,* 25–30.

Kotter, J., & Rathgeber, H. (2005). *Our iceberg is melting.* New York: St. Martin's Press.

Leape, L. (2009). Errors in medicine. *Clinica Chimica Acta, 404,* 2–5.

Leape, L., Berwick, D., Clancy, C., Conway, J., Gluck, P., Guest, J., et al. (2009). Transforming healthcare: A safety imperative. *Quality and Safety in Health Care, 18,* 424–428.

Leape, L. L., & Berwick, D. M. (2005). Five years after To Err Is Human: What have we learned? *Journal of the American Medical Association, 293*(19), 2384–2390.

Leonard, M. (2010). Patient safety and quality improvement: Medical errors and adverse events. *Pediatrics in Review, 31,* 151–158.

Leonard, M., Graham, S., & Bonacum, D. (2004). The human factor: The critical importance of effective teamwork and communication in providing safe care. *Quality and Safety in Health Care, 13,* 85–90.

Locke, A. (Ed.). (2002). *LTD team coordination course (r). Instructor guide.* Andover, MA: Dynamics Research Corporation.

Marshall, D. A., & Manus, D. A. (2007). A team training program using human factors to enhance patient safety. *AORN Journal, 86*(6), 994–1011.

Marshall, S., Harrison, J., & Flanagan, B. (2008). The teaching of a structured tool improves the clarity and content of interprofessional clinical communication. *Quality and Safety in Health Care, 18,* 137–140.

Maxfield, D., Grenny, J., McMillian, R., Patterson, K., & Switzler, A. (2005). *Silence kills: The seven crucial conversations for healthcare.* Vital Smarts™ Industry Watch. Retrieved from www. silencekills.com

McConaughey, E. (2008). Crew resource management in healthcare, the evolution of teamwork training and MedTeams®. *Journal of Perinatal and Neonatal Nursing, 22*(2), 96–104.

O'Connor, E., Coates, H. M., Yardley, I. E., & Wu, A. W. (2010). Disclosure of patient safety incidents: A comprehensive review. *International Journal for Quality in Health Care.* Retrieved August 25, 2010, from http://intqhc.oxfordjournals.org

Pronovost, P., Holzmueller, C. G., Needham, D. M., Sexton, J. B., Miller, M., et al. (2006). How will we know patients are safer? An organizational approach to measuring and improving safety. *Critical Care Medicine, 34*(7), 1988–1995.

Pronovost, P., & Sexton, B. (2005). Assessing safety culture: Guidelines and recommendations. *Quality and Safety in Health Care, 14,* 231–233.

Pronovost, P., & Vohr, E. (2010). *Safe patients, smart hospitals: How one doctor's checklist can help us change health care from the inside out.* New York: Penguin Group.

Reason, J. (2000). Education and debate, human error: Models and management. *BMJ, 320,* 768–770.

Reina, M. L., Reina, D. S., & Rushton, C. H. (2007). Trust: The foundation for team communication and healthy work environments. *Advanced Critical Care, 18*(2), 103–108.

Rose, J. S., Thomas, C. S., Tersigni, A., Sexton, J. B., & Pryor, J. (2006). A leadership framework for culture change in healthcare. *Journal on Quality and Patient Safety, 32*(8), 433–442.

Salas, E., DiazGranados, D., Klien, C., Burke, C. S., Stagl, K. C., Goodwin, G. F., et al. (2008). Does team training improve team performance? A meta-analysis. *Human Factors, 50*(6), 903–933.

Salas, E., Weaver, S. J., DiazGranados, D., Lyons, R., & King, H. (2009). Sounding the call for team training in healthcare: Some insights and warnings. *Academic Medicine, 84*(10), 128–131.

Salas, E., Wilson, K. A., Burke, C. S., & Priest, H. A. (2005). Using simulation-based training to improve patient safety. *Journal on Quality and Patient Safety, 31*(7), 363–371.

Salas, E., Wilson, K. A., Lazzara, E. H., King, H. B., Augenstein, J. R., Robinson, D. W., et al. (2008). Simulation-based training for patient safety: 10 principles that matter. *Journal of Patient Safety, 4*(1), 3–8.

Sammer, C. E., Lykens, K., Singh, K. P., Mains, D. A., & Lackan, N. A. (2010). What is patient safety culture? A review of the literature. *Journal of Nursing Scholarship, 42*(2), 156–165.

Sax, H. C., Browne, P., Mayewski, R. J., Panzer, R. J., Hittner, K. C., Burke, R. L., et al. (2009). Can aviation-based team training elicit sustainable behavioral change? *Archives of Surgery, 144*(12), 1133–1137.

Sexton, J. B., Helmreich, R. L., Neilands, T. B., Rowen, K., Vella, K., Boyden, J., et al. (2006). The safety attitude questionnaire: Psychometric properties, benchmarking data, and emerging research. *BMC Health Services Research, 6*(44). doi:10.1186/1472–6963-6–44

Sexton, J. B., Paine, L. A., Manfuso, J., Holzmueller, C. G., Martinez, E. A., Moore, D., et al. (2007). A check-up for safety culture in "my patient care area." *Joint Commission Journal on Quality and Patient Safety, 33*(11), 699–703.

Singer, S. J., Falwell, A., Gaba, D. M., Meterko, M., Rosen, A., Hartmann, C. W., et al. (2009). Identifying organizational cultures that promote patient safety. *Health Care Management Review, 34*(4), 300–311.

Smetzer, J. L., & Cohen, M. R. (2005). Intimidation: Practitioners speak up about this unresolved problem. *Joint Commission Journal on Quality and Patient Safety, 31*(10), 594–599.

Spath, P. L. (2003, December). Can you hear me now? Providers must give voice in efforts to reduce medical errors. *Hospitals and Health Networks, 77*, 36–49.

Starfield, B. (2000, July 26). Is US health really the best in the world? *Journal of the American Medical Association, 284*(4), 483–485.

Thomas, E. J., Sherwood, G. D., & Helmreich, R. D. (2003). Lessons from aviation: Teamwork to improve safety. *Nursing Economics, 21*(5), 241–243.

Trbovich, P. L., Pinkney, S., Cafazzo, J. A., & Easty, A. C. (2009). The impact of traditional and smart pump infusion technology on nurse medication administration performance in a simulated inpatient unit. *Quality and Safety in Health Care.* Retrieved May 28, 2010, from qshc.bmj.com

Usprung, R., & Gray, J. (2010). Random safety auditing, root cause analysis, failure mode and effects analysis. *Clinics in Perinatology, 37*, 141–165.

Veltman, L. (2007). Getting to havarti: Moving toward patient safety in obstetrics. *Obstetrics & Gynecology, 110*(5), 1146–1150.

Voelker, R. (2009). Medical simulation gets real. *Journal of the American Medical Association, 302*(20), 2190–2193.

Weaver, S. J., Rosen, M. A., DiazGranados, D., Lazzara, E. H., Lyons, R., Salas, E., et al. (2010). Does teamwork improve performance in the operating room? A multilevel evaluation. *Joint Commission Journal on Quality and Safety, 36*(3), 133–142.

Weinschreider, J., & Dadiz, R. (2009). Back to basics: Creating a simulation program for patient safety. *Journal for Healthcare Quality, 31*(5), 29–37.

Weinstock, M. C., Taekman, J. M., Kleinman, M. E., Grenier, B., Hickey, P., Burns, J. P. (2005). Toward a new paradigm in hospital based pediatric education; the development of an onsite simulator program. *Pediatric Critical Care Medicine, 6*, 635–641.

Will, S. B., Hennicke, K. P., Jacobs, L. S., O'Neill, L. O., & Raab, C. A. (2006). The perinatal patient safety nurse: A new role to promote safe Care for mothers and babies. *Journal of Obstetric, Gynecologic, and Neonatal Nursing, 35*(3), 417–423.

Woodward, H. I., Mytton, O. T., Lemer, C., Yardley, I. E., Ellis, B. M., Rutter, P. D., et al. (2010). How have we learned about interventions to reduce medical errors? *Annual Review of Public Health, 31*, 479–497.

CHAPTER 11

Cultural Sensitivity and Competency in Human Simulation

Souzan Hawala-Druy and Mary H. Hill

INTRODUCTION

The health care system today is facing a variety of challenges as it strives to meet the presenting and emerging health care needs of a growing and diverse population. The Sullivan Commission (2004) report, *Missing Persons: Minorities in the Health Professions*, addressed growing concerns over health care quality and access for this population. According to the commission, the U.S. population is rapidly becoming a dynamic mixture of diversity, which is defined by socioeconomics, gender, race, age, ethnicity, culture, abilities, and language. The commission embraced the broader perspective of not only increasing minority representation in health professions: it further identified that health profession schools must provide multicultural education built on the ideals of social justice and civic responsibility, and prepare individuals to deliver culturally competent care.

THE IMPORTANCE OF STRIVING TOWARD CULTURAL COMPETENCY

Now, more than ever, health professionals are considering issues of race, ethnicity, and cultural competence in the preparation for practice. The United States is becoming increasingly ethnically and racially diverse (U.S. Census Bureau, 2000), and the percentage of minorities in the United States will increase 90% from 1995 to 2050 (U.S. Census Bureau, 1996). Moreover, evidence has suggested significantly higher rates of health disparities and disability among people of color (Brach & Fraser, 2000). Over the past few decades, the United States has exhibited a growing understanding and respect for the diverse cultures, religions, ethnicities, and values within its society. Given these trends, health professionals are more likely than ever to have to provide care for individuals from diverse ethnic backgrounds and yet may not be prepared to adapt, adjust, or to modify their practices to the specific cultural values, beliefs, and needs of that population. The American Association of Colleges of Nursing issued a position statement in 1997 stating that anticipation of a progressively more diverse population would make issues relating to cultural diversity increasingly central to nursing education (American Association of Colleges of Nursing, 1997). Therefore, excellence in nursing education is very difficult to achieve in a culturally limited environment, and health profession education programs must recognize that missing the experience of cultural diversity diminishes the overall quality of health profession education, and could only adversely affect the future health status of the individuals and populations served.

THE SIGNIFICANCE OF CULTURALLY SENSITIVE AND COMPETENT HEALTH PROFESSIONS

Being culturally competent is the understanding that individuals from different cultures have different values that affect the way health and health care are viewed and how the world is viewed. As stated in the Institute of Medicine (IOM 2000; 2002) reports, *To Err is Human* and *Unequal Treatment,* and the U.S. Department of Health and Human Services, (2005) *Healthy People 2010,* cultural competence of health professionals is a necessity in today's health care arena and plays a critical role in reducing health disparities and improving health outcomes. To this end, one critical aspect of reducing health disparities is moving health care providers, staff, administrators, and practices toward increased cultural competence and proficiency (IOM, 2002; U.S. Department of Health and Human Services, 2000). The IOM recommended implementing cultural competency curricula so that health care professionals could acquire the knowledge and develop the appropriate cultural skills and attitudes for working with diverse groups (IOM, 2002). As stated by Barrera, Corso, and Macpherson (2002, p. 103), "...the key to culture competence lies in our ability to craft respectful, reciprocal and responsive effective interactions across diverse cultural parameters."

CULTURAL COMPETENCY VERSUS CULTURAL SENSITIVITY

In ancient Greece, a certain academy gave a three-year course: Students in the first year of that course were called "Wise Men." In the second year they were called "Philosophers," meaning persons who wanted to be wise men. In the third year they were called simply "Students," meaning that they had been in school long enough to know how much they needed to learn.

Wilbur Schramm, 1907–1987
Father of Communication Studies

Despite the widespread agreement about the importance of cultural competency, there is little consensus among scholars about how best to define, approach, conceptualize, or measure it. Therefore, a brief description of the ways cultural sensitivity, communication, and competency have been defined, developed, and applied is presented in an effort to answer if achieving culture sensitivity and culture competency hinges on our knowledge, our behavior, or both.

SENSITIVITY

Sensitivity as it relates to culture can be categorized as intercultural sensitivity and cultural sensitivity. Chen and Starosta (2000) define intercultural sensitivity as "the affective" aspect of intercultural competence and "a readiness to understand and appreciate" cultural differences in intercultural communication. Cultural sensitivity is the knowledge and positive attitudes of health professionals toward health traditions of diverse cultural groups that are exhibited by health professions in the delivery of health care. Culturally sensitive health care is a phrase used to describe systems that are accessible to diverse populations and health professionals that respect the beliefs, attitudes, and cultural lifestyles of their clients. As a concept, cultural competency and sensitivity mean moving beyond stereotypes but remaining sensitive to one's own culture and the culture of other persons. Health professionals need to understand that during interactions with clients from diverse cultural backgrounds, "intercultural sensitivity does not come naturally" (Olson & Kroeger, 2001, p. 116) and is not a natural human quality. However, intercultural sensitivity can best be developed through planned learning experiences that afford health profession students opportunities to develop a heightened sensitivity to cultural differences.

COMPETENCY

There is no consensus on a definition for cultural competence that exists for all disciplines, and the meaning may vary depending on how and by whom it is used. Many definitions have evolved from diverse disciplines, perspectives, interests, and needs. Therefore, to truly understand cultural competency, further analysis is necessary.

Culture itself is a complex concept that can be defined in many different ways. Sometimes it is useful to think of it in terms of its characteristics rather than as a definition. Culture entails one's values, beliefs, traditions, customs, knowledge, ethics, and practices. It is learned, shared, and transmitted from generation to generation and is dynamic in nature (Leininger 1991; Leininger & McFarland, 2006).

The term *competence* (effectiveness, success, understanding, or adjustment) has roots in sociolinguistic traditions as well as in intercultural communication, which gives it greater credibility (Koester, Wiseman, & Sanders, 1993). Chen and Starosta (2003) conceptualize and define competence from an intercultural communication perspective as "the ability to acknowledge, respect, tolerate, and integrate cultural differences that qualifies one for enlightened global citizenship" (p. 344). The term *competency* is widely used by health professionals in curricula, training, and research rather than the term *sensitivity*. However, debate remains in the educational arena regarding whether education programs provide experiences to increase cultural sensitivity, and whether the development of cultural competency is a result of a myriad of experiences in providing care to diverse populations.

CULTURAL COMPETENCY

W. J. Starosta (personal communication, January 7, 2011) defines cultural competency as thoroughly understanding certain aspects of someone's culture and intercultural competency as putting understanding into sensitive, competent, perceptive, receptive, and effective practice, while inviting someone of another culture to engage in the reciprocal process.

Starosta continues, saying that intercultural communication moves from the personal to the interpersonal, and from the one to the several, from the within to the between. "Culture One" is the birth culture that is learned without trying by its members. They play it without having to construct in their minds "how to do it." An outsider who is going to participate in that culture can start acquiring skills that will make survival more possible. The urge to know about some other culture moves one immediately toward "Culture Two." In short, the person who finds reason to know the Culture One of another is on the road toward gaining intercultural competence (W. J. Starosta, personal communication, January 7, 2011).

Cultural competence is an experiential understanding and acceptance of the beliefs, values, and ethics of others, as well as the intercultural skills necessary to provide care effectively and efficiently for diverse individuals and groups. Therefore, the development of cultural competence within nursing and health professions is a requirement and a necessity. It is an essential component of health professionals' clinical practice, which is increasingly emphasized in nursing education and research (Clark, Zuk, & Baramee, 2000), and is highlighted by Jeffreys (2006, 2010) as dynamic and ongoing rather than an end product. It is also affirmed by Suarez-Balcazar and Rodakowski (2007, p. 15) that "becoming culturally competent is an on-going contextual, developmental, and experiential process of personal growth," and the process can happen through repetitive engagement with individuals who are different from us. Therefore, cultural competence cannot be achieved simply by learning how to act toward a particular cultural group, but involves considering all aspects of the surrounding circumstances and adapting health practice to fit each individual's needs (moving toward congruent care). Health professionals need to gain an understanding of each client's values as well as their own personal biases and stereotypes so that quality and equality can be reached during the delivery of culturally sensitive and competent care. Furthermore, for health professionals, in their efforts to become competent while interacting with culturally diverse individuals, families, and communities, they need to possess self-awareness, to demonstrate knowledge of the client's culture, to accept and respect differences, and to adapt care to be congruent with the client's cultural needs and expectations (Jeffreys, 2006; Leininger & McFarland, 2006).

Because there are multiple definitions and terminologies for cultural competence and no single agreed upon definition in the context of health care, it is recommended that health professions adopt their own definition for cultural competence to better understand the term and how to measure it. This is done by taking into consideration specific history and needs while avoiding the use of stereotypes and personal biases. Effective culturally competent communication subsequently improves health outcomes that would otherwise be hindered by the influence of differing cultural perspectives (clients and health professionals).

COMMUNICATION

Most people conceptualize communication primarily as just "talk," "chat," or "conversation." Sometimes we overlook its importance and complexity, but in truth it is a "universal human experience" that is integral to human society and culture (Littlejohn & Foss, 2005, p. 2). Furthermore, communication is "a process by which information is exchanged between individuals through a common system of symbols, signs, or behavior" (Merriam-Webster's Collegiate Dictionary, 1983, p. 266) and thus includes both written and oral language, gestures, facial expressions, body language, and space (Giger & Davidhizar, 2008; Littlejohn & Foss, 2004). Another important aspect of communication is the level of context in which the message is passed, where high-context communication is one in which most of the information is either in the physical context or internalized in the person, while very little of the message is actually in words, as in Eastern culture (Hall, 1976, p. 79). Conversely, low-context communication is where most of the information is verbalized. For example, the United States is considered a low-context culture. Therefore, when we discuss communication and culture of health professionals and their diverse clients, we should be aware of the total range of communication, including language, nonverbal communication, customs, perceived values, and concepts of time and space that could create cultural conflict and misunderstanding. To minimize such misunderstandings during interactions with clients, Ruben (1976) has emphasized the importance of behavioral elements such as display of respect, interaction posture, knowledge, empathy, role behaviors, interaction management, and tolerance of ambiguity. By consciously applying these practices, health care professionals can learn to foster effective intercultural communication that adapts to cultural differences in a respectful and yet functional manner. In conclusion, we could say that culture and communication are inseparable (Chen & Starosta, 2003). Because culture is the foundation of communication, when cultures vary, communication practices must also vary accordingly.

NONVERBAL COMMUNICATION

Proximity, Gesture, Eye Contact, and Touch

Communication is a dynamic process that is made up of the interacting components of sending, receiving, and responding. According to Hall, Chia, and Wang (1996), 65% of messages received in communication are nonverbal. In addition, silence during communication may itself be a significant part of the message. Nonverbal cues also influence how we perceive and are perceived. In clinical settings, for instance, a nervous facial expression hinders others' perception of our competence, persuasiveness, sincerity, power, or vulnerability. Nonverbal cues may be unconsciously acted and reacted upon, regulating proximity (space), gestures (body language), eye contact, and touch.

Nonverbal communication has many functions in the communication process, and it may support or replace verbal communication. Moreover, nonverbal communication can be equally problematic in health care, as language barriers affect communication and hinder health outcomes. For example, the "OK" gesture that is so commonly used in the United States is derogatory in many other cultures. Also, eye contact can be a source of confusion because many cultures avoid eye contact as a sign of respect. In addition, African, Arab, Hispanic, and Italian patients may prefer to engage at close range, while patients from Asia, Europe, and North America may desire extra interpersonal distance (Witte & Morrison, 1995). Therefore, Africans and Arabs may view American health care professionals as cold and uncaring. Touch is another nonverbal variable that can cause problems in health care settings. In some cultures, the use of touch is viewed as warm and friendly, whereas in other cultures, it is viewed as intrusive and inappropriate. Finally, the patient's orientation to time may affect when he or she will show up for appointments and how consistently they will follow medical advices. Differences in time orientation can also influence the amount of time the health care professional spends with the patient.

For practical application, health care professionals should be aware that certain cultural groups are often characterized as having a present orientation of time and being unable or reluctant to incorporate the future into their plans (polychromic-time culture). As in polychromic-time cultures, patients would expect the health professional to spend more time establishing rapport and explaining both the causes of illness and the treatment in lengthy, detailed ways (Giger & Davidhizar, 2004; Hall et al., 1996; Spector, 2004, 2009). It is important for health professionals to remember that personal ethnocentric attitudes toward time may negatively affect the planning of care for such cultural groups. Individuals may be late for appointments not because of reluctance or lack of respect, but because they may be more concerned with a current activity than with the activity of planning ahead to be on time (Davidhizar, 2001; Hall et al., 1996).

All of the previously cited scholars assert that individuals are rarely aware of their nonverbal behavior that, like culture, tends to be elusive, spontaneous, and often unconsciously executed.

Theories and Models of Culture Competency

In this section, Madeleine Leininger's Theory of Cultural Care Diversity and Universality (and Sunrise Enablers), Giger and Davidhizar's Transcultural Assessment Model, the Purnell Model for Cultural Competence, and Papadopoulos, Tilki, and Taylor's Model for Developing Cultural Competence are briefly introduced. Then, Campinha-Bacote's *The Process of Cultural Competence in the Delivery of Healthcare Services* is briefly described. The key elements of each are presented, and their applications are briefly outlined. The conclusion of this section features scenarios that represent cultural competency constructs and are designed to be used in human simulation laboratories of health professions and nursing.

Several models of transcultural care have emerged over the last three decades (Giger & Davidhizar, 1999, 2004, 2008). As with other models of nursing, they have been constructed with concepts that are already found in the biological, behavioral, and human sciences.

Culture Care Diversity and Universality Theory

Leininger is an anthropologist, a nurse, and a theorist who founded the transcultural nursing movement in education, research, and practice. She developed the Theory of Culture Care Diversity and Universality (Figure 11.1) as a means to providing culturally congruent holistic care. The theory was born of Leininger's clinical experiences and recognition that culture, a holistic concept, was the missing link in nursing knowledge and practice. Its concept of culture is derived from anthropology, and its concept of care is derived from nursing (Leininger & McFarland, 2006). Early in her nursing career, she recognized the importance of the concept of "caring" in nursing. The central purpose of Leininger's theory is to discover and to explain the diverse and universal culturally based care factors influencing the health, well-being, illness, or death of individuals or groups (Andrews & Boyle, 2008, p. 8). Later, Leininger added the term "culturally congruent care" as the primary goal of transcultural nursing practice. The theory proposes three modes of action for congruent care that are predicted to lead to health and well-being and to help clients face disabilities, illness, and death (Leininger, 2002, p. 76). The three modes are as follows:

1. Cultural care preservation or maintenance: This refers to nursing care activities that help people of particular cultures to "retain, preserve, or maintain beneficial care beliefs and values or to face handicaps and death" (Leininger & McFarland, 2006, p. 8).

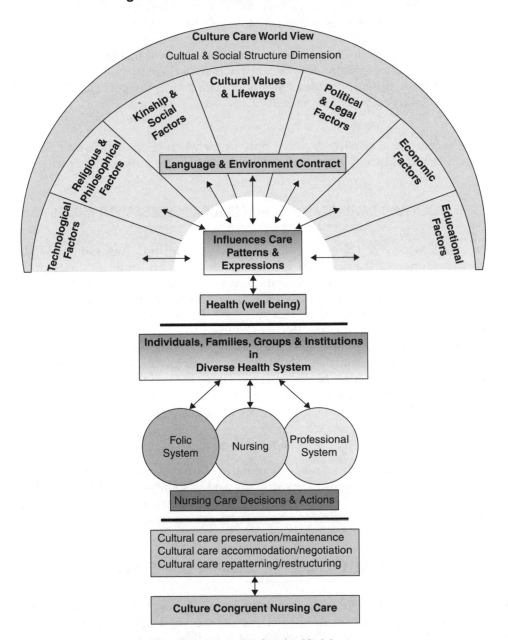

Figure 11.1 *The Sunrise Model.*
Source: From Leininger, M., & McFarland, M. (2006). Reprinted with permission.

2. Cultural care accommodation or negotiation: This refers to creative nursing actions that help people of a particular culture "adapt to or negotiate with others for culturally congruent, safe, and effective care for their health, well-being, or to deal with illness or dying" (p. 8).

3. Cultural care repatterning or restructuring: This refers to therapeutic actions taken by culturally competent nurses or family that assist a client to modify personal health behaviors toward beneficial outcomes while respecting the client's cultural values (Andrews & Boyle, 2008; Leininger, 2002).

Culturally competent nursing care can only occur when client beliefs and values are thoughtfully and skillfully respected and incorporated into nursing care plans.

GIGER AND DAVIDHIZAR'S TRANSCULTURAL ASSESSMENT MODEL

Giger and Davidhizar (2008) developed the Transcultural Assessment Model in 1988 in "response to the need for nursing students in an undergraduate program to assess and provide care for patients that were culturally diverse" (Douglas & Pacquiao, 2010, p. 1105). It was then refined in 1991 to "minimize the time needed to conduct comprehensive assessment" (Giger & Davidhizar, 2008, p. 5). The model includes six cultural phenomena that can be used to assess the cultural uniqueness of each individual. The phenomena are time, space, communication, social organization, environmental control, and biological variations (three of these are fully discussed in a previous section of this chapter; Giger & Davidhizar, 2008). This model provides a framework for patient assessment from which culturally sensitive care can be designed.

Applications

This model can be applied to a majority of health care professions (nursing, medicine, dentistry, education and training departments, and hospital administration) and is also applicable to the analysis of current trends in multiculturalism in health care (Giger & Davidhizar, 2008, p. 16).

PURNELL MODEL FOR CULTURAL COMPETENCE

The Purnell Model for Cultural Competence is a concept based on multiple theories and research and that defines circumstances that affect a person's cultural worldview. It also provides a framework for health care providers to learn concepts and characteristics of culture while reflecting human characteristics, such as "motivation, intentionality, and meaning" (Douglas & Pacquiao, 2010, p. 107S). The model acknowledges many culturally influenced health beliefs (Figure 11.2) and distinguishes between primary characteristics of culture—which are usually unchangeable—and secondary characteristics, which are often more flexible and influenced by time, family, community, society, and location. On the macro level, Purnell's model conceptualizes society as hierarchically divided into four metaparadigm concepts: global society, community, family, and person. On the microlevel, there exist 12 domains, which are common to all cultures (Purnell, 2002; Purnell & Paulanka, 2003; Douglas & Pacquiao, 2010):

1. Overview, Inhabited localities, and topography
2. Communication
3. Family roles and organization
4. Workforce issues
5. Biocultural ecology
6. High-risk behaviors

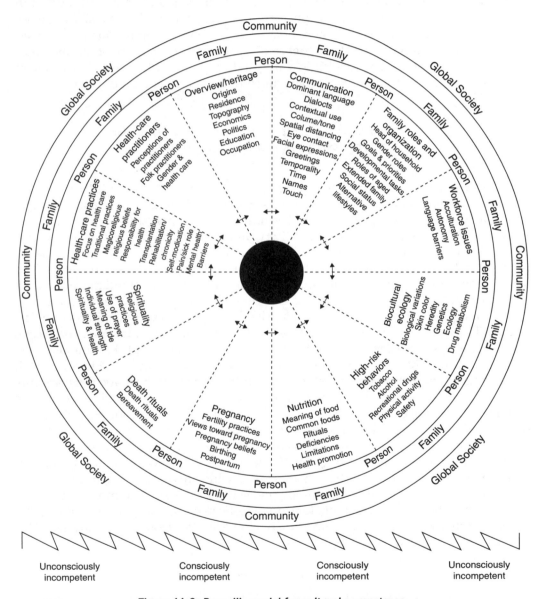

Figure 11.2 *Purnell's model for cultural competence.*
Source: Reprinted from Purnell (2002). With permission.

7. Nutrition
8. Pregnancy and child bearing
9. Death rituals
10. Spirituality
11. Health care practice
12. Health care practitioners

Applications

All health care providers in any practice setting can use the model, which makes it desirable in today's team-oriented health care environment and across all health care disciplines (nurses, physicians, and physical and occupational therapists). In practice, the model can guide the development of assessment tools and individualize interventions. As an educational tool, the model can be used within a variety of disciplines, in both staff development and academic settings. It can be used in research, as well, by using both primary and secondary characteristics to collect demographic data.

THE PAPADOPOULOS, TILKI, AND TAYLOR MODEL FOR DEVELOPING CULTURAL COMPETENCE

This European model's purpose is to promote the development of culturally competent health care professionals, where cultural competence is both a process and an output (Douglas & Pacquiao, 2010). The model has four constructs and stages: cultural awareness, cultural knowledge, cultural sensitivity, and cultural competence. The first stage in the model is cultural awareness, which begins with an examination of the health professional's "self-awareness" and his or her own personal values and beliefs. This stage is composed of three steps to cultivate this awareness: understand the importance of one's own "heritage adherence" and that of others, acknowledge "ethnocentricity" and "stereotypes" as contributing factors to health disparities and discrimination, and "cultural identity" and its influence on people's heath beliefs and practices. The second stage, cultural knowledge, is cultivated by experiencing meaningful encounters with people from different cultural groups, which then enhances knowledge about their health beliefs and behaviors. Other elements of the cultural knowledge stage are similarities and differences, health inequalities, and psychological, social, political, and biological knowledge. Stage three is cultural sensitivity. This stage supports the development of appropriate interpersonal relationships between clients and health care professionals by employing culturally competent communication skills that include trust, acceptance, and respect of clients' beliefs and values, while accepting them as true partners. Stage four is cultural competence, which requires the application of all previously gained awareness, knowledge, and sensitivity. The most important components of this stage are assessment skills, diagnostic skills, clinical skills, and the ability to recognize and challenge discrimination and racism (Douglas & Pacquiao, 2010; Papadopoulos, Tilki, & Taylor, 1998).

Applications

Because of the simplicity of the model, it can be extremely effective in nursing and medical education (as curriculum, and in development of cultural competence assessment tools) and research.

CULTURAL COMPETENCY AND HUMAN SIMULATION

Constructs for Developing Cultural Competency

One of the greatest challenges facing health professions and nursing education today is to ensure that students (Nursing, Medicine, Dentistry, Pharmacy & Allied Health) have experiential learning activities that promote the development of critical thinking and decision making for the provision of safe and effective quality health care. In addition, the novice health professional that enters today's workforce also must be educated to develop the requisite knowledge and skills to be able to provide culturally sensitive and competent care. Just as clinical simulations using medium- or high-fidelity manne-quins have helped students apply theoretical knowledge, case scenarios should include teaching and learning activities that foster the development of culturally sensitive and culturally competent behaviors for approaches to providing care for patients from vul-nerable populations.

The acquisition of the knowledge and skills to provide conscious care, however, evolves over time as health professionals engage in a wide variety of experiences dur-ing health care delivery. Therefore, because the development of cultural competency is an ongoing process, approaches to teaching such competencies using simulation should focus on guiding students through the different stages of acquiring cultural competence. In her study, *The Process of Cultural Competence in the Delivery of Healthcare Services*, Campinha-Bacote (2002) identifies five cultural constructs—desire, aware-ness, knowledge, skill, and encounters—and examines how these constructs can be applied to promote culturally competent health care providers and practices. These five constructs cannot be approached individually; they are designed to build upon one another and only when approached as an integrated, holistic framework do they effectively lead to cultural competence: *cultural desire* erupts, motivating the profes-sional to seek *cultural awareness* by obtaining *cultural knowledge*; this then yields *cultural skill*, which is then used during *cultural encounters* (Campinha-Bacote, 2003a, 2003b, 2007). The following discussion will focus on ways to incorporate each construct using clinical simulation.

Desire

In this construct, Campinha-Bacote (2007) explains the concept of cultural desire as the desire to learn and practice cultural sensitivity and equality in health care. She suggests that, when genuine, it is desire that drives an individual to truly embrace the concepts of cultural competence, where desire is defined as "the motivation of the healthcare pro-fessional to 'want to' engage in the process of becoming culturally competent; not the 'have to'" (p. 21). Along with this, the construct stresses the importance of the individ-ual's capacity for sacrifice, in that one must be willing to sacrifice prejudice and biases to develop this cultural desire. For example, this could be used in human simulation and standardized patient (SP) scenarios by simulating the relationship between a health care provider who possesses cultural desire and is willing to care for a patient even when his or her sexual orientation, religious beliefs, and so forth are in contrast to their own. The author then examines the role that social justice plays, asserting that "true cultural competence necessitates an understanding of social inequalities and how they affect individuals and communities" (p. 23). The last element that Campinha-Bacote touches on is humility, arguing that "health care professionals who are humble possess a genuine desire to discover how their patients think and feel differently from them" (p. 25). Each of these elements—caring and love (humanistic and spiritual), sacrifice (one's prejudice and biases), social justice (inequity and inequality), and humility—is essential to developing a strong sense of cultural desire, which can then fuel one's own personal journey toward cultural competence (Campinha-Bacote, 2003a, 2003b, 2007).

Awareness

Campinha-Bacote (2003a, 2003b, 2007) defines cultural awareness as "the deliberate self-examination and in-depth exploration of our personal biases, stereotypes, prejudices and assumptions that we hold about individuals who are different from us" (Campinha-Bacote, 2007, p. 27). Under this construct, the author explores the different ways in which health care professionals interact with patients from other cultures and how varying degrees of cultural sensitivity can affect success. In addition, she proposes four levels of cultural competence: unconscious incompetence (unaware of lacking cultural knowledge), conscious incompetence (aware of lacking necessary cultural knowledge), conscious competence (aware of accommodating and respecting cultural differences), and unconscious competence (spontaneous cultural response), in which one possesses an intuitive ability to effectively communicate in cross-cultural encounters. Furthermore, the author outlines the different styles of interaction between health care professionals and their patients and explains how a health care professional's own cultural and ethnic background can "affect interpreting, assigning meaning to, and creating value judgments about their patients" (Campinha-Bacote, 2007, p. 35). Thus, it is extremely important for health care professionals to be able to interact appropriately and sensitively with patients from different cultural backgrounds to provide the greatest diagnostic clarity (Campinha-Bacote, 2007). Educators can incorporate this construct into human simulation by assigning students SPs who exhibit cultural traits that are different from their own and assessing the level to which students are aware of their own competence or incompetence.

Knowledge

Campinha-Bacote (2007) explores what it means to have cultural knowledge and why it is particularly important when considering health care provider–patient relationship. According to Campinha-Bacote, "cultural knowledge is the process of seeking and obtaining a sound educational base about culturally diverse groups" (p. 37). When aiming to acquire this knowledge, health care professionals should focus on three specific issues: health-related beliefs and values, disease incidence and prevalence, and treatment efficacy. The following scenario demonstrates how to apply the construct of knowledge in practice: A Mexican mother brings her 1-year-old child to the clinic for immunization. While there, a nurse remarks that the child is beautiful and adorable. The day after receiving the shot, the mother returns to the clinic, complaining that her child is sick and accusing the nurse of having given the baby the evil eye, or *mal ojo*. In this case, the culturally competent health care provider should know that in Mexican culture, babies are considered very weak and even a slight compliment without touching the child can bring on the evil eye. The client confused a routine reaction to immunization with a culture-bound illness.

The integration of these three elements is extremely important to obtaining diagnostic clarity among cultural groups. This includes the role of health care professionals and their ability to maintain diagnostic objectivity in cross-cultural situations, as cultural incompetence is often the cause for misdiagnoses. The author also stresses the importance of being able to determine the extent to which the client identifies with his or her cultural background because although someone who is entirely immersed in their cultural beliefs and traditions may appreciate culturally relevant services, one who is acculturated to mainstream American culture may be offended by such an offer.

Skills

Cultural skill is a health care professional's ability to obtain and apply information from the client that will result in a culturally relevant and acceptable treatment plan. Thus, it is the ability to perform accurate cultural assessment, which Leininger (1978) defines as "a systematic appraisal or examination of individuals, groups, and communities as to their cultural beliefs, values, and practices to determine explicit needs and intervention practices within the context of the people being served" (Campinha-Bacote, 2007, pp. 85–86). To do so, one must use a wide range of cultural assessment tools, such as Purnell and Paulanka's (2003) 12 domains to assess a client's cultural background, and Giger and Davidhizar's (2008) Transcultural Assessment Model. Campinha-Bacote (2007) reviews a series of methods that health care professionals can use to gain insight into their client's background, current life status, and the way they view their medical condition. The experienced health care professional will know how to use these methods and models in a supportive and sensitive manner that will ensure the client is comfortable and feels as though he or she is truly being listened to and respected. To implement this construct in human simulation scenarios, while interviewing and conducting cultural assessment, the nurse or health care provider could ask, "Are there foods to be avoided because of your cultural origin, health status, or illness?" or "Do you rely on any self-care or traditional medicine practices?" in an effort to gain culturally relevant information from the client.

Encounters

As eloquently elaborated by Kim and Ruben (1988), in our complex intercultural world:

> Most people who struggle to find their way into intercultural encounters are quite likely to "profit" by that struggle. In becoming intercultural, there is a special privilege to think, feel, and behave beyond parameters of any single culture. This accomplishment, regardless of the accompanying psychological and social "cost" has a merit in dealing with our increasingly complex intercultural world. (p. 317)

Health care professionals cannot be expected to deliver culturally sensitive care without having a wide variety of their own experiences interacting with people from different races, sexual orientations, genders, economic statuses, and so forth. In discussing cultural encounters, Campinha-Bacote (2007) explains methods for effectively gaining a deep respect and understanding of a variety of cultures and traditions in a sensitive and humanistic manner, and citing Howard's (as cited in Campinha-Bacote, 2007) affirmation that methods should be designed to develop a "deep respect for differences and equally intentional openness to the possibility of connection" (Campinha-Bacote, 2007, p. 81). Campinha-Bacote touches on how encounters can be difficult when dealing with linguistic barriers, or even non-face-to-face situations, and how barriers can be overcome to yield the most beneficial and culturally aware health outcomes. The author concludes by cautioning against the use of untrained interpreters or family members because they often lack knowledge of medical terminology and disease entities.

In a nutshell, throughout their career and as life-long learners, health professionals should be aware of their own culture as well as well as clients' cultures (awareness), be able to recognize what cultural practice is appropriate (knowledge), have the ability to perform that practice (skill), "want" to communicate in an effective and appropriate way (desire), and strive to experience numerous and frequent interactions with culturally diverse clients and other health care professionals (encounter) to become culturally competent care providers.

Applications

The model is widely used by all health professions in clinical practice, education, research, administration, health policy, and nursing assessment and intervention. It can be used in clinical practices such as, but not limited to, home care, rehabilitation, spiritual care, and care to a special population; in education during curriculum, training, and faculty development; in research when organizing framework and tool development; and in assessment and interventions for nursing and ethnic pharmacology (for the pictorial model, see www.transculturalcare.net/Cultural_Competence_Model.htm).

HUMAN SIMULATION

Today's health care professionals are faced with the twofold dilemma of an increasingly complex and intricate health care system, along with an ever-growing variety of medical, ethical, and social challenges. Modern concepts such as patient rights, confidentiality regulations, and higher acuity levels of patients have led to limited access to appropriate clinical venues for quality student learning experiences, making it difficult for nursing programs to train their novice students. As a result, innovative, simulation-enhanced education was developed worldwide and presently is being used in many health care curricula. Traditionally, health professions and nursing educators have used the term simulation to include a variety of experiential learning techniques including games, case studies, role-playing, skills practice using models or mannequins, multimedia presentations, and computer-assisted instruction (Gaberson & Oermann, 1999; Jeffries, 2005; Shearer & Davidhizar, 2003; Tomasulo, 1999). Infante (1985, p. 90) defined simulation as a "replication of the essential aspects of reality so that the reality can be better understood, controlled and practiced," then Jeffries (2005) added that simulation can be detailed, mimicking reality or some components of reality such as SP and human simulation.

The effective use of simulation may reduce and provide better use of the time required in clinical settings. In addition, training through simulation scenarios—before "face-to-face" interaction with "real" patients—in a "mistake-forgiving" environment allows students to make, recognize, and correct errors in a nonthreatening environment. As mentioned in previous chapters, SP encounters are used extensively in medical education and have recently been adopted by nursing programs worldwide. SP is becoming one of the most renowned expanding practices in health professions education and an educational approach to helping students develop appropriate clinical skills, along with culturally sensitive encounters and communication skills. These encounters emphasize personal strengths while improving student confidence, clinical communication, and cultural competency.

Furthermore, simulation provides a setting for the teaching, learning, and evaluation of multidisciplinary education and training, and more than often for multicultural professionals through scenarios rich with sensitive cultural competence issues and elements such as communication, safety, critical thinking, decision making, and other valid disciplinary program objectives and outcomes in a safe environment (Haskvitz & Koop, 2004; Jeffries, 2005).

STANDARDIZED PATIENT SIMULATION

SP scenarios should be based on presentations of real patient scenarios commonly encountered in the same community where training takes place (demographic and ethnographic data). Standardized patients can be designed not only as evaluation tools, but also as learning tools for sensitive patient care issues (problem-based Learning). Furthermore, Buenconsejo-Lum and Maskarinec (2004) stated that SP simulation can be designed as an "effective element of cultural competence instruction", and used as "teaching tools for sensitive patient care issue" (Buenconsejo-Lum & Maskarinec, 2004, p. 23). Therefore, scenarios should be specifically tailored to teach and to evaluate intercultural and cross-cultural issues with a focus on curriculum, student discipline (e.g., nursing, medicine, occupational therapy), and diverse clients.

SCENARIOS FOR STANDARDIZED PATIENT SIMULATION TO TEACH AND EVALUATE CULTURAL COMPETENCY

Hana is a 52-year-old married, Middle Eastern female with very little English proficiency who lives in a suburban community with her family (husband, five children, three grand children and mother-in-law). Hana is here today, accompanied by her 22-year-old daughter who is fluent in English, to follow-up on the Pap smear result from 4 weeks ago (her appointment was 2 weeks ago, but because she was not very worried about the results, she rescheduled it for today).

This is Hana's first Pap smear because she recently arrived from her country of origin where there are no routine cancer screening programs (vaginal or breast) except when signs and symptoms are exhibited. At her last visit, Hana was complaining of some vaginal bleeding "now and then" in the last "2 months" and "too weak to care for grand children and old mother-in-law," so the female nurse practitioner did a Pap smear and pelvic examination. Hana stated that she was not very concerned because "that is OK" and that most women back home "have it."

At the end of the last visit, the nurse practitioner seemed very concerned and made sure that the patient kept this follow-up appointment so that they could discuss the test results. That nurse practitioner is not here today, so Hana is being seen by a young male nurse practitioner whom she has never seen before. The patient does not suspect that anything is wrong, which is why she did not bother to show up to the clinic 2 weeks ago. Today's practitioner will need to give the patient the diagnosis of advanced cancer of the cervix and discuss some general treatment plans (referral to specialty physician(s), more tests, therapy in stages [surgery, chemotherapy, radiation therapy, or all three]). The practitioner should also begin discussions with the patient regarding end-of-life issues. The practitioner will not be doing a physical examination.

Practitioners are assessed based on the following abilities:

- Deliver very bad news (advanced cervical cancer) in a manner appropriate for the patient.
  - Middle Eastern patients are not accustomed to discussing anything related to female anatomy and sexual issues.
- React appropriately to patient's religious, spiritual, and fate beliefs.
  - In this scenario, the practitioner should be prepared to respectfully react to the patient's perception of her illness. In Middle Eastern culture, it is common to accept life changes, including terminal illnesses and death, as being preordained by God (fate).
- Adjust to a situation where there might be conflicts between the patient and the practitioner.
  - In this case, the gender of the practitioner may make the patient extremely uncomfortable because most Middle Eastern females are uncomfortable discussing issues of female sexuality and anatomy with the opposite sex.
  - In addition, the young age of the practitioner may make it hard to convince the older patient to consider end-of-life decisions, who may see the younger professional as lacking in life experience and wisdom.
- Determine the client's understanding and ability to communicate in English, talk slowly and clearly, use a translator to facilitate communication if needed, but not a family member.
  - In this case, it is important not to rely on the daughter; although she is fluent in English, she does not possess the appropriate medical terminology.
  - In Middle Eastern culture, family members often hide the true extent of bad news from the patient.
- Recognize that canceling, missing, or being late for appointments is not a sign of disrespect toward health care providers but is simply a reflection of how many cultures place other responsibilities, such as family and work, before individual health issues. Health care providers should be sensitive to this and be aware of their own verbal and nonverbal communication.
  - The health care provider should not chastise Hana for having rescheduled her original appointment.
- Communicate with the patient with no confusion by clearly explaining any use of medical jargons.
- Establish rapport with family members, assess family members' understanding of the client's condition, and encourage expression of feelings.

MODIFYING EXISTING SCENARIOS TO ASSESS VARYING CULTURAL ISSUES

When using human simulation and standardized patients in education, it is important to recognize that even simple manipulations of developed scenarios, such as modifying the cultural background, needs, experiences, and diverse social and environmental support system of the patient or health care provider, can create entirely new scenarios in which students can be assessed on a variety of cultural competency and communication skills. For example, when using the previously mentioned scenario, simple changes can make it applicable to various disciplines, curricula, and cultural groups. Possible modifications could include the following:

- Replace the 22-year-old daughter with Hana's mother-in-law (Camphina-Bacote model).
- Exchange Hana's daughter with a son (Purnell model).
- Replace the nurse practitioner with a physician (Camphina-Bacote model).
- Change the age, the gender, and the cultural background of the practitioner (Giger and Davidhizar's model).
- Replace the cultural group (Middle Eastern) with another group (Hispanic).
- Ask students to discuss not only the diagnosis but also the treatment options (Leininger theory—negotiation and repatterning).

DEVELOPING SCENARIOS FOR EDUCATIONAL USE

The following discussion examines different elements that health care educators should keep in mind when developing new scenarios for student use. Educators should be aware of the contributions and effects of communication skills, attitudes, and knowledge, as well as cultural predispositions of students.

Communication Knowledge

Health profession students should demonstrate knowledge of culturally relevant values and practices. For example, such knowledge should be applied when discussing end-of-life decision making, taking into account patient attitudes toward suffering and death and the possibility of spiritual concerns of patients and their families. Likewise, students should be aware of the possibilities of complementary and alternative medicine use by patients (e.g., such as in chronic pain disorders). Educators are encouraged to develop scenarios that include variety of topics and discussion areas that will add breadth to students' level of knowledge. Topics include, but are not limited to, the following: vulnerable population and persons living with HIV/AIDS, deaf culture and person with disability, generation differences, sexual orientation and gay and lesbian culture, homeless persons with mental illness, grief and loss in different cultures, and social justice awareness.

Communication Skills

Health profession students should exhibit appropriate to excellent use of culturally sensitive interviewing and communication styles that include effective information gathering (cultural history), appropriate levels of eye contact and body posture (nonverbal communication), appropriate active listening skills, demonstration of empathy and rapport building, and appreciation and respect of patient's perception regarding cause of illness. Culturally competent care and ideal health care outcomes can only be achieved when this communication is done in an effective and efficient manner.

Communication Attitudes

Health profession students should show professional manners and attitudes, appropriately and responsibly accommodating patient and family needs while negotiating patient care, and repatterning care plans to accommodate the patient's cultural background and social needs without jeopardizing the appropriate treatment. Student attitudes should demonstrate high levels of professionalism (respect, patience, adherence to policies, civility, accountability, ethical principles, and so forth). Furthermore, future health professionals should strive to expand the level of knowledge regarding professionalism and what it entails, as exhibited through a commitment to fulfill professional responsibilities toward diverse patient populations by cultivating and maintaining a culturally sensitive and competent health care practice.

Literature review and research results, as documented throughout this chapter, have shown that an individual health professional's ability to offer culturally sensitive and responsive care is directly related to one's level of cultural competence. In turn, this will ultimately improve the quality and the equality of the care provided and will help reduce health care disparities among culturally and ethnically diverse populations.

It is vital that all health professionals, regardless of their level of training, whether a first year nursing student or an experienced practitioner, be educated and trained to manage patients with varying health care beliefs and needs. Effective training in cultural competency should be included and infused throughout the curriculum of all health care professionals (cognitive, practical, and affective learning). The focus has to be on improving the awareness and knowledge regarding diverse populations, improving communication skills and practices, and increasing the encounters the students have with diverse populations. Before encounters with real patients, health professional students may benefit from training through standardized patient simulation. Training sessions with standardized patients, in a safe and nonthreatening environment, will help build students' confidence, improve their communication skills, and increase their overall level of cultural sensitivity and competency.

REFERENCES

American Association of Colleges of Nursing. (1997). *Diversity and equality of opportunity.* Retrieved October 16, 2010, from http://www.aacn.nche.edu/publications/positions/diverse.htm

Andrews, M. M., & Boyle, J. S. (2008). Transcultural concepts in nursing care (5th ed.). Philadelphia: Lippincott Williams & Wilkins.

Barrera, I., Corso, R. M., & Macpherson, D. (2002). *Cultural competency as skilled dialogue. Topics in Early Childhood Special Education,* 22(2), 103–113. Retrieved June 21, 2008, from http://tec.sage-pub.com/content/22/2/103

Brach, C., & Fraser, I. (2000). Can competency reduce racial and ethnic health disparities? A review and conceptual model. *Medical Care Research and Review, 57,* 181–217.

Buenconsejo-Lum, L., & Maskarinec, G. (2004). Using standardized patients to enhance cross-cultural sensitivity. *Asia Pacific Family Medicine, 3,* 23–27. Retrieved December 18, 2010, from http://www.apfmj-archive.com/3rd_issues/afm_007.pdf

Campinha-Bacote, J. (2002). The process of cultural competence in the delivery healthcare services: A model of care. *Journal of Transcultural Nursing, 3,* 181–184.

Campinha-Bacote, J. (2003a). Many faces: Addressing diversity in health care. *Online Journal of Issues in Nursing,* 8(1), Manuscript 2. Retrieved April 20, 2009, from http://www.nursingworldorg/

MainMenuCategories/ANAMarketplace/ANAPeriodicals/OJIN/TableofContents/
Volume82003/No1Jan2003/AddressingDiversityinHealthCare.aspx

Campinha-Bacote, J. (2003b). *The process of cultural competence in the delivery of health care services* (4th ed.). Cincinnati, OH: Transcultural CARE Associates.

Campinha-Bacote, J. (2007). *The process of cultural competence in the delivery of health care services: The journey continues.* Cincinnati, OH: Transcultural CARE Associates.

Chen, G.-M., & Starosta, W. J. (2000). Intercultural sensitivity. In L. A. Samovar & R. E. Porter (Eds.), *Intercultural communication: A reader.* Belmont, CA: Wadsworth.

Chen, G.-M., & Starosta, W. J. (2003). Cultural awareness. In L. A. Samovar & R. E. Porter (Eds.), *Intercultural communication: A reader* (pp. 344–354). Belmont, CA: Wadsworth.

Clark, L., Zuk, J., & Baramee, J. (2000). A literature approach to teaching cultural competence. *Journal of Transcultural Nursing, 11,* 199–203.

Davidhizar, R. (2001, Spring). So your patient is Latino. *Journal of practical Nursing, 51*(1), 18–20.

Douglas, M. K., & Pacquiao, D. F. (Eds.). (2010). Core curriculum in transcultural nursing and health care. *Journal of Transcultural Nursing, 21*(Suppl. I), 5S–417S.

Gaberson, K. B., & Oermann, M. H. (1999). *Clinical teaching strategies in nursing.* New York: Springer Publishing.

Giger, J., & Davidhizar, R. (1999). *Transcultural nursing: Assessment and intervention* (3rd ed.). St. Louis, MO: Mosby.

Giger, J., & Davidhizar, R. (2004). *Transcultural nursing: Assessment and intervention* (4th ed.). St. Louis, MO: Mosby.

Giger, J., & Davidhizar, R. (2008). *Transcultural nursing: Assessment and intervention* (5th ed.). St. Louis, MO: Mosby.

Hall, E. (1976). *Beyond culture.* Garden City, NY: Anchor.

Hall, C. W., Chia, R., & Wang, D. (1996). Nonverbal communication among American and Chinese students. *Psychological Reports, 79,* 419–428.

Haskvitz, I. M., & Koop, E. C. (2004). Students struggling in clinical? A new role for the patient simulator. *Journal of Nursing Education, 43*(4), 181–184.

Howard. G. (2003). Speaking of difference: Reflections on the possibility of culturally competent conversation. New Horizons for Learning Online Journal, 9(2). Retrieved May 25, 2011, from http://home.blarg.net/~building/strategies/multicultural/howard.htm

Infante, M. S. (1985). *The clinical laboratory in nursing education* (2nd ed.). New York: John Wiley & Sons.

Institute of Medicine of the National Academies. (2000). To Err is Human. Retrieved May 15, 2010 from http://www.nap.edu/books/0309068371/html/

Institute of Medicine of the National Academies. (2002, March 20). Unequal treatment: Confronting racial and ethnic disparities in health care. Retrieved April 16, 2008, from http://www.iom.edu/

Jeffreys, M. R. (2006). Teaching cultural competence in nursing and health care: Inquiry, action, and innovation (2nd ed.). New York: Springer Publishing.

Jeffreys, M. R. (2010). *Teaching cultural competence in nursing and health care: Inquiry, action, and innovation* (2nd ed.). New York: Springer Publishing.

Jeffries, P. R. (2005). A framework for designing, implementing, and evaluating simulations used as teaching strategies in nursing. *Nursing Education Perspectives, 26*(2), 96–103.

Kim, Y. Y., & Ruben, B. D (1988). Intercultural transformation: A systems theory. In Y. Y. Kim & W. B. Gudykunst (Eds.), *Theories in intercultural communication. International and intercultural communication annuals, XII* (pp. 299–321). Newbury Park, CA: Sage.

Koester, J., Wiseman, R. L., & Sanders, J. A. (1993). Multiple perspective of intercultural communication competence. In R. L. Wiseman & J. Koester (Eds.), *Intercultural communication competence. International and intercultural communication annuals, XVII* (pp. 3–15). Newbury Park, CA: Sage.

Leininger, M. (1978). Transcultural nursing: Theories, concepts, and practices. New York: John Wiley & Sons.

Leininger, M. (1991). *Culture care diversity and universality: Theory of nursing.* New York: National League for Nursing.

Leininger, M. (2002). The theory of culture care and the ethnonursing research method. In M. Leininger & M. McFarland (Eds.), Transcultural nursing: Concepts, theories, research and practices (3rd ed., pp. 71–116). New York: McGraw-Hill.

Leininger, M., & McFarland, M. (2006). *Culture care diversity and universality: A worldwide theory of nursing* (2nd ed.). Sudbury, MA: Jones and Bartlett.

Littlejohn, S. W., & Foss, K. A. (2005). Theories of human communication (8th ed.). Belmont, CA: Thomson/Wadsworth.

Merriam-Webster's collegiate dictionary (9th ed.). (1983). Springfield, MA: Merriam-Webster.

Olson, C. L., & Kroeger, K. R. (2001). Global competency and intercultural sensitivity. *Journal of Studies in International Education, 5*(2), 116–137.

Papadopoulos, I., Tilki, M., & Taylor, G. (1998). *Transcultural care: A guide for health care professionals.* Wilts: Quay Books. Information retrieved December 10, 2010, from http://www.ieneproject. eu/download/Outputs/intercultural%20model.pdf

Purnell, L. (2002). The Purnell model of competency. *Journal of Transcultural Nursing, 13*(3), 193–196. Retrieved November 12, 2010, from http://etna.middlesex.wikispaces.net/file/view/The+Pur nell+Model+for+Cultural+Competence%5B1%5D.pdf

Purnell, L. D., & Paulanka, B. J. (2003). *Transcultural health care: A culturally competent approach* (2nd ed.). Philadelphia, PA: F. A. Davis.

Shearer, R., & Davidhizar, R. (2003). Using role-play to develop cultural competence. *Journal of Nursing Education, 42*(6), 273–276.

Spector, R. E. (2004). Cultural diversity in health and illness (6th ed.). Upper Saddle River, NJ: Pearson/Prentice Hall.

Spector, R. E. (2009). Cultural diversity in health and illness (7th ed.). Upper Saddle River, NJ: Pearson/Prentice Hall.

Starosta, W. J., & Chen, G.-M. (2003). Intercultural Awareness. In L. A. Samovar & R. E. Porter (Eds.), *Intercultural communication: A reader* (pp. 344–354). Belmont, CA: Wadsworth.

Suarez-Balcazar, Y., & Rodakowski, J. (2007). Becoming a culturally competent occupational therapy practitioner. *OT Practice, 12*(17), 14–17.

Sullivan Commission. (2004). *Missing persons: Minorities in the health professions.* Retrieved April 23, 2009, from http://www.aacn.nche.edu/mrdia/pdf/sullivanreport.pdf

Tomasulo, D. (1999). Action methods of teaching cultural diversity awareness. In *Issues of education at community colleges: Essays by fellows in the mid-career fellowship program at Princeton University 1998–1999.* Retrieved August 27, 2010, from http://eric.ed.gov:80/PDFS/ED437118.pdf

U.S. Census Bureau. (1996). *Population projections of the United States by age, sex, race, and Hispanic origin: 1995 to 2050.* Washington, DC: U.S. Bureau of the Census, Current Population Reports, P25–1130, U.S. Government Printing Office. Retrieved September 20, 2010, from http://www. census.gov/prod/1/pop/p25–1130/p251130.pdf

U.S. Census Bureau. (2000). *Projections of the resident population by race, Hispanic origin, and nativity: Middle series, 2025–2045.* Washington, DC: Author. Retrieved April 20, 2004, from www. census.gov/population/projections/nation/summary/np-t5-c.pdf

U.S. Department of Health and Human Services. (2000). With understanding and improving health and objectives for improving health. *Healthy people 2010* (2nd ed.). Washington, DC: U.S. Government Printing Office.

U.S. Department of Health and Human Services. (2005). *Healthy People 2010.* Retrieved April 16, 2010, from http://www.healthypeople.gov/About/hpfact.htm

Witte, K., & Morrison, K. (1995). Intercultural and cross-cultural health communication. In R. L. Wiseman (Ed.), Intercultural communication theory (pp. 216–246). Thousand Oaks, CA: Sage.

CHAPTER 12

Human Simulation/Standardized Patient Business Plan

Denise LaMarra and Gayle Gliva-McConvey

INTRODUCTION

*T*he use of standardized patients (SPs) is widely supported in literature, and those in the field of SP education know the value of SPs from both an instructional and a fiscal perspective. However, many SP educators hesitantly approach the business aspects of their positions, and are more comfortable focusing on educational design and implementation. This chapter is written for the SP educator who is required to have a foot in both the SP methodology and the business and financial worlds.

Whether the SP program is in the nascent stage or well-established, it is critical to the long-term success of any SP program to have an operations plan and, as needed, a business plan. An operations plan guides the staff in achieving day-to-day program requirements and outlines the program's existing financial commitments. A business plan moves the program ahead and toward specific goals; it may be used to garner interest from external groups or generate investment for growth by key decision makers.

If not already done, the SP educator needs to develop and understand their operations plan before a business plan can be created. They must also realize that once the business plan has accomplished its specific goal, it becomes part of their operations plan. Therefore, a solid operations plan will serve as a foundation for developing goal-oriented business plans. A dynamic template, the business plan should be updated to meet individual programs' changing needs, such as to (1) increase staff to cover increased workload or areas of involvement, (2) expand or build dedicated space, (3) create new revenue-generating projects, or (4) request a technology upgrade.

As SP educators, we have learned the value of a comprehensive and well-thought-out plan, as compared with data that are pulled together quickly in a reactive manner, in response to an imposed deadline. An operations plan gives the SP educator leverage with key decision makers, and adds credibility to the profession and program. An operations plan highlights the educational design and curricular/development aspects of the position, and dispels the notion that our sole responsibilities are to hire actors and tally supplies.

Although creating operations and business plans are no small tasks, the good news is that most SP educators and administrators have much of the information they need already at their fingertips. In the planning stages, it is important to establish a team to pull it all together in an organized way and to maintain the operational plan so the content remains up-to-date. The up-to-date operations plan information can then be quickly inserted into the business plan template when needed. The following is a thumbnail sketch of the contents of each to illustrate the areas of overlap.

THE OPERATIONS PLAN

As stated earlier, an operations plan provides the leadership a greater understanding of how the SP program functions on a continuing basis. It provides a snapshot of the program's status, states priorities and responsibilities, tracks progress, monitors financial commitments and expenses, and manages growth proactively. It also provides milestones and measurable objectives, which keep staff on task and focused collectively on the program's overall goals.

Operations plans should contain key elements such as an overall program description, mission statement, objectives, financial review, performance matrix, personnel infrastructure, facilities overview, and appendices. Each of these elements is explained in detail on the following pages.

	Operations	Business
Overall description	X	
Mission statement	X	X
Objectives	X	X
Financial review	X	X
Performance matrix	X	X
Introduction		X
Executive summary		X
SWOT (Strengths, Weaknesses, Opportunities, Threats) analysis		X
Leadership/personnel		X
Quality control/assurance plan		X
Marketing strategies		X
Facility overview	X	X
Goal statement		X
Timelines		X
Appendices		
SP history/benefits	X	X
Testimonials	X	X

Program Description

The overall program description should succinctly highlight the breadth and depth of one's program. Important points to include the following:

- Range of roles and definition of SPs (SPs vs. physical-teaching associates vs. standardized participants, clients, students, family members, team members, faculty, et al.)
- When and how the program originated
- How it is being used in the curriculum and various formats (Appendix 12.A)
- Users and clients (medical and nursing students, residents, fellows, other health professionals, and nonmedical trainees)
- External perception of the program (regional or national recognition, unique contributions to the field of education)
- Detailed descriptions of methodology and when learners work with SPs throughout their education, types of programs, formative vs. summative, involvement of faculty, etc.

For emerging programs, this section may be brief but should be informative to the leadership and key decision makers.

Mission Statement

Two separate mission statements should be included in the operations plan: an educational mission statement for the operations plan, which supports all goals of the program (Appendix 12.B), and a business mission statement (Appendix 12.C) that addresses the revenue-generating facet of one's program. The educational mission statement is a crucial building block in creating a program's operations plan.

To create rich, meaningful mission statements, it is recommended that all staff be involved (including faculty representation from the leadership) rather than drafting them in a vacuum behind one's desk. This will ensure that all views are represented, and provide buy-in needed as groups collectively work toward the program missions. Posting mission statements in offices and on Web sites encourages program leaders and staff to be intimately familiar with the language. To avoid stagnancy, mission statements should be revisited every 3 to 5 years, and the operations plan modified regularly to ensure it is still in alignment with the program's missions.

Goals and Objectives

"Unless there are clearly defined SP program goals and objectives, it is difficult to measure whether a given program is successful in achieving its outcomes and thus in justifying its costs" (King, Perkowski-Rogers, & Pohl, 1994). To operationalize the mission, one must generate functional, achievable goals and objectives. As with mission statements, it is recommended that all staff be involved in the creation of goals and objectives, including faculty and students. The terms *goals* and *objectives* are often used interchangeably. However, for the purposes of this chapter, goals will be defined as broad, less structured, long-term intentions, whereas objectives will be defined as narrow, precise, and concrete attainments. Goals cannot be validated, but objectives can usually be measured and validated.

For example, a goal to develop a workshop for SP educators might be achieved by meeting these objectives: participants will gain a foundation of SP methodology and understand the difference between standardization and simulation. Appendix 12.B offers another example, illustrating goals and objectives in the context of a mission statement.

Financial Review

Whether the SP program is fully supported by the institutional leadership or is solely responsible for generating funding, it is important for the viability of SP programs to document the specific fiscal usage per user group, per individual learner, and the comparative costs over several years. The operations plan may also be a vehicle to demonstrate the cost-saving value of SPs (i.e., how SPs save faculty time doing basic instruction), illustrate the revenue-generating potential of SPs, and also to detail ways in which running an SP program can become more cost-effective. These ways may include consolidating efforts among SP educators and other medical education experts, sharing resources, improving technology, and maximizing workflow, to name a few.

Tracking resources and maintaining detailed records of time spent on various tasks and courses can be downright tedious. Taking the time to incorporate recordkeeping spreadsheets into a business plan initially, then updating quarterly, will make this task much more painless. Appendices 12.D and 12.E provide sample methods of tracking SP usage and student contact hours, respectively; Appendix 12.F provides a sample budget report.

Performance Matrix (Quality and Control): "How Do You Know You're Getting There?"

To illustrate how objectives are being accomplished, the operations plan should include subjective data (such as testimonials from faculty and learners that SP experiences are useful) as well as objective, measurable data supporting the effectiveness of the SP program (such as improved patient satisfaction data and higher student test scores). Other measurement instruments include the following:

- Student evaluation forms (to assess student satisfaction; Appendix 12.H)
- SP performance evaluation data
- Faculty and client satisfaction
- SP training evaluations (both SP satisfaction with the training as well as trainer evaluation of SP learning ability)
- Student self-evaluations
- Faculty evaluation of students longitudinally
- Interrater reliability data (between SPs and faculty, and faculty and faculty)
- Intrarater reliability data (SP reviewing their own recordings)
- SP job satisfaction data, which demonstrates low turnover, and high stability and experience of SPs (which translates into less time spent on recruiting and training SPs; Appendix 12.I)

Leadership/Personnel

Faculty and staff profiles are an effective way to illustrate the breadth and credibility of one's program, as well as to balance the business aspects with a human element. Profiles of SPs should not be overlooked. It is important to explain that SPs are highly trained professionals from various fields. Highlighting the talent, education, experience, and intelligence of SPs is an important way to enhance the credibility of one's program.

It also substantiates the need for SPs to be hired through the SP program, rather than simply hiring actors independently.

Facilities and Resources Overview

The facilities and resources overview should list and describe current facilities and capabilities, including case bank, facility size, number of designated examination rooms, support rooms (reception, student orientation, SP dressing rooms, bathrooms, conference, etc.), training rooms, office space, technology (web-based simulation-center software systems), student classrooms, clinical simulators/models, et cetera.

THE BUSINESS PLAN

"Successful implementation of a business plan to generate revenue requires two crucial elements: appropriate financial support and commitment, and the ability to form partnerships with other health care institutions or organizations within the community" (Peteani, 2004). Once the operational plan has been developed, much of the information can be extracted and inserted within the business plan. However, some information will need to be customized for the goal-specific business plan (for example, pitching a new collaboration with leadership at another institution).

Honig and Karlsson (2004) defined a business plan as "a written document that describes the current state and the presupposed future of an organization." A formal statement of a set of business goals, the business plan also prescribes how to reach those goals. The business plan offers a foundation for exploring potential areas for growth or change, and may inspire program leadership and staff to be more creative in their approach to cultivating these opportunities.

A business plan is typically geared toward a specific initiative. Once the intended audience and focus have been identified, the business plan can be quickly adapted as necessary. This may require deleting or inserting certain sections. For example, a plan geared toward external groups such as a board of trustees, a granting foundation, or a private donor should include an overview of the history of SPs—in general and within one's institution—whereas a plan geared toward developing a new source of revenue or internal leadership would not include the overview. The following are just a few examples of target audiences to consider:

- Granting organizations, potential donors, alumni
- Senior administrators who are working on a higher level business plan (e.g., university wide)
- Project manager hired to work with architects or engineers to plan new space or technology implementation for SP program
- Any internal or external party who is interested in partnering with the SP program to develop new programs or curriculum

Structure of the Business Plan

As a rule, all business plans should include, in this order:

1. Title page
2. Table of contents
3. Introduction

4. Executive summary
5. Body of plan
    a. Introduction
    b. Goal statement
    c. SWOT analysis
    d. Financials
    e. Timelines
    f. Leadership and personnel
    g. Marketing analysis and strategies
6. References/bibliography
7. Appendices

Business plans should not exceed 15 to 20 pages in length, excluding appendices. Unlike a comprehensive operations plan used as an ongoing reference for staff, a business plan needs to be succinct enough to ensure that it will be read.

Executive Summary

The executive summary provides a concise overview of the business plan, including a clear statement describing the goals and objectives of the business plan. The summary's purpose is to aid in decision making by summarizing key points, preparing for the upcoming content, and enticing the reader to read the rest of the business plan. It is often called the most important part of the business plan, and if it does not do what it is intended to do, the business plan may be set aside unread.

Although it appears at the beginning of the business plan, it is the last part of the business plan written. It should make a conclusion, make a recommendation(s), and summarize more than one document (Appendix 12.J).

Body of Plan: Introduction
The introduction of the business plan integrates previously developed information from the program description section of the operations plan. The program description highlights the program's current state, whereas the introduction of the business plan is geared toward a specific project(s) linked to a desired state of change.

Body of Plan: Goal Statement(s)
Unlike a mission statement for the program, a goal statement identifies the focus and concept of the more short-term business plan.

Sample goal statement: *To create a revenue-generating course for practicing physicians.*

Objectives
- To fulfill an identified need not available in other venues
- To create work for SPs to maintain skills
- To support the SP trainer's salary
- To create a curriculum that can be reproduced in other programs
- To bring in a revenue goal of $100,000

Body of Plan: SWOT Analysis

A SWOT analysis is a standard business tool, giving readers a quick glance at an organization's strengths, weaknesses, opportunities, and threats. Even if a business plan is geared toward internal staff, a SWOT analysis should still be implemented to highlight staff needs and development opportunities. Data from a SWOT analysis will guide the content within each section of a business plan. For example, if one's goal is to receive funding to upgrade to a new software system from an existing paper-based system (weakness), it would be beneficial to illustrate the potential implementation of additional programs if the proper resources were in place (opportunity). For example, a graph showing the number of hours spent by staff doing menial tasks can effectively convey the potential benefits of a time-saving system. Other topics to be highlighted are staff experience and expertise, as well as the breadth of programs (strengths) and the potential revenue loss incurred by turning down requests for new programs (threat).

The following SWOT analysis illustrates a snapshot of past and current positions, which lay the groundwork for developing strategies to work toward future goals.

Strengths
- High industry recognition
- Experience in operating large and diverse training programs
- Experience in conducting large-scale clinical skills assessments
- Experience in designing assessment programs
- Possess an accumulated wealth of materials, procedures, and practices that enables smooth and efficient operations
- Record of frequent collaboration with other institutions
- Existing infrastructure in place for project

Weaknesses
- Staff fatigue: staff working beyond expected hours while adding additional responsibilities and clients
- Risk of losing of high-quality, well-trained personnel without additional support

Opportunities
- Provide additional funding stream for core budgets, and skills center
- Maintain continued support of the MD curriculum
- Meet the increasing need of students/clients
- Provide collection of data for comparative benchmarks that students must meet
- Provide a state-of-the-art end-of-third-year assessment with a remediation component to all students
- Provide detailed feedback to students/clients using enhanced software

Threats
- Loss of valuable, well-trained personnel due to burnout and to recruitment by other new programs coming online as this type of training and testing becomes more universal
- Lengthy training of new personnel because the program's technically demanding nature puts a strain on resources
- Loss of market share as other institutions and for-profit vendors meet the demand for course

Body of Plan: Financial Reviews—Revenue and Costs

If one's goal is to receive support from investors or institutional administrations, an illustration of potential return on investment is advisable. A request for a technology upgrade, for example, would be facilitated using charts to demonstrate the current time spent on various administrative tasks compared with projected estimates using the desired system.

The proliferation of SPs brings with it a need to outline the many resources and tasks involved to develop and implement an SP session. These include, but are not limited to, identifying learning goals, curriculum design, creating assessment instruments, generating score reports, briefing and debriefing learners, conducting program satisfaction evaluations, and casting and training SPs.

How an individual SP program is funded will determine how readily these data need to be produced. Some SP programs use a chargeback system, generating an invoice for payment after each program. In that case, payors will want to see a detailed cost breakdown. A business plan will guide programs in calculating fair and appropriate service fees. For those fortunate enough to have a substantial SP program budget as part of their home organization, it is still important to maintain these records for forecasting purposes (Appendix 12.G).

Body of Plan: Timelines, Milestones, or Key Stages

Timelines that identify and support project implementation and progress will be important to project investors. This section and depth of information should be based on who will be reviewing the plan, the time span of the project, the amount of money requested, etc. Essentially, it should be considered the "checklist of progress."

The following sample timeline outlining projected program expansion lists very high-level goals and objectives. It is intended to show a concise overview of milestones during a 5-year period. For operational purposes, of course, the tasks would be delineated in much greater detail.

Goal: *12 months—develop a 6-station clinical skills assessment for our graduating students.*

Objectives

- Secure dedicated space
- Outfit existing (borrowed) examination rooms for 6-station examination
- Form faculty committee to develop 6 cases
- Recruit and hire SPs
- Create SP training materials
- Train SPs
- Administer examination
- Deliver score reports to faculty and students

Goal: *18 months—expand to 12-station assessment for our students (150) and 1 visiting class (100).*

Objectives

- Outfit and renovate space with new technology—AV/hardware, software
- Hire additional staff, SPs
- Draft policies and procedures for new space
- Increase case bank; assign faculty committee to develop at least 6 additional cases
- Create SP training materials

■ Train SPs
■ Administer examination
■ Deliver score reports to faculty and students

Goal: *Within 5 years—expand to 12 stations for students (150) plus 2 other schools, and expand case bank.*

Objectives

■ Continue to build case bank (at least 4 additional cases) via faculty committees
■ Continue to build pool of SPs
■ Conduct quality assurance, data analysis to assure reliability and validity of assessment
■ Administer professional development programs for staff and SPs (e.g., train-the-trainer sessions, administer exercises for SPs to improve recall)
■ Increase usage among Graduate Medical Education (GME) and other external groups by publicizing space and program
■ Partner with area institutions, conducting needs assessment (e.g., remediation after examination or preparation for examination)
■ Establish chargeback system for program costs, including curriculum development, space rental, administration, etc.
■ Upgrade hardware and software as necessary

Body of Plan: Marketing Analysis and Strategies

The products of an SP program may not be as tangible (or as ubiquitous) as those sold by a local bookstore or home goods outlet, but SP educators nonetheless have a unique commodity and need to determine the best way to market those services. A marketing analysis and strategy for any new course or program is an essential component of the business plan. When thinking about marketing needs, SP educators must start by asking, "Who is the competition?"

It would be a mistake to surmise that because there is only one SP program in one's institution or region there is no competition. SP educators are often in the position of pitching the concept of SPs to course directors who are either unfamiliar with SPs, or who see the value of SPs but lack the funding or time to build SPs into the curriculum.

In that sense, the SP educator is competing with core funds or scheduling constraints. The viability of the SP program depends on the educator's ability to show why SPs are better than—or are necessary adjuncts to—other teaching tools. If, on the other hand, the SP educator is in direct competition with other area programs, it is crucial to position one's program as superior to others. In either case, advertising and promotion strategies (print media, Internet, and direct mail campaign) need to be established (Appendix 12.K).

Some institutions may have a surplus of faculty buy-in and technological resources (dedicated space, software, and audiovisual capability), but are seeking full-time training staff or SPs. In that case, program directors will want to develop a plan for reaching out to the community to recruit SPs or simply to increase the local visibility of their program. Depending on factors such as the location of one's program, or how long it's been in existence, some SP programs may be competing with other SP programs for experienced SPs. One way to remedy this is to cultivate a pool of less experienced SPs by enhancing the training methodology. SP educators should also consider the retention of good SPs; if one's budget won't allow for pay increases, other perks may include inexpensive promotional giveaways, snacks and meals, or covering travel expenses.

The marketing plan may also cover the benefits of using SPs. Testimonials from faculty and learners are effective; data supporting the effectiveness of the SP program (e.g., improved patient satisfaction data, higher student test scores), are even more so. The Appendices should include scholarly articles showing the cost–benefit ratio of using SPs (Hasele, Anderson, & Szerlip, 1994), the link between poor physician communication skills and malpractice claims (Levinson, Roter, Mullooly, Dull, & Frankel, 1997), or any other timely, relevant topic that will strike a chord within one's institution.

SP educators should be aware of opportunities to synergize marketing efforts with other departments—admissions, marketing, development, continuing medical education, for example. The marketing plan is a good place to describe how the SP program will adapt to current trends or anticipated changes in the field of SP education. The field is growing rapidly. SP educators must stay abreast of changes and embrace opportunities for innovation not only to sustain operations, but also to flourish and have a meaningful impact on the profession.

REFERENCES

Hasele, J. L., Anderson, D. S., & Szerlip, H. M. (1994). Analysis of the costs and benefits of using standardized patients to help teach physical diagnosis. *Academic Medicine, 69*(7), 567–570.

Honig, B., & Karlsson, T. (2004). Institutional forces and the written business plan. *Journal of Management, 30,* 29–48.

King, A. M., Perkowski-Rogers, L. C., & Pohl, H. S. (1994). Planning standardized patient programs: Case development, patient training and costs. *Teaching and Learning in Medicine, 6*(1), 6–14.

Levinson, W., Roter, D. L., Mullooly, J. P., Dull, V. T., & Frankel, R. M. (1997). Physician–patient communication: The relationship with malpractice claims among primary care physicians and surgeons. *Journal of the American Medical Association, 277,* 553–559.

Peteani, L. A. (2004). Enhancing clinical practice and education with high-fidelity human patient simulators. *Nurse Educator, 29*(1), 25–30.

APPENDICES

Appendix 12.A: Use of SPs

We use SPs in a variety of programs that are expanding yearly to serve learners across the medical education continuum: undergraduate, graduate, and continuing medical education. Some of our programs teach new skills, some provide opportunities to practice and refresh skills, and some are tests designed to evaluate learners' performance.

We implement our SP programs in the following formats:

One-on-one: These cases usually teach or test interpersonal, history-taking, physical examination, and diagnostic skills. They take place either in the classroom or in clinical examination rooms. They often require the SP to fill out a checklist after the encounter. These cases may or may not have a physical examination component, and they may or may not require the SP to provide the student with feedback after the encounter.

Small group: This format is used for teaching both interpersonal and physical examination skills. The SP goes into a room of 3 to 12 medical students with 1 to 3 faculty members. These cases require the SP to offer feedback to the students.

Large group: Some cases involve one SP being interviewed or examined by a physician in front of an entire class of medical students (~150 students).

Appendix 12.B: Educational Mission Statement

The mission of the SP program is to deliver high-quality SP programming to train and test learners at various stages in their medical education.

GOAL: Using a creative and collaborative approach to program development, the SP program fosters a partnership with faculty and learners to integrate innovative humanistic training with traditional science-based medical education.

Objectives

- Offers learners a safe, controlled environment where they can develop and refine their own unique approach to patient care with honest and nonjudgmental feedback from a diverse group of SPs.
- Administers reliable, valid examinations using conscientiously trained SPs and rigorous quality assurance to grade learners on their progress and prepares them for licensing exams.
- Aims to cultivate our resources, develop our programming, and keep our institution at the forefront of the rapidly growing field of clinical skills education.

Appendix 12.C: Business Mission

The external business mission is to develop service-oriented, revenue-producing programs for external clients. This endeavor leverages current and proposed infrastructure while contributing to the primary mission. Supplying services to external clients can enhance the primary mission in a number of ways. It can serve as an external source of funds, ensure a stable long-term workforce that would guarantee the highest professional standards for SPs, and facilitate the promotion of the university in the local business community.

Business Objectives

- To contribute to the overall mission of the university by providing resources to a variety of organizations with the potential for promoting health care in our region and nation.
- To provide high-quality services for external business that promotes positive relationships for the university and generates revenue for program expansion.

Appendix 12.D: SP Usage

Hours of Standardized Patient Usage UME FY99–02 for Operations Plan

Year and Course	FY99	FY00	FY01	FY02
M1 Clinical Medicine	1,152	1,179	1,689	1,954
M2 Clinical Medicine	568	846	795	1,019
M3 Family Medicine Clerkship	504	784	471	962
M3 Internal Medicine Clerkship	442	570	601	700
M3 Surgery Clerkship	309	372	365	383
M3 OB/GYN Clerkship	160	160	168	200
M4 Clinical Skills Assessment	571	646	869	865
Demonstrations	118	140	139	90
Total UME hours	3,824	4,697	5,097	6,173

(continued)

Appendix 12.D (continued)

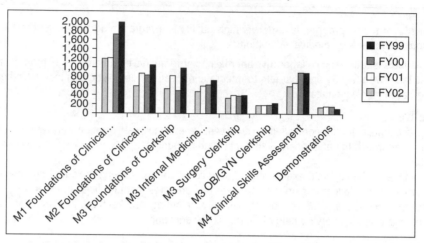

Appendix 12.E: Student Contact Hours

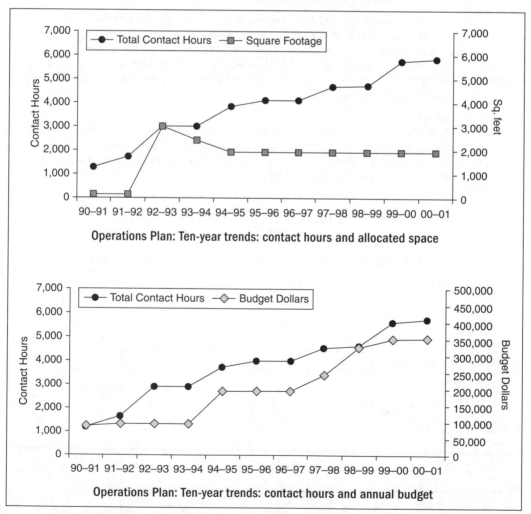

Operations Plan: Ten-year trends: contact hours and allocated space

Operations Plan: Ten-year trends: contact hours and annual budget

Appendix 12.F: Budget Report

Budget Reporting for Operations Plan

FY00	Operating Budget	Actual Expenditures
Staff salaries and wages	$131,152.00	$155,001.00
Standardized patients	$66,969.00	$100,130.00
Fringe benefits	$30,728.00	$39,571.00
Supplies	$8,400.00	$8,400.00
Contractual	$12,760.00	$13,560.00
General expenses	$8,594.00	$8,594.00
Rent	$58,836.00	$58,836.00
Equipment	$7,000.00	$9,000.00
Total	$324,439.00	$393,092.00

3-Year Projected Expenditures for Operations Plan

	1 year	2 years	3 years
Staff salaries and wages	$166,651.00	$174,441.00	$174,441.00
Standardized patients	$100,130.00	$100,130.00	$100,130.00
Fringe benefits	$40,292.00	$41,035.00	$41,800.00
Supplies	$8,400.00	$8,400.00	$8,400.00
Contractual	$18,760.00	$22,760.00	$32,000.00
General expenses	$8,594.00	$8,594.00	$8,594.00
Rent	$58,836.00	$58,836.00	$58,836.00
Equipment	$15,000.00	$9,000.00	$17,000.00
Total	$416,663.00	$423,196.00	$441,201.00

Appendix 12.G: Project-Specific Budget

Sample Proposed New Workshop for Business Plan: Project-Specific Budget

New Workshop Proposed		
Revenue per workshop	$ Per Workshop	$ Annual
Number of workshops	1	12
Participants per workshop	16	192
Price per person	$800.00	$800.00
Total revenue	$12,800.00	$153,600.00
Expense per workshop		
Standardized patients	$2,540.00	$30,480.00
Personnel and administration	$3,158.00	$37,896.00
Supplies	$1,440.00	$17,280.00
Ongoing expenses—technology support	$955.00	$11,460.00
Total expenses	$8,093.00	$97,116.00
Excess/(deficit)	$4,707.00	$56,484.00
Margin (%)	36.77%	36.77%

Appendix 12.H: Student Satisfaction Data

N	Mean	Questions	
120	3.63	1. The portrayal by the SP portraying a cancer patient was convincing.	1 = Strongly Disagree
120	3.71	2. The portrayal by the SP portraying an HIV patient was convincing.	2= Disagree
120	3.38	3. The feedback from the cancer SP was valuable.	3= Agree
120	3.40	4. The feedback from the HIV SP was valuable.	4= Strongly Agree
120	3.53	5. The objectives of the SP interview were clear.	
120	3.46	6. The cases were appropriate for my level of training.	
120	3.48	7. This session will help me be more comfortable and/or skillful in breaking bad news to a patient.	

8. What did you like most about this experience? *

* "SPs give great feedback. It's excellent to practice breaking news to SPs rather than an actual patient."
* "Great to practice this and see how to deal with these issues before we need to do this in the hospital."

* "Actually going through an experience like this is much better than just reading or talking about it. I thought I knew what I was going to say, but it was much harder actually getting thoughts and words out."
* "Very realistic portrayals. It was very uncomfortable, but this was not necessarily a bad thing, as these interactions will always be difficult."

Appendix 12.I: SP Job Satisfaction Data

SP JOB SATISFACTION SURVEY RESULTS—60 respondents

Answer Key:

   5 = *Strongly agree*
   4 = *Agree*
   3 = *Neutral*
   2 = *Disagree*
   1 = *Strongly disagree*

1. I enjoy coming to work. 4.30
2. The institution uses my time and talents well. 4.20
3. Staff members treat me with respect. 4.37
4. I am recognized for my efforts. 4.03
5. The training prepares me well to perform in the programs. 4.62
6. Training instructions are consistent among trainers. 3.88
7. I receive feedback on how I am performing on the job. 3.80
8. I am held to the same standards of performance as my peers. 4.20
9. I am encouraged to communicate questions or concerns about my job. 4.12
10. I get prompt answers to my questions. 4.33
11. I am paid fairly for the work that I do. 3.67
12. I am satisfied with the amount of work for which I am scheduled. 3.45
13. I have a safe workplace. 4.62
14. The locations of the training sessions and programs are convenient. 4.03
15. Snacks/refreshments are adequate. 3.62
16. Management shares information about the organization. 3.48
17. Information from staff about organization policies and procedures (e.g., scheduling, payroll, and other job protocols not related to training or performance) is clear and consistent. 3.90
18. I understand the impact of my role in the organization as a whole. 4.05
19. I feel that my work contributes to the greater good of the community. 4.38

Appendix 12.J: Executive Summary (Goal: to increase space)

This document provides decision makers with an accurate picture of the current status of the SP program. Among other issues, this document addresses the critical shortage of space available in the Clinical Medical Education Building. Although present curricular demands are being met, this aging facility, for which the university does not hold a lease, is exceeding maximum capacity to deliver these vital services.

Currently, the program is being asked to expand its role in the curriculum. This request is a natural extension into the third year, allowing the university to better prepare students for the implementation of the USMLE step 2 CS, SP Exam. The latest information regarding implementation of this examination calls for live testing in 2004, with the requirement that the graduating class of 2005 complete the examination as part of the licensure sequence. It is also probable the examination will be a prerequisite for step 3. The increased teaching and assessment demand exceeds the capabilities of the existing facility.

In addition, the mandates of the Accreditation Council for Graduate Medical Education for a competency-based core curriculum will begin to affect the institution's graduate medical education community in the near future. The most recent timeline suggests that programs will be held responsible for these new competency-based requirements in July 2002. Academic institutions must begin planning and/or piloting integration of the core competencies and implement new and/or improved assessment tools now to be ready for these changes.

We have the expertise, experience, and human capital to benefit from these trends. The personnel, systems, and procedures are in place for continued growth, which is necessary if the SP program is to keep up with nationwide academic trends and requirements. However, it is impossible to deliver expanded programs under the current physical conditions.

The university was an early leader in the use of SPs for medical education, a process that is now endorsed and expanding. Our position of leadership and capability is now in jeopardy. Now is the time to take advantage of the developed expertise, steep learning curve, and the growing market demand for the benefit of the School of Medicine, the university, and the community at large.

Appendix 12.K: Marketing Strategies

The initial success of the course will depend on the marketing of this program. Although the program is currently unique in its venture, the immersion into the market will need support from several venues. We can depend on our reputation as having quality programs to entice participants. Active marketing and advertising is essential to inform the medical education community of the program and its mission. A mechanism to advertise to individual students is essential to attract the external clients. The quality of the program and the innovative approach to refining skills will enhance our reputation and its positive value will be spread by word of mouth.

The proposed marketing strategies for the course include but are not limited to:

- Web site with URL address advertising the course
- Professionally designed web site by a webmaster who specializes in medical web pages
- Brochures designed for the course to be distributed
- Telephone or e-mail request
- Student Affairs offices
- Assistance from Deans of Education and Student Affairs
- Letters of introduction to counterparts at select institutions
- Notification to potential partners

CHAPTER 13

Human Simulation Mini Cases for
Undergraduate Nursing

Mary Gallagher Gordon

*T*he use of simulation in the undergraduate nursing program has proven to be an asset to nursing students. The process of thinking in action is easier said than done. Thus, when the concept of recording and grading is added to the curriculum, students tend to get unnerved. However, after the students experience simulation as a part of the coursework, they often have a common reaction: that was not as bad as I thought it was going to be.

HISTORY OF THE MINI CASE USE IN AN UNDERGRADUATE PROGRAM

In the winter of 2005, the first class of co-op students was entering their senior year. At this time, the vision of introducing simulation into the traditional co-op senior nursing curriculum could finally be implemented. In the course, the students participated in a cumulative review of all the previously learned clinical content from the beginning of the curriculum through lectures, National Council Licensure Examination for Registered Nurses (NCLEX)-style questions, and case studies. The intent of weaving simulation into this review course was to create a means of evaluating the students' clinical skills and their ability to integrate theory knowledge into caring for patients in the clinical setting.

MINI CASE

The simulation faculty along with the didactic faculty needed to review how simulation would advance the course objectives. Important in the development of the simulation experience are the outcomes important for the learner to take away after the experience. At Drexel, the undergraduate simulation faculty member is the case developer for the student experience. The cases are developed based on core content from the curriculum to simulate a realistic situation that a new graduate nurse may encounter. The faculty initially completes a needs assessment of the students and then develops learning objectives for the simulation session. Ideally, there should be a clinical, patient safety as well as a behavioral objectives core to the case. Currently, there are approximately 20 adult content areas that the faculty can pull from to develop a case. This case content list is shared with the students' who are encouraged to use this list while they practice and prepare for the simulation experience. No new content is integrated into the simulation—its purpose is for practical, hands on, thinking in action review. The simulation content list was formulated by looking at the core material taught in the curriculum. The cases chosen also aim to evaluate the students' ability to integrate skills that are taught in the curriculum in a simulated clinical environment. Allowing the students to enter the patient room for the simulation experience gives the students the opportunity to act on the clinical skills, knowledge, and hone their communication skills without the risk of "patient" harm.

For example, four mini case options drawn from skills the students develop while in the undergraduate nursing program include: (1) a focused health history, (2) focused physical assessment, (3) patient education, or (4) an ethical dilemma. These mini cases are independent of each other during the simulated experience.

Currently, the simulation format is structured as a 1-hour simulation session. Each student will have the opportunity to be involved in two cases during their simulation experience: (1) a history or a physical assessment, and (2) a patient education or ethical case. The students will not know what case they are assigned until they enter into the simulation waiting area immediately before the encounter.

By utilizing the "gold standard" fundamental textbook that the students use as they advance through the program, the faculty can develop a clear and accurate physical assessment, patient education, or health history case. The ethical case is developed using the 21 clinical content areas and then consulting current literature to determine the common ethical dilemmas facing practicing nurses. Recall that as the cases are being developed, the students are not tested on new knowledge, but on content that has been the foundation for the undergraduate program. Traditionally, although nursing students are generally well-prepared in theory, there are still gaps in the transition into the clinical area and the ability of the students to think on their feet. This area in which students commonly struggle is known as clinical decision-making.

Overall, case development must include key points. These key points include the *type* and *content* of case to be developed; the *name* of the client, particularly a name that can be used for either an actor or an actress; a specific *setting* for the experience, such as the medical surgical patient room or an outpatient clinic; the *scenario*, or the story line which is the problem that brought the client to the room (this portion will be longer and more detailed to assist the actor with training and preparing for the case). The *door sign* is a synopsis of the scenario. The door sign should be approximately three or four sentences and posted on the door so the student can read it before entering the room. It gives the student a clear and concise summary of the simulation so that they may begin preparing for the experience before entering the simulation room. The students tend to have approximately three to five minutes to stand at the door, use their resources in their mobile device, and plan out their session. The *opening line* is an introduction to the case when the student enters the room. This is the introduction the actor will use when the student begins the dialogue and is not visible to the students.

In addition to those requirements listed above, there may be *challenge questions* that are developed to test the student's ability to think on their feet. These are questions the actor can ask the student at the appropriate point in the simulation and should be based on specific case content, the patient's situation, and the common experiences in the field. For example, during the simulation, the patient may ask the student, "Why do I continue to get this chest pain if I take the nitroglycerin as I was told to?"

Training questions are developed to attempt to standardize the experience for all of the students. Training questions are an area that will improve each time training sessions occur between the actor and the faculty. If the faculty member is training an actor for full days of student encounters, there should be required blocks of time to allow for a standardized training to occur before the student encounters. This extended time frame will allow faculty to review the content specific to each of the mini cases. Actors tend to ask excellent questions about the mini cases that allow the faculty member to improve and standardize the case. For example, a training question would state, "The father is deceased." The actor may then want additional information, like the father's age, cause of death, and how this family history correlates to the experience. The training questions are developed in relation to the type of simulation experience, such as a focused physical assessment, but also include other possible questions that the student may ask during the experience. An example may be with a focused physical assessment patient experience, in which the student may want to get a bit of history before beginning their physical assessment. Therefore, to standardize the experience, when developing a case, the faculty member will want to think of the multiple angles that the student may explore and communicate these to the actor.

While completing the actor training, if there are specific *skills* that the students are expected to demonstrate, the actors will be educated on the specifics of the skill. If there is equipment that will be used for the case, this must be communicated to the staff responsible for preparing the laboratory for the sessions. The actors should have the time to practice using the equipment and understand how it relates to the experience.

The *summary* section following the training questions is where information on how the actor should be positioned and dressed is discussed. If there are any additional items that will be necessary for the room, they are also included in this section. Once the case has been developed, the faculty member will want to have it reviewed by peers who are proficient in the content for reviews all of the cases.

Student grading for the mini cases depends on the experience content. For example, in a health history case, communication and patient safety will be the primary grading components. Specifically:

> Did the student introduce his or herself?
> Did the student validate the name and date of birth verbally, as well as check the ID band?
> Did they ask about allergies?
> Did the student ask about alleviating factors?
> Did the student ask about family history?

For the focused physical assessment case, the student's ability to complete an assessment, use therapeutic communication, as well as identify patient safety criteria, are core components. For example:

> Did the student offer assistance when asking the patient to change positions?
> Did the student check pulses bilaterally in upper extremities?
> Did the student check capillary refill in both lower extremities?

Patient safety is integrated into the development of the cases and should be included in the simulation. The types of patient safety elements used are dependent on the particular case scenario. For example, all cases should have criteria that have the student identify the client by name and date of birth. The student should also be required to ask about allergies. Other patient safety criteria can be built into the case as each specific simulation allows.

The faculty member, using the course objectives as well as learning outcomes, develops the *grading* criteria for the cases. On the basis of whether the experience is formative or summative, the faculty member will need to decide on the best way to grade the experience. If this is a summative experience, a "passing" grade for the experience must be defined. One option for the grading criteria may be that the student either completed the item on the checklist, or did not complete the item. Then, based on the number of items in the mini case, the passing grade can be established. If the outcome is focused on looking at how well the student completed each of the criteria, there may be additional options that should be included, such as: completed correctly, completed but missed steps, did not complete, or did not complete successfully. This process would require the faculty member to weigh the items accordingly. The faculty member may also decide that some criteria are particularly critical, such as patient identifiers, that if the student misses any of these criteria, the system will flag them as failing the experience.

Students are given detailed information regarding the simulation experience in the course syllabus on day one of the term. In addition, the simulation faculty member attends a portion of a class in the weeks before the student simulation encounter to give an overview of the standardized patient experience and answer any specific questions the students may have. Over the years, students have offered suggestions to improve the preparation for the experience, and many of these students' suggestions have been implemented in the simulation experience. One former student requested to hear from students who had completed the simulation experience to garner advice about the sessions. Thus, an available graduate will attend class and spend time with the seniors discussing the standardized patient experience, as well as answer general questions the students may have. A class of graduating seniors had their suggestions videotaped so that future students could hear the voice of students who have completed the experience. Another class developed a "Pearls of the SPL experience" and has given permission to share this project with future classes. These "pearls" are statements the students made in their self-reflections that offered good insight to future students.

When developing the cases, the faculty will need to keep in mind what reference and papers the students will be allowed to bring into the experience with them. Drexel nursing students have a program-issued mobile device loaded with their core reference books. These references include a drug guide, a nursing procedure manual, a dictionary, disease guide, and a health assessment guide. The students are encouraged to use these resources as needed during the experience. The students are also allowed to bring in one large index card that has been prepared before they enter the simulation area. This index card can have whatever information the student feels will be important to them during the experience. However, students may not have an index card for each of the content areas and then pull out the one that pertains to the course after they read the sign on the door. In years past, the students could bring in as many papers as they wanted, but the shuffling of all the papers was found to be very distracting to the actors, as well as waste student encounter time, and has been discontinued.

The experience allows the student the ability to think on their feet, use the tools provided to them, and gain important experience that mirrors the clinical practice. The students would attend a 1-hour mini case simulation session during the midterm week of the term. This 1 hour was broken down to allow for two 15-minute cases, time to allow the actors to complete the checklist criteria that are specific to the case, debriefing time with the student and the actor or actress after the session, and then time to prepare for the next case. After the debriefing in the second session, the students are excused for the day. At the end of the day, the video of the experience is available for the student to review. They are required to sit, view their video, and answer questions to allow for self-reflection. Any student who was not successful in the experience is required to remediate with the nursing laboratory educational staff to prepare for the second and final experience. There is then an additional time when the student will again complete their encounter. This second attempt will require that the faculty develop 2 new mini cases, as well as additional training time with the actors.

Students have commented that the experience has made them a better nurse, given them the opportunity to use their therapeutic communication skills, allowed them to self-reflect via the video review, and reinforced that they have the ability to think in action.

SAMPLE MINI CASES

NAME: Kelly/Kelli M.

SETTING: Outpatient office

SCENARIO: Kelly/Kelli M. has not been feeling well for the past few hours with some fatigue, severe sunburn, and a bit of a headache. The sunburn pain and headache was progressively getting worse so the patient went to the local shore outpatient clinic.

DOOR SIGN: Kelly/Kelli M. has not been feeling well for the past few hours, with some fatigue, severe sunburn, and a headache. The sunburn pain was progressively getting worse so the patient went to local shore outpatient clinic. Your assignment is to do a complete history. You have 15 minutes for the encounter.

OPENING LINE: I just feel terrible. My head hurts and this sunburn is horrible!

TRAINING QUESTIONS

What is your date of birth or your age? Use your own

Are you married? Use your own

Occupation? Works at Drexel.

When did the sunburn pain start? Around 4 hours ago.

When did the severe headache start? Late this morning.

Does anything make it better/worse? No, I don't think so.

Have you had any fever or chills? Yes, I did have chills.

Have you had any sensitivity to light (photophobia)? No.

Have you had any feeling of disorientation? No.

Have you ever had anything similar in the past? No.

Did you use sunscreen today? Yes, I had some left over from last year; it is an SPF 5, I think.

Were you sitting in the sun all day today? Yes, it was so hot; I was sitting at the water's edge.

Did you reapply the sunscreen today? No, I did a really good job this morning.

Did you drink any water today? No, I was drinking diet soda this morning.

Do you have any stressors or are you experiencing any stress? Yes, the sunburn and this headache are really stressing me out.

Have you ever used any recreational drugs? No.

Have you ever been hospitalized? Use your own

Have you ever had surgery? Use your own

Have you ever been pregnant? Use your own, if applicable

Do you have any chronic illnesses? No.

Are you taking any medications? No.

How is your father? Use your own

How is your mother? Use your own

How is/are your sibling(s)? Healthy if you have siblings—can use your own

Past health history (none)

Neurological (none)

> Integumentary (many previous sunburns as a child)
> Cardiovascular (none)
> Respiratory (none)
> Gastrointestinal (none)
> Genitourinary (none)
> Gynecological (none)
> Obstetrical (use your own if applicable)

Diet—I eat anything I want.

MEDICATIONS

> Prescription medications (none)
> Over the counter medications (none or your own)
> Medication allergies—none
> Seasonal allergies—use your own

PSYCHOSOCIAL HISTORY

> Smoking history none
> Alcohol history (social, one or two drinks a week if I have a party)
> Recreational drug history (none)
> Sexual history (use your own)
> Stress history

You should be in your clothes, sitting on the edge of the table. You will have a moulage on your nose, shoulders, ears, and forehead to represent bubbling sunburn.

STUDENT GRADING

Communication

1. Introduces self (name and title)
2. Identified you using ID band as well as date of birth
3. Asked About Allergies
4. Good eye contact (50% or greater of the time)
5. Spoke clearly in terms the patient can understand
6. Active listener
7. Asked about your medical history
8. Asked about your family's medical history
9. Asked about previous hospitalizations
10. Asked about current medications I am taking
11. Asked about sunscreen history
12. Asked about sun safety guideline knowledge
13. Asked about reapplication of sunscreen

10. Asked about what you did after coming out of the sun
11. Asked about hydration
12. Asked about previous activities for the day
13. Performed a pain assessment
14. Asked about the onset of the headache and sunburn
15. Asked you to rate your headache and sunburn pain on pain scale (0–10)
16. Asked about nausea
17. Created an atmosphere that put the patient at ease (Ignatavicius, 2010)

FOCUSED PHYSICAL ASSESSMENT

NAME: Jo/Joe J.

SETTING: Medical Surgical Unit (Inpatient Hospital Room)

SCENARIO: Patient came into the emergency room complaining of problems with breathing since last night. The patient was placed on oxygen via a nasal cannula, received a dose of IVP Lasix, had a 12-lead EKG, and was sent up from the ER to the floor with a diagnosis of congestive heart failure (CHF).

INSTRUCTIONS/DOOR SIGN: Complete a focused assessment/cardiac assessment on this patient. You have 15 minutes to complete the encounter.

OPENING LINE: This is a (use your own age) patient who has been admitted to the Medical Surgical Unit (an inpatient room) from the Emergency Department with a diagnosis of CHF.

PATIENT BACKGROUND INFORMATION:

(Student is NOT required to do a history for this experience—but provide this information as an answer to any questions that may be posed during the physical examination)

Use your own age.

The shortness of breath started last night and you feel better when you are sitting up and worse when you expend energy or lie flat.

You had this problem 1 week ago and came to the ER then. You were admitted and told you had CHF. You have no significant PMH prior to last week. You have had no surgery or previous hospitalizations. You were not on any medications prior to last week.

You do not use any recreational medications, but do smoke off and on (if asked, since you were in high school, and three packs a week). You are only a social drinker, around one glass or one beer a week or every 2 weeks.

The current medication you are on is a "water pill" called Lasix. "They started me on it when I was in the ER last week. I am supposed to take it every day. I hate taking the medication because it makes me run to the bathroom too often."

Your parents died of natural causes, and your siblings are all healthy.

You should be in a hospital gown, bras and underwear OK, sitting on the edge of the table. You will be on oxygen at 2 L via nasal cannula, but the nasal cannula will be around your neck, not in the proper position.

STUDENT GRADING

1. Introduced self
2. Checked name, DOB, allergies, and verified name band
3. Washed hands before examination
4. Used terms that were appropriate for me
5. Explained to me what she/he was doing with each step of exam
6. Established eye contact
7. Helped to position me
8. Was professional in manner
9. Maintained modesty during exam

10. Blood pressure sitting or laying correctly
11. Counted my pulse and respiratory rate
12. Palpated my point of maximum impulse
13. Listened to my heart in at least four places
14. Listened to my lungs in at least eight places
15. Checked O_2 for correct amount and repositioned nasal cannula for correct administration of oxygen
16. Examined bilateral lower extremities for edema (no swelling)
17. Palpated bilateral lower extremity pulses
18. Observed the right sternocleidomastoid area for neck vein distention
19. Auscultated carotid artery (Potter and Perry, 2008)

■ **SP will also provide feedback**

PATIENT TEACHING CASE

SETTING: Inpatient Hospital Room

SCENARIO: The patient came to the emergency room with a complaint of difficulty catching their breath and was given a diagnosis of reactive airway disease. Patient is going to be discharged today and you will need to review discharge teaching.

INSTRUCTIONS/DOOR SIGN: The patient came to the emergency room with visible complaints of respiratory distress and was given a diagnosis of reactive airway disease. Patient is going to be discharged today and you will need to review discharge teaching. You have 15 minutes to complete appropriate patient teaching.

OPENING LINE: This is a (use your own age) patient who has been admitted to the Medical Surgical Unit (an inpatient room) from the emergency department.

CHALLENGE QUESTIONS:
Can you tell me what reactive airway disease is?
Discuss with the actors this disease

TRAINING QUESTIONS:

1. Discussed the importance of good asthma control by teaching you about what an asthma attack is.

2. Discussed the importance of medication administration, differences between types of asthma medications such as rescue and daily medications.

3. Discussed care of an inhaler. The actor will not know how to use an inhaler or the care of an inhaler.

4. Discussed the importance of identifying triggers. The actor will have a trigger of perfume, smoking, and exercise.

5. Discussed the asthma symptoms that require emergency interventions.

6. Discussed the importance of infection prevention. Explain this to the actors.

STUDENT GRADING

1. Introduces self (name and title)
2. Identified you using ID band as well as date of birth
3. Asked about any allergies
4. Used terms that were appropriate for me
5. Good eye contact
6. Active listener
7. Created an atmosphere that put the patient at ease
8. Asked you about your knowledge of asthma
9. Discussed the importance of identifying triggers

10. Discussed the importance of medication administration
11. Discussed the importance of quick relief or rescue medications
12. Discussed the asthma symptoms that require emergency interventions
13. Discussed the importance of early recognition of infection (Lewis, Heitkemper, & Dirksen, 2004)

ETHICAL DILEMMA

NAME: Jack/Jackie M.

PERSON IN ROOM: Mother or father of patient

SCENARIO: Your daughter was in a cheerleading accident and has been in the intensive care unit for a week. Earlier today, the physician told you the daughter is "brain-dead" and wants you to consider donating her organs. You are still confused after having been given information from the professionals regarding your daughter condition when she still has a heartbeat.

DOOR SIGN: The patient's father or mother is in the room, waiting to speak to the nurse. The parents were informed that their child is brain-dead. The parents were asked if they wanted to donate their daughter's organs. Please speak to the patient's family member in this private waiting room. You have 15 minutes to complete the encounter.

OPENING LINE: "Thank you for coming."
  My daughter was in a cheerleading accident. Today the physician told me my daughter is brain-dead. The doctor also said I should consider donating her organs. A representative from the organ donation site spoke to me, but I am still confused. I do not understand how my daughter can be dead when she still has a pulse. This is horrible!" (upset/anxious)
  Patient can be in regular clothes, sitting on the chair in the room.

TRAINING QUESTIONS:

Discuss with the actors what brain death means? It means the brain is injured or not working.

When asked if the actor understand the process of organ donation, state, No. Discuss this concept with the actors, so they do understand the topic if the student educates them.

If asked about their daughter being an organ donor and if it is stated on her license, the actor will say, No.

If asked if you would like to speak with any of the following offered by the student: a doctor, the organ donation representative, your family, a clergy or counselor.

CHALLENGE QUESTION: "Are you sure my daughter is brain-dead? I need to be absolutely sure."

STUDENT GRADING

1. Introduced self
2. Good eye contact
3. Spoke clearly in terms the patient can understand
4. Did the student allow you to speak without interruption after asking you a question?
5. Did the student tell you about organ donation in an informative way?
6. Did the student basically explain the process of organ donation?
7. Did the student try to find out what you know or your perceptions of brain death?
8. Did the student explain what brain death means?
9. Did the student acknowledge your emotions?
10. Was the student supportive?
11. Was the student an attentive listener?
12. Did the student exhibit comforting body language?
13. Did the student create an atmosphere that you put at ease?
14. Did the student use silence appropriately?
15. Did the student determine what your support systems are?
16. Did the student suggest speaking to your other family members or suggest a family meeting?

17. Did the student offer to call the physician for you to speak to him again?
18. Did the student offer to call someone else beside the physician or a family member for your support? (clergy, social worker, etc.)

The SP will also provide feedback after the encounter. This feedback only relates to therapeutic communication and the therapeutic relationship. How did the student nurse make the SP feel as a patient? Private waiting room on a medical surgical unit.

In summary, as a faculty member integrating simulation into your program, you will want to complete a needs assessment of the students, determine outcomes for the course and program, write and refine a case, reserve a date for the training of the actors, as well as a date for the experience, and if necessary, a date for an additional experience for those students who may be ill or unsuccessful during the first experiences, share critical information with the students in a timely manner to allow for them to review before the experience, train the actors, and review critical elements with the simulation staff the week before the experience.

On the day of the experience, be sure you review your final checklist of the supplies for each room. You should have a copy of the correct door signs, a hard copy of the experience grading checklist, the student assignment list that says when and where each student is scheduled, and the sign-in sheet, which will help you make sure to cover the key components of the simulation.

REFERENCES

Ignatavicius, D. D., & Workman, M. L. (2010). *Medical-surgical nursing: Patient-centered collaborative care* (6th ed.). St. Louis, MO: Elsevier.

Lewis, S. M., Heitkemper, M. M., & Dirksen, S. R. (2004). *Medical surgical nursing: Assessment and management of clinical problems* (6th ed.). St. Louis, MO: Mosby.

Potter, P., & Perry, A. (2008). *Fundamentals of nursing* (7th ed.). St. Louis, MO: Mosby.

CHAPTER 14

Human Simulation Comprehensive Cases for Undergraduate Nursing

Linda Wilson and Mary Ellen Smith Glasgow

Dr. Howard Barrows, a neurologist, raised eyebrows in medical education in 1963 by using an artist-trained model in his class to depict a paralyzed patient with multiple sclerosis. His innovative idea was not viewed as an academic innovation by his physician colleagues, but rather as a scandalous teaching modality. In fact, Dr. Barrows was told that he was maligning the dignity of medical education by using such actors. Although an esteemed neurologist, he was asked to speak on neurological subjects but requested to not discuss simulated patients (University of Kentucky College of Medicine, 2008; Wallace, 1997). In an effort to legitimize his work, Dr. Burrows responded personally to each dean or associate dean that criticized his use of simulated patients. In 1964, he published a paper with his colleague on the topic, "The programmed patient: A technique for appraising student performance in clinical neurology" (Barrows & Abrahamson, 1964). Dr. Barrows is to be commended for his creativity and tenacity in the face of a cold reception from his medical colleagues, thereby allowing his innovation to grow and thrive.

It is remarkable to think that today, this type of simulation, known as an objective structured clinical examination or SP experience, has been embraced by academic medicine and become an important tool for teaching and evaluation for medical students, as well as a requirement for medical school graduation and licensure (Wallace, 1997; Wartman, 2006).

However, despite the fact that medical schools have used standardized patients (SPs) to facilitate learning and evaluation for many years, nursing education has been a slow adopter of this innovative teaching tool, particularly in undergraduate nursing programs. Although graduate nursing programs have used SP experiences to evaluate nurse practitioner students' history-taking and physical examination skills for the last 11 years, the literature is limited with descriptions of the use of SP experiences in undergraduate nursing programs (Rentschler, Eaton, Cappiello, McNally, & McWilliam, 2007).

Nonetheless, the benefits of SP experiences, which provide an opportunity for students to be evaluated on their interpersonal and interview skills, problem-solving abilities, assessment skills, patient teaching, and clinical decision making, are detailed in the literature (Redfern, Norman, Calman, Watson, & Murella, 2002). So why have undergraduate nursing faculty been reticent to adopt this innovative teaching methodology? Perhaps the cost and resources involved in such an endeavor were barriers. Also, some faculty may not have been able to see beyond using the SP within the medical model.

In this chapter we will discuss how a human simulation using SPs was incorporated in a large undergraduate nursing program and how it evolved in 10 short years.

THE ORIGINS OF HUMAN SIMULATION WITH SP AT DREXEL UNIVERSITY

In 1999, Drexel University began to develop a five-year BSN cooperative program (BSN Co-op Program). Drexel, a noted leader in technology and innovation, would be the second cooperative nursing program in the country. At the time, Dr. Mary Ellen Smith Glasgow saw the value of the SP experience in graduate nursing and medical education and decided to have several SP experience requirements in the BSN Co-op Program. Realizing that the competencies for the BSN graduate are unique, Dr. Smith Glasgow developed SP cases to evaluate the competencies specific to the BSN graduate. These cases did not involve differential diagnosis. Rather, they involved competencies such as history-taking, data interpretation, physical examination skills, procedure skills, therapeutic communication, and dealing with difficult subjects, including domestic violence or substance abuse. The cases often incorporated ethical dilemmas as novice nurses need knowledge and skills to effectively deal with complex issues.

From the beginning, nursing faculty were emphatic that the program was not educating undergraduate students to become advanced practice nurses, but rather educating professional nurses to have expert health assessment and superior communication skills to ensure that they provided quality, highly skilled nursing care. At that time as well, the undergraduate nursing SP experience took place in the university's medical school simulation lab, with the nursing program paying a fee to use the lab space, hire patient actors, and utilize the medical school's administrative staff. The most challenging aspect of this arrangement was changing the mindset of the actors and administrative staff to recognize the competencies of the undergraduate nursing student and how they differed from those of a medical student.

In 2002, Drexel University's Accelerated BSN Program had its first SP experience as a 45-minute summative end-of-program experience, which included history-taking skills, physical examination skills, and patient teaching. Mini-SP experiences were incorporated into the BSN Co-op Program along with the comprehensive SP experience for the summative end of program experience. The mini-SP experiences in the BSN Co-op Program included a focused exam on one system, dealing with an ethical dilemma, history-taking, and patient teaching (see chapter 13). Since its inception, the SP experience program has evolved and is now included in multiple courses, formats, and disciplines. Drexel University is now planning to incorporate SP experiences in its undergraduate leadership course to enhance conflict resolution, delegation, collaboration, and change of shift report or hand off communication.

The evidence to date suggests that the SP experiences have taken root at Drexel University and are an integral part of its undergraduate nursing education. Faculty can construct their own learning environments, students can make a mistake in a controlled safe surrounding, faculty can view the entire patient–student interaction digitally, and, lastly, the patient can give feedback to the student. The innovation continues as faculty members construct new learning situations for students to teach and evaluate clinical competence. In summary, the early development of the SP experiences was not always smooth. The nursing faculty innovators did not always receive a warm reception from their colleagues about their ideas related to simulation in undergraduate education. Like Dr. Barrows, however, they were tenacious and trusted that this disruptive innovation could improve student learning and ultimately patient care.

Simulation Cases

The comprehensive simulation cases are labeled by diagnosis name or the primary focus of the case. Some of the Drexel University undergraduate nursing program cases include the following: angina, congestive heart failure, chronic obstructive pulmonary disease, diabetes, headache, hypertension, meningitis, pancreatitis, peptic ulcer disease, stroke, and vascular disease. A few brief examples of these case scenarios follow.

HYPERTENSION

NAME: Pat V.

SETTING: Medical Surgical Unit (Inpatient Hospital Room)

SCENARIO: The patient has a 2-day complaint of severe headache. On arrival to the emergency room (ER), the patient was diagnosed with severe hypertension. The patient's initial blood pressure in the emergency department was 200/120. (BACKGROUND) The patient had been to the emergency department about 6 months ago with a similar complaint and was diagnosed with hypertension at that time. The patient was given a prescription for a hypertension medication, Lopressor. The patient was taking the medication as prescribed until he or she went to a health fair at their church about 1 week ago. His or her blood pressure at the health fair was "normal." Since the blood pressure was normal and the patient was feeling great, the patient decided to just stop taking the medication. Plus, the medication was very expensive and the patient can certainly use that money for something else. The patient started getting a severe headache about 2 days ago and thought he or she should get checked at the ER. The patient is pleasant and talkative.

DOOR SIGN: Mr./Mrs. Pat V. was admitted to the medical surgical unit from the ER today. The patient has a 2-day complaint of severe headache. On arrival to the ER, the patient was diagnosed with severe hypertension. Do a complete history, focused physical examination, and appropriate patient teaching. You have 45 minutes for the encounter.

OPENING LINE: This is a (use your own age) patient who has been admitted to the Medical Surgical Unit (an inpatient room) from the emergency department.

CHALLENGE QUESTIONS:

The blood pressure medicine that the doctor had me on . . . can you tell me how that medication works?
The med acts on certain receptors in the body and decreases blood pressure and heart rate.

Why was my blood pressure normal at the health fair?
The medication was working or was in your system, so that made your blood pressure within normal range when you went to the health fair.

TRAINING QUESTIONS

What is your date of birth? Use your own

Are you married? Use your own

Occupation? Worked in a factory (or store or office, etc.), left on disability due to back injury. Currently under a lot of stress because having a difficult time making "ends meet" on the income you are receiving.

When did the severe headache start? 2 days ago.

Does anything make it worse? No. I don't think so.

Does anything make it better? No—I tried the usual over-the-counter medication that I take for headache but it did not help at all.

Have you had any fever or chills? No, not that I know of, but I haven't taken my temperature.

Have you ever had anything similar in the past? Yes, I came to the emergency department about 6 months ago with a similar headache. At that time, they said I had high blood pressure. They gave me a prescription for a blood pressure medication called Lopressor.

Have you ever used any recreational drugs? No.

Have you ever been hospitalized? No (or use your own if necessary but nothing related to current complaint).

Have you ever had surgery? Use your own

Have you ever been pregnant? Use your own

Do you have any chronic illnesses? Yes, I guess the high blood pressure could be considered a chronic illness, but I did not think I had it anymore.

Are you taking any medications? Yes, I was taking a medication after my last visit to the emergency department. It was a medication for my high blood pressure. I stopped taking the medication after I had my blood pressure checked at the health fair at church. My pressure was normal when they took it there, so I knew I did not need the medication any longer. I also felt great! Plus, that medication was very expensive!

How is your father? Died from a stroke a few years ago. Father also had hypertension.

How is your mother? Alive, if appropriate, or deceased.

How is/are your sibling(s)? Healthy

Health history (none or your own)

> Neurological (none)
> Cardiovascular—high blood pressure
> Respiratory (none)
> Gastrointestinal (none)
> Genitourinary (none)
> Gynecological (none)
> Obstetrical (use your own)

Diet—I eat anything I want. I love potato chips, dill pickles, I love anything that tastes salty.

Medications
> Prescription medications—I was taking Lopressor once a day when I had the high blood pressure, but before coming to the ER today, I was not taking any medications.
> Over-the-counter medications (none or your own)
> Medication allergies—None
> Seasonal allergies—Use your own

Psychosocial History
> Smoking history (yes—smoked 1 pack a day for as long as I can remember)
> Alcohol history (like to have a few beers with my friends on the weekend)
> Recreational drug history (none)
> Sexual history (use your own))
> Stressors—(stressed about finances—difficulty making ends meet on disability salary)

You should be in a hospital gown, bra, and underwear, sitting on the edge of the table.

STUDENT GRADING

Communication

__ Introduced self (name and title)
__ Good eye contact (50% or greater of the time)

__ Spoke clearly in terms the patient can understand (three strikes rule)
__ Active listener
__ Asked patient's age or date of birth
__ Asked about patient's marital status
__ Asked about patient's work history
__ Asked about previous hospitalizations
__ Asked about allergies
__ Asked about your medical history
__ Asked about your family's medical history
__ Asked about current medications
__ Asked about a history of chest pain
__ Asked about a history of palpitations
__ Asked about smoking history
__ Asked about alcohol history
__ Asked about my diet
__ Asked about exercise
__ Asked about stresses in life
__ Created an atmosphere that put the patient at ease
__ Answered patient's question about blood pressure medication Lopressor
__ Answered patient's question about why BP was normal at the health fair

PHYSICAL EXAMINATION

__ Washed hands before examination
__ Explained to me what she/he was doing with each step of examination
__ Helped to position me
__ Was professional in manner
__ Maintained modesty during examination
__ Checked blood pressure in both arms
__ Blood pressure sitting or lying
__ Blood pressure standing
__ Counted my pulse
__ Counted my respiratory rate
__ Took my temperature
__ Listened to my heart in at least 4 places anterior on skin
__ Listened to my lungs in at least 4 places (2 pairs) bilateral anterior on skin
__ Listened to my lungs in at least 4 places (2 pairs) bilateral posterior on skin

PATIENT TEACHING

__ Discussed the importance of taking medicines as prescribed
__ Discussed the importance of a low-salt diet
__ Discussed the importance of exercise
__ Offered information or suggested some options for stress management
__ Offered information or suggested some options for smoking cessation
   ■ **SP will also provide feedback**

CHRONIC OBSTRUCTIVE PULMONARY DISEASE

NAME: Jamie W.

SETTING: Medical Surgical Unit (Inpatient Hospital Room)

SCENARIO: The patient was admitted from the emergency department with a 2-day complaint of shortness of breath. Patient is pleasant and talkative.

DOOR SIGN: Mr./Mrs. Jamie. W. was admitted to the medical surgical unit from the ER today. The patient came to the ER with a complaint of shortness of breath and has a previous diagnosis of COPD.

Do a complete history, focused physical examination, and appropriate patient teaching. You have 45 minutes for the encounter.

OPENING LINE: This is a (use your own age) patient who has been admitted to the Medical Surgical Unit (an inpatient room) from the emergency department.

CHALLENGE QUESTIONS:

Can you tell me how the Pulmicort Turbuhaler works?
The inhaler acts as an anti-inflammatory and immune modifier. It decreases the severity of asthma attacks. It also improves asthma symptoms.

Can you tell me how the Proventil HFA inhaler works?
The medication acts on the receptors in the body and cause relaxation of airway smooth muscle and bronchodilation.

TRAINING QUESTIONS:

What is your date of birth? Use your own

Are you married? Use your own

Occupation? Retired, worked in a cigar factory/or currently work in a factory.

When did the shortness of breath start? 2 days ago.

Does anything make it better/worse? No. I don't think so.

Does anything make it worse? Yes—exercise, walking up stairs, increased activity.

Have you had any fever or chills? No, not that I know of, but I haven't taken my temperature.

Have you ever had anything similar in the past? Yes.

Have you ever used any recreational drugs? No.

Have you ever been hospitalized? A few months ago with shortness of breath...and that is when the doctor said I had COPD.

Have you ever had surgery? No or use your own if necessary due to scar etc.

Have you ever been pregnant? Use your own

Do you have any chronic illnesses? Yes, COPD.

Are you taking any medications? Yes, I was, but I just stopped taking them about 2 weeks ago because they made my heart beat fast.

How is your father? Alive, if appropriate, or deceased.

How is your mother? Alive, if appropriate, or deceased.

How is/are your sibling(s)? Use your own—Healthy if you have siblings.

Health history (none or your own)

> Neurological (none)
> Cardiovascular (none)
> Respiratory—COPD—diagnosed about 6 months ago
> Gastrointestinal (none)
> Genitourinary (none)
> Gynecological (none)
> Obstetrical—Use your own

Medications

> Prescription medications—I was taking Pulmicort Turbuhaler and Proventil HFA inhaler
> Over-the-counter medications (none or your own)
> Medication allergies—None
> Seasonal allergies—Use your own

Psychosocial history

        Smoking history (usually smoke about 1 pack per day)

        Alcohol history (one beer or one small glass of wine at a social gathering once or twice a month)

        Recreational drug history (none)

        Sexual history (use your own)

        Stressors (sometimes stressed about making ends meet financially)

You should be in a hospital gown, bra, and underwear, sitting on the edge of the table.

STUDENT GRADING

Communication

___ Introduced self (name and title)

___ Good eye contact (50% or greater of the time)

___ Spoke clearly in terms the patient can understand (three strike rule)

___ Active listener

___ Asked patient's age or date of birth

___ Asked about patient's marital status

___ Asked about patient's work history

___ Asked about the onset of shortness of breath

___ Asked about relieving factors

___ Asked about aggravating factors

___ Asked about a cough

___ Asked about your medical history

___ Asked about your family's medical history

___ Asked about previous hospitalizations

___ Asked about allergies

___ Asked about current medications you are taking

___ Asked about smoking

___ Answers patient's question about Pulmicort Turbuhaler

___ Answers patient's question about Proventil HFA inhaler

PHYSICAL EXAMINATION

___ Washed hands before examination

___ Explained to me what she/he was doing with each step of exam

___ Helped to position me

___ Was professional in manner

___ Maintained modesty during exam

___ Blood pressure sitting or lying correctly (only 1 BP required)

___ Counted my pulse

___ Counted my respiratory rate

___ Took my temperature

___ Listened to my heart in at least 4 places anterior on skin

___ Listened to my lungs in at least 4 places (2 pairs) bilateral anterior on skin

___ Listened to my lungs in at least 4 places (2 pairs) bilateral posterior on skin

___ Tapped on my back from side to side

___ Assessed mucous membranes for cyanosis or pallor

___ Examined extremities for clubbing or cyanosis

PATIENT TEACHING

___ Discussed the importance of taking medicines as prescribed

___ Offered information or suggested some options for stress management

___ Offered information or suggested some options for smoking cessation

    ■ **SP will also provide feedback**

ANGINA

NAME: Fran H.

SETTING: Medical Surgical Unit (Inpatient Hospital Room)

SCENARIO: The patient was admitted from the emergency department with a 3-day complaint of chest pain, which was unrelieved by sublingual nitroglycerine. The chest pain was off and on frequently for the past 3 days, but today the chest pain was up to an 8/10 and was radiating to the patient's left arm and all the way through to the back—so the patient thought he should come to the ER. Patient was given medication in the ER to relieve the chest pain and is admitted for additional cardiac testing. Patient has a history of unstable angina (chest pain) for the past year. The patient does not follow any special diet and does not do any additional exercise. In the ER, the patient was given morphine for pain, sublingual nitroglycerine, and oxygen. The patient is pleasant and talkative. The chest pain at the time of encounter is a dull ache (3–4/10).

DOOR SIGN: Mr./Mrs. Fran H. was admitted to the medical surgical unit from the ER today. The patient has a 3-day complaint of chest pain and has a medical history of unstable angina. Complete a full history, a focused physical examination, and appropriate patient teaching. You have 45 minutes for the encounter.

OPENING LINE: This is a (use your own age) patient who has been admitted to the Medical Surgical Unit (an inpatient room) from the emergency department.

CHALLENGE QUESTIONS:

The doctor referred to risk factors for cardiac disease—what are those?
There are risk factors that you can control and those that you cannot control.
    Those that you can control are poor diet, lack of exercise, stress, smoking, high cholesterol, weight, high blood pressure, substance abuse.
    Those that you cannot control are heredity, race (African Americans more at risk), gender (men more at risk), and age (over 65).

I know that I take those little sublingual nitroglycerine tablets when I get chest pain, but can you tell me how they work?
They increase coronary blood flow by dilating the coronary arteries and improving collateral flow to ischemic regions. They also reduce myocardial oxygen consumption.

Is there a proper way to take the nitroglycerine tablets?
Place one tablet under your tongue. Can repeat the pill if pain continues every 5 minutes, for a maximum of 3 tablets.

TRAINING QUESTIONS:

What is your age or date of birth? Use your own

Are you married? Use your own

Occupation? Retired or work in "sales."

When did the chest pain start? 3 days ago.

Does anything make it better? Taking the nitro under my tongue makes it better—usually after I take 3 or so of those little pills, it makes the chest pain go away.

Does anything make it worse? Sometimes, it increases when I get stressed.

Have you had any fever or chills? No, not that I know of, but I haven't taken my temperature.

Do you have any shortness of breath? No.

Have you ever had anything similar in the past? Yes, I have had these episodes more frequently over the past 6 months, but this morning, even the sublingual nitroglycerine pills that I put under my tongue did not work.

Have you ever used any recreational drugs? No.

Have you ever been hospitalized? Use your own plus.... Yes, I was admitted to the hospital for the same problem about 1 year ago (initial diagnosis).

Have you ever had surgery? Use your own

Have you ever been pregnant? Use your own

Do you have any chronic illnesses? I guess you would call this chest pain a chronic illness.

Are you taking any medications? Yes, I take one aspirin every day, and I take Isordil, and I also take those nitro pills under my tongue when I get the chest pain.

FYI—Isordil is classified as an "antianginal" or "nitrate" medication. The drug produces vasodilation. It increases coronary blood flow by dilating coronary arteries and improving collateral flow to ischemic regions. Dose is 40 mg every 6 hours.

How is your father? Father died from heart attack.

How is your mother? Alive, if appropriate, or deceased.

How is/are your sibling(s)? Use your own—if you have siblings they are healthy.

Health history (none or your own)

>   Neurological (none)
>   Cardiovascular (chest pain that "happens every once in a while")
>   Respiratory (none)
>   Gastrointestinal (none)
>   Genitourinary (none)
>   Gynecological (none)
>   Obstetrical (use your own)

Medications

>   Prescription medications (aspirin, Isordil, and nitro under the tongue for chest pain)
>   Over-the-counter medications (Use your own)
>   Allergies to medications—None
>   Seasonal allergies—Use your own

Psychosocial history

>   Smoking history (a pack or more per day for a very long time)
>   Alcohol history (pick your beverage, but you have some every night or every other night)
>   Recreational drug history (none)
>   Sexual history (Use your own)
>   Stress (sometimes you get stressed worrying about finances and making ends meet)

Diet—I eat anything I want.

Exercise No way!

Chest pain questions

__ Asked about the onset of chest pain (the pain started about 3 days ago)
__ Asked about the location of the pain (it hurts in the middle of my chest)
__ Asked about the quality of the pain (it is sharp, like a knife going through me)
__ Asked about the radiation of the pain (sometimes radiates to my left arm the pain goes all the way through my back)
__ Asked about the severity of the pain (on a scale of 0 to 10, with 10 the worst, my pain at the worst point was an 8/10). Now the pain is a 3–4/10.
__ Asked if you have any sweating with the chest pain (yes)
__ Asked if you have any heartburn with the chest pain or at other times (yes, sometimes with the chest pain and sometimes without it)

__ Asked about any association with nausea or vomiting (none)
__ Asked what you do when you get the chest pain (I took 3 of those Nitro pills under my tongue)
__ Do you ever have chest pain when you are at rest? (yes, sometimes)

You should be in a hospital gown, bra, and underwear, sitting on the edge of the table.

STUDENT GRADING

Communication

__ Introduced self (name and title)
__ Good eye contact (50% or more of the time)
__ Spoke clearly in terms the patient can understand (three strikes rule)
__ Active listener
__ Asked patient's age or date of birth
__ Asked about patient's work history
__ Asked about shortness of breath
__ Asked about the description of the chest pain (location, quality, severity)
__ Asked about radiation of the chest pain
__ Asked about sweating with the chest pain
__ Asked about heartburn
__ Asked about relieving or alleviating factors
__ Asked about aggravating factors
__ Asked about pain at rest
__ Asked about previous hospitalizations
__ Asked about allergies
__ Asked about your medical history
__ Asked about your family's medical history
__ Asked about current medications I am taking
__ Asked about how the patient takes the sublingual Nitroglycerine (how many/how often)
__ Asked about my diet
__ Asked about exercise
__ Asked about a history of chest pain
__ Asked about a history of palpitations
__ Asked about smoking history
__ Asked about alcohol history
__ Asked about cocaine or recreational drug use
__ Asked about family history
__ Asked about lifestyle stresses or stress in general
__ Answered patient's question about how nitroglycerine works
__ Answered patient's question about the proper way to take nitroglycerine tablets
__ Answered patient's question about the risk factors for cardiac disease

PHYSICAL EXAMINATION

__ Washed hands before examination
__ Explained to me what she/he was doing with each step of exam
__ Helped to position me
__ Was professional in manner
__ Maintained modesty during exam
__ Blood pressure sitting or lying correctly (only 1 BP required)
__ Counted my pulse
__ Counted my respiratory rate
__ Took my temperature
__ Listened to my heart in at least 4 places anterior on skin
__ Listened to my lungs in at least 4 places (2 pairs) bilateral anterior on skin
__ Listened to my lungs in at least 4 places (2 pairs) bilateral posterior on skin
__ Palpated the PMI
__ Observed the right sternocleidomastoid area for neck vein distention
__ Auscultated carotid artery
__ Palpated carotid artery one side at a time

PATIENT TEACHING

__ Discussed the importance of a proper diet
__ Discussed the importance of exercise
__ Offered information or suggested some options for stress management
__ Offered information or suggested some options for smoking cessation
   ▓ **SP will also provide feedback**

REFERENCES

Barrows, H., & Abrahamson, S. (1964). The programmed patient: A technique for appraising student performance in clinical neurology. *The Journal of Medical Education, 39,* 802–805.

Redfern, S., Norman, L., Calman, L., Watson, R., & Murells, T. (2002). Assessing competence to practice in nursing: A review of the literature. *Research Papers in Education, 17,* 51–77.

Rentschler, D. D., Eaton, J., Cappiello, J., McNally, S. F., & McWilliam, P. (2007). Evaluation of undergraduate students using objective structured clinical evaluation. *Journal of Nursing Education, 46*(3), 135–139.

University of Kentucky College of Medicine. (2008). *Origin of standardized patients in the United States.* Retrieved September 4, 2008, from http://www.mc.uky.edu/meded/cstac/sphistory.asp

Wallace, P. (1997). Following the threads of an innovation: The history of standardized patients in medical education. *Caduceus, 13*(2), 5–28.

Wartman, S. A. (2006). My mother, a professional patient: When a physician's aging mother starts visiting lots of specialists and often being unsatisfied with the results, the son comes with a cleaver, life-enhancing solution. *Health Affairs, 25*(5), 1407–1411.

CHAPTER 15

Human Simulation Team Cases for Undergraduate Nursing

Linda Wilson, Fabien Pampaloni, John Cornele, and Robert Feenan

The purpose of this chapter is to provide an overview of the Sim Team Project at Drexel University. *SimTeam: The Joint Education of Health Professionals and Assistive Personnel Students in a Simulated Environment* was a three-year project at Drexel University funded by the Barra Foundation, Inc (Wilson, 2010). The purpose of the Sim Team project was to improve teamwork, communication, and coordination of quality of care delivered by registered nurses, practical nurses, and medical assistants through human simulation experiences with standardized patients (Wilson, 2010). Drexel University College of Nursing and Health Professions undergraduate nursing students worked with the Prism Career Institute medical assistant students and practical nurse students throughout this project.

The primary objectives of the Sim Team project included the following:

1. Develop a collaborative relationship with the Prism Institute to incorporate medical assistants in individual and multidisciplinary health professions training using simulation strategies
2. Implement an educational experience specific to the needs of the medical assistant, emphasizing their crucial relationship with licensed health providers
3. Evaluate the communication, delegation, evaluation, and conflict resolution competencies of nurses and health professionals working with assistive personnel
4. Evaluate team competencies of the MAs, MOAs, and practical nurse students with emphasis on their ability to take direction, report incidents, and accept monitoring and feedback on their performance from health professional supervisors
5. Document and disseminate the strategies, successes, and challenges of the project so that other schools might use the Sim Team approach in their nursing and health professions students' clinical learning experiences. (Wilson, 2010, p. 10)

Drexel University College of Nursing and Health Professions faculty worked with the Prism Career Institute faculty to develop the Sim Team Cases for this project (Wilson, 2010). All cases were developed to meet the needs of all the student participants. The simulation cases included history-taking skills, physical examination skills, patient teaching, teamwork, delegation, and conflict resolution (Wilson, 2010).

The Sim Team cases are labeled by diagnosis name or the primary focus of the case. Some of the Sim Team cases included the following: asthma, depression, cough, cough and rinorrhea, diabetes, heartburn, homeless mental illness, myocardial infarction and cocaine, and shortness of breath and the postoperative patient (Wilson, 2010). A few examples of these cases are included at the end of this chapter.

SIMULATION CASES

SIM TEAM Case—Chronic Cough and Rinorrhea—Passing Grade 76%
(Reprinted with Permission)

NAME: Mr./Mrs. Pat K.

SETTING: Medical Surgical Unit (Inpatient Hospital Room)

SESSION DETAILS:

> 30-minute encounter with patient
> 13 minutes for SP to complete checklist
> 12 minutes for feedback
> 5 minutes for turnaround

SESSION TEAM APPROACH:

- This is a team experience including a nursing student and a medical assistant student.
- The medical assistant will enter the room first and will ask you demographic questions (which you can make up).
- The medical assistant will do your vital signs.
- The nursing student will enter the room 5 minutes later.
- The nursing student and medical assistant student will discuss the information that was collected thus far, including vital signs.
- The nursing student will then proceed to do a complete history, focused physical, and appropriate patient teaching.
- The nursing student reviews the physician's orders and will ask the medical student to draw blood or do a blood glucose finger stick (which varies for each case).
- If the case includes a dressing change, we hope the nursing student and medical assistant work together to change the patient dressing (which is not included in all cases).
- In the remaining time, we hope the nursing student and medical student will work together to care for the patient.
- At the end of the encounter, during feedback time, both students will re-enter the room to receive feedback together.
- You will provide feedback to the nursing student and to the nursing assistant.
- You will also provide feedback based on how they worked as a team.

GRADING CHECKLISTS:

- In this case information, you will see two types of detailed checklists (which both contain the same information).
- The first grading checklist, which comes right at the end of the scenario information, clearly separates the categories of grading items for the medical assistant, the nursing student, and the team.
- The second grading checklist (combined grading list), which comes at the very end of the scenario, is just one long list without headers. Each of the items begins with either "MA" for medical assistant, "SN" for student nurse, or "TEAM" for team items. This is probably the format the checklist will be in because at this point we are not sure if the system can take three separate checklists.

SCENARIO: The patient is being seen in the medical surgical unit with a complaint of chronic cough and requests an antibiotic. The patient does not have a primary physician and comes to the ER for any medical problems. The patient was admitted to the medical surgical unit for further evaluation.

DOOR SIGN: Mr./Mrs. Pat Keifer came in to the ER today and was admitted to the medical surgical unit for further evaluation. The patient does not have a primary physician and has presented a complaint of chronic cough. You have 30 minutes to complete a history, focused physical examination, and appropriate patient teaching.

Please refer to patient chart for any specific patient orders.

OPENING LINE: This is a (use your own age) patient who came in because of a chronic cough.

CHALLENGE QUESTIONS: (The nursing student may use PDA to answer these questions)

I've heard that it's not good to take an antibiotic if you have a virus. Why not?
Antibiotics only kill bacteria, not viruses. Taking an antibiotic when you don't need one can lead to the development of bacteria that are antibiotic-resistant.

They took a blood sample. What was that for?
A complete blood count checks the levels of red blood cells, white blood cells, and platelets in your blood. If you have an infection, your white blood cell count will go up.

TRAINING QUESTIONS:

What is your age or date of birth? Use your own

Are you married? Use your own

Occupation? Retired or work in "sales" (or you can pick your favorite profession).

When did the cough start? A little more than 2 months ago.

Are you coughing up any sputum? No.

Does anything make it better? No.

Does anything make it worse? When I smoke, or am around people that are smoking, or am around a lot of dust.

Have you had any fever or chills? No, not that I know of, but I haven't taken my temperature.

Do you have any other symptoms? Some sneezing and runny nose.

What color is your nasal drainage? Clear.

Have you ever had anything similar in the past? I get a cough sometimes when the ragweed comes out.

Have you ever used any recreational drugs? No.

Have you ever been hospitalized? Use your own

Have you ever had surgery? Use your own

Have you ever been pregnant? Use your own

Do you have any chronic illnesses? No.

Are you taking any medications? No.

How is your father? Alive, or deceased, if appropriate.

How is your mother? Alive, or deceased, if appropriate, but did have asthma.

How is/are your sibling(s)? Use your own—if you have siblings they are healthy

Health history (none or your own)

Neurological (none)

> Cardiovascular (none)
> Respiratory—(seasonal allergies)
> Gastrointestinal (none)

Genitourinary (none)
Gynecological (none)
Obstetrical (use your own)

Medications

Prescription medications—(none)
Over the counter medications (use your own)
Allergies to medications—none

Psychosocial History

Smoking history (a pack or more per day for a very long time)
Alcohol history (use your own)
Recreational drug history (none)
Sexual history (Use your own)

Diet Nothing special

Exercise No way!

SP should be in a hospital gown, bra, and underwear, sitting on the edge of the table.

MEDICAL ASSISTANT STUDENT GRADING

CHECKLIST GRADING OPTIONS: Done/Not Done/N/A

COMMUNICATION

__ Introduced self (name and title)
__ Good eye contact (50% or more of the time)
__ Spoke clearly in terms the patient can understand (three strikes rule)
__ Active listener
__ Created an atmosphere that put the patient at ease
__ Collected demographic information in an organized manner
__ Asked patient questions clearly
__ Communicated demographic information to the student nurse clearly
__ Communicated vital signs to the student nurse clearly

PHYSICAL EXAMINATION

__ Washed hands before examination
__ Explained to me what they were doing with each step of exam or procedure
__ Helped to position me (if applicable)
__ Was professional in manner
__ Maintained modesty during exam (if applicable)
__ Blood pressure sitting or lying correctly (only one BP required)
__ Counted my pulse
__ Counted my respiratory rate
__ Took my temperature
__ Drew a blood sample (if directed by the nursing student)
__ Put on gloves before drawing blood
__ Applied tourniquet as gently as possible
__ Selected purple tube for blood draw
__ Removed tourniquet after blood draw completed
__ Labeled specimen tube with patient's name
__ Disposed of needle properly after blood draw
__ Washed hands after removing gloves

NURSING STUDENT GRADING

CHECKLIST GRADING OPTIONS: Done/Not Done/N/A

COMMUNICATION

__ Introduced self (name and title)
__ Good eye contact (50% or more of the time)
__ Spoke clearly in terms the patient can understand (three strikes rule)
__ Active listener
__ Asked about cough
__ Asked about the presence of a fever
__ Asked about the presence of other symptoms
__ Asked about relieving or alleviating factors
__ Asked about aggravating factors
__ Asked about previous hospitalizations
__ Asked about allergies
__ Asked about your medical history
__ Asked about your family's medical history
__ Asks about current medications you are taking
__ Asked about your diet
__ Asked about exercise
__ Asked about smoking history
__ Asked about alcohol history
__ Asked about cocaine or recreational drug use
__ Answered patient's question about antibiotics
__ Answered patient's question about the blood sample

PHYSICAL EXAMINATION

__ Washed hands before examination
__ Explained to me what she/he was doing with each step of exam
__ Helped to position me (if applicable)
__ Was professional in manner
__ Maintained modesty during exam (if applicable)
__ Reviewed vital signs obtained by medical assistant student
__ Listened to my heart in at least four places anterior on skin
__ Listened to my lungs in at least four places (two pairs) bilateral anterior on skin
__ Listened to my lungs in at least four places (two pairs) bilateral posterior on skin
__ Directed medical assistant student to draw a complete blood count

PATIENT TEACHING

__ Offered information or suggested some options for smoking cessation
__ Offered information regarding the appropriate time to take an antibiotic
__ Discussed the importance of a proper diet
__ Discussed the importance of exercise

TEAM GRADING

CHECKLIST GRADING OPTIONS: Done/Not Done/N/A

Did the nursing student and the medical assistant student work well together as a team?

Did the nursing student and the medical assistant demonstrate mutual respect for each other?

Did the nursing student and the medical assistant have good eye contact with each other?

Did the nursing student and the medical assistant demonstrate good listening skills with each other?

Did the nursing student demonstrate good delegation/leadership skills?

Did the medical assistant defer to the nursing student for direction?

■ **SP will also provide feedback**

FEEDBACK TO NURSING STUDENT/FEEDBACK TO MEDICAL ASSISTANT STUDENT/ FEEDBACK TO BOTH ON TEAM FUNCTION

SIM TEAM Case—Diabetes—Passing grade 76%
(Reprinted with Permission)

NAME: Mr./Mrs. Toni T.

SETTING: Medical Surgical Unit (Inpatient Hospital Room)

SESSION DETAILS:

> 30-minute encounter with patient
> 13 minutes for SP to complete checklist
> 12 minutes for feedback
> 5 minutes for turnaround

SESSION TEAM APPROACH:

- This is a team experience including a nursing student and a medical assistant student.
- The medical assistant will enter the room first and will ask you demographic questions (which you can make up).
- The medical assistant will do your vital signs.
- The nursing student will enter the room five minutes later.
- The nursing student and medical assistant student will discuss the information that was collected thus far, including vital signs.
- The nursing student will then proceed to do a complete history, focused physical examination, and appropriate patient teaching.
- The nursing student reviews the physician's orders and will ask the medical student to draw blood or do a blood glucose finger stick (which varies for each case).
- If the case includes a dressing change, we hope the nursing student and medical assistant work together to change the patient dressing (which is not included in all cases).
- In the remaining time, we hope the nursing student and medical student will work together to care for the patient.
- At the end of the encounter, during feedback time, both students will re-enter the room to receive feedback together.
- You will provide feedback to the nursing student and to the nursing assistant.
- You will also provide feedback based on how they worked as a team.

GRADING CHECKLISTS:

- In this case information, you will see two types of detailed checklists (which both contain the same information).
- The first grading checklist, which comes right at the end of the scenario information, clearly separates the categories of grading items for the medical assistant, the nursing student, and the team.
- The second grading checklist (combined grading list), which comes at the very end of the scenario information, is just one long list without headers. Each of the items begins with either "MA" for medical assistant, "SN" for student nurse, or "TEAM" for team items. This is probably the format the checklist will be in because at this point, we are not sure if the system can take three separate checklists.

SCENARIO: The patient came to the emergency room with complaints of increased thirst, increased urination, and hunger, and is now admitted with a diagnosis of hyperglycemia due to poorly controlled diabetes. Patient is pleasant and talkative. Patient is in total denial of the seriousness of the diagnosis of diabetes.

INSTRUCTIONS/DOOR SIGN: Mr./Mrs. Toni T. came to the emergency room with complaints of increased thirst, increased urination, and hunger, and is now admitted to the medical surgical unit. You have 30 minutes to complete a history, focused physical examination and appropriate patient teaching. Please refer to patient chart for any specific patient orders.

OPENING LINE: This is a (use your own age) patient who has been admitted to the Medical Surgical Unit (an inpatient room) from the emergency department.

CHALLENGE QUESTIONS: (nursing student may use PDA to answer these questions)

Can you tell me how insulin works?
Lowers blood glucose by increasing transport into cells and promoting the conversion of glucose to glycogen, which helps control blood glucose in diabetic patients.

Why do I get thirsty when my blood sugar is high?
When blood sugars go up, water is pulled out of the cells, including those in the thirst center. Dehydration of the cells also causes dry mouth.

TRAINING QUESTIONS:

What is your age? Use your own

Are you married? Use your own

Occupation? Use your own

Have you ever had anything similar in the past? Yes, I was seen in the ER approximately 6 months ago with the same problem.

Have you ever used any recreational drugs? No.

Have you ever been hospitalized? No, or use your own if necessary, due to scar, etc.

Have you ever had surgery? No, or use your own if necessary, due to scar, etc.

Have you ever been pregnant? Use your own.

Do you have any chronic illnesses? When I was seen in the ER 6 months ago, the doctor said I had diabetes.

Are you taking any medications? When I came to the ER 6 months ago, the doctor prescribed 70/30 insulin, which I have to give myself with a needle every morning.

How is your father? Died a few years ago from a stroke.

How is your mother? Alive, has a history of an above-the-knee amputation, history of diabetes, just started on dialysis a few months ago.

How is/are your sibling(s)? Healthy

Health history ("none, until the visit to the ER 6 months ago")

> Neurological (none)
> Cardiovascular (none)
> Respiratory (none)
> Gastrointestinal (none)
> Genitourinary (none)
> Gynecological (none)
> Obstetrical (use your own)

Immunizations up to date? All immunizations are up to date. Last tetanus shot was 2 years ago.

Diet I eat anything I want to—no restrictions. I love chocolate! I like all kinds of candy.

Activity/exercise I get enough exercise at work every day.

Medications

> Prescription medications—Humulin 70/30 insulin, 20 units, subcutaneous injection every morning
> Over the counter medications—none
> Medication allergies—none
> Seasonal allergies—use your own

Comfortable with giving insulin injections You don't have any trouble with those—the needle is very small—you are totally comfortable with this. You give the shot in your outer arm or abdomen and you do rotate (alternate) the injection sites.

Psychosocial history

> Smoking history (one pack per day for 10 years)
> Alcohol history (I only drink on the weekends when I go out with a few of my friends—I usually drink about six beers (or your preferred beverage) when I go out)
> Recreational drug history (none)
> Sexual history (use your own)
> Stress history (sometimes get stressed, finances are tough trying to make ends meet)

Do you check your blood sugar at home on a regular basis (use a glucometer)? Sometimes.

Are you comfortable with the procedure of using a glucometer? Yes.

When you do your blood sugar with a glucometer, what does it usually run? 250–300.

Are you having any problems as a result of your diabetes? No.

Do you have any numbness or tingling in your feet? No tingling, but I really can't feel my feet very well. I walk around in my house without my shoes on most of the time, and I'm always stepping on things.

SP should be in a hospital gown, bra, and underwear, sitting on the edge of the table.

SP will keep their socks on and have a gauze dressing on one leg.

MEDICAL ASSISTANT STUDENT GRADING

CHECKLIST GRADING OPTIONS: Done/Not Done/N/A

COMMUNICATION

__ Introduced self (name and title)
__ Good eye contact (50% or greater of the time)
__ Spoke clearly in terms the patient can understand (three strikes rule)
__ Active listener
__ Created an atmosphere that put the patient at ease
__ Collected demographic information in an organized manner
__ Asked patient questions clearly
__ Communicated demographic information to the student nurse clearly
__ Communicated vital signs to the student nurse clearly

PHYSICAL EXAMINATION

__ Washed hands before examination
__ Explained to me what she/he was doing with each step of exam or procedure
__ Helped to position me (if applicable)
__ Was professional in manner
__ Maintained modesty during exam (if applicable)
__ Blood pressure sitting or lying correctly (only one BP required)
__ Counted my pulse
__ Counted my respiratory rate
__ Took my temperature
__ Checked blood glucose (if directed by nursing student)
__ Put on gloves before checking the blood glucose
__ Washed hands after removing gloves after blood glucose check
__ Disposed of needle correctly after checking blood glucose
__ Put on gloves before assisting the SN with the dressing change
__ Washed hands after removing gloves after assisting the SN with dressing change

NURSING STUDENT GRADING

CHECKLIST GRADING OPTIONS: Done/Not Done/N/A

COMMUNICATION

__ Introduced self (name and title)
__ Good eye contact (50% or greater of the time)
__ Spoke clearly in terms the patient can understand (three strikes rule)
__ Active listener
__ Created an atmosphere that put the patient at ease
__ Asked about the dressing on the patient's leg
__ Asked about your medical history
__ Asked about your family's medical history
__ Asked about previous hospitalizations
__ Asked about allergies
__ Asked about diet
__ Asked about activity/exercise
__ Asked about current medications
__ Asked about smoking history
__ Asked about alcohol history
__ Asked about the patient's vision
__ Asked about date of last eye exam
__ Asked about numbness or tingling in the hands or feet
__ Asked about excessive thirst
__ Asked about excessive urination
__ Asked about having to urinate in the middle of the night
__ Asked about the use of a glucometer
__ Asked about usual blood sugar ranges
__ Asked if patient is comfortable with giving their insulin injections
__ Answered patient's question about insulin
__ Answered patient's question about thirst

PHYSICAL EXAMINATION

__ Washed hands before examination
__ Explained to me what she/he was doing with each step of exam
__ Helped to position me (if applicable)
__ Was professional in manner
__ Maintained modesty during exam (if applicable)
__ Reviewed vital signs obtained by medical assistant student
__ Listened to my heart in at least four places anterior on skin
__ Listened to my lungs in at least four places (two pairs) bilateral anterior on skin
__ Listened to my lungs in at least four places (two pairs) bilateral posterior on skin
__ Checked pulses in both feet (pedal pulses)
__ Checked capillary refill of both lower extremities
__ Examined both feet for any sores (must look at bottom of both feet)
__ Removed dressing and examined leg
__ Put on gloves before removing dressing
__ Washed hands after removing gloves after checking patient's leg dressing
__ Assessed sensation in both legs
__ Examined both lower extremities for pitting edema
__ Directed medical assistant student to check the patient's blood sugar

PATIENT TEACHING

__ Discussed the importance of checking blood sugar regularly
__ Discussed the importance of proper diet
__ Discussed the importance of regular foot care and inspection
__ Discussed the importance of not going without shoes/wearing well-fitting shoes
__ Discussed the importance of regular eye exams
__ Discussed the danger signs of hypoglycemia (dizziness, light-headedness, shaky, and heart pounding)

__ Discussed the danger signs of hyperglycemia (increased thirst, urination, vomiting, nausea, and disorientation)

__ Discussed the long-term consequences of poor blood sugar control (vascular disease, loss of limbs, loss of eyesight, and kidney disease)

__ Discussed the impact of excessive alcohol intake on blood sugars

__ Offered information or suggested some options for stress management

__ Offered information or suggested some options for smoking cessation

TEAM GRADING

CHECKLIST GRADING OPTIONS: Done/Not Done/N/A

Did the nursing student and the medical assistant student work well together as a team?

Did the nursing student and the medical assistant demonstrate mutual respect for each other?

Did the nursing student and the medical assistant have good eye contact with each other?

Did the nursing student and the medical assistant demonstrate good listening skills with each other?

Did nursing student demonstrate good delegation/leadership skills?

Did medical assistant defer to the nursing student for direction?

Did the team handle the conflict situation well?

■ **SP will also provide feedback**

Feedback to nursing student/feedback to medical assistant student/feedback to both on team function.

REFERENCE

Wilson, L. (2010). *SimTeam: The joint education of health professionals and assistive personnel students in a simulated environment.* Philadelphia, PA: Drexel University College of Nursing and Health Professions.

CHAPTER 16

Human Simulation: Comprehensive Cases for Graduate Nursing

Amy Flanagan Risdal

*I*ncorporating the use of standardized patients (SPs) into graduate nursing education has been generally well-received by learners in the last few years. Nurses appreciate the ability to interact with "real people" while still in the learning environment. Well-written cases provide faculty with an excellent opportunity for students to demonstrate skills learned in the classroom and in the clinic, performed in the same way that will be expected of them after graduation. Comprehensive cases written for graduate nursing students do an excellent job of allowing the student to demonstrate a wide range of skills, while also giving faculty valuable feedback on individual student performance as well as the overall program.

GOALS AND OBJECTIVES

When beginning to write a case using SPs, the overall goals and objectives of the simulated encounter must first be outlined. Faculty often feel driven by the need to get their students "in" for a simulation experience and then get them "assessed," rather than first identifying the educational goals and objectives they want to achieve through simulations with Standardized Patients. Creating an effective case, however, requires going through all of the skills a learner is expected to know at this point and then identifying only a few to be evaluated through each encounter. Is this encounter solely for the student's benefit to give them additional learning experience? Or is the encounter going to be a demonstration of skills and techniques, perhaps for a grade?

Sample Goals and Objectives—Formative event (for practice only)

PSYCHIATRIC INTERVIEW (PATIENT "ERIC A."—DEPRESSION, SUICIDAL IDEATION)

GOAL: To allow student nurse practitioners to conduct a thorough intake interview with a patient under stress from possible mental illness.

OBJECTIVES:
1. Given a standardized patient portraying the affect of depression, a student nurse practitioner will be able to practice interview skills, including interview pace, transitions, organization of evaluative components (MMSE and SIGECAPS), and building patient rapport.

2. Given statements of suicidal ideation by the patient, a student nurse practitioner will demonstrate their ability to respond to the patient's statements with appropriate questioning and will show awareness on the appropriate next steps for a patient at this level.

Sample Goals and Objectives—Summative Event
(for Assessment and/or a Grade)

FAMILY MEDICINE CASE (PATIENT "WILLOW R."—HEADACHES)*
GOAL: To assess student nurse practitioner history taking, physical examination, and interpersonal communication skills in an adult patient.

OBJECTIVES:
1. Given a standardized patient presenting with a chief complaint of headaches, a student nurse practitioner will conduct a competent focused history and physical examination, including a focused neurological examination.
2. Given a challenge by the standardized patient on the efficacy of prescription medicine for migraines, a student nurse practitioner will give a competent explanation of at least two different medications, including side effects.

The SP Checklist

Whether the simulation experience is for practice or for a grade, you must next decide what information you want to receive from this event. In the goals and objectives presented earlier, the word *competent* appears several times. How will you know if a student performs these tasks with competence? How will competence from a first-year and second-year student be different? Standardized patients can reliably report on several aspects of the encounter, but first, each exact task that you expect must be outlined.

Sample SP Checklist—Patient "Willow R." (Headaches)

History	YES	NO
Upon questioning by the student, I responded that:		
1. I've had headaches for 10 years.	O	O
2. I have 4–5 severe headaches a month.	O	O
3. I am nauseated with my headaches and sometimes I do vomit.	O	O
4. Before a headache starts, I get a sensation of flashing lights in my eyes.	O	O
5. The headaches are more often on the right side of my head than the left. The pain is usually behind my eye and bores through my head.	O	O
6. Headaches last, I don't know, about 6–8 hours, but it varies.	O	O
7. Lying down with a cool cloth on my forehead sometimes will help.	O	O
8. I've tried Tylenol every 4 hours, but it doesn't help much.	O	O
9. I haven't hit my head or lost consciousness.	O	O
10. None of my family members have had problems with headaches.	O	O
11. Light really bothers me when I have one of these headaches.	O	O
12. I haven't had any recent sinus congestion.	O	O

* "Willow R[...]" (Headaches). **Diane Padden, NP, Richard Hawkins, MD, Graceanne Adamo, MA, CMA, Aileen Zanoni. Adapted from** A Day in the Office: Case Studies in Primary Care. **Jeffrey A. Eaton, Joyce D. Cappiello, Mosby, 1998.**

PHYSICAL EXAMINATION

The Student:	YES	NO
13. Washed his/her hands in my presence before examining me or putting on gloves.	O	O
14. Pressed on my head for tenderness.	O	O
15. Pressed on my sinuses.	O	O
16. Looked into my open mouth with a light.	O	O
17. Examined my eyes with an ophthalmoscope.	O	O
18. Checked my neck for stiffness and range of motion.	O	O

CIRCLE: PASSIVE *(student moved my head)* or ACTIVE *(I moved my head)*

Checked the Following:

	YES	NO
19 Followed an object/finger with my eyes.	O	O
20. Asked me to bite down and clench teeth.	O	O
21. Touched my face to check sensation.	O	O
22. Used tongue depressor and asked me to say, "AH."	O	O

Checked Strength:

	YES	NO
23. Both shoulders.	O	O
24. Both arms.	O	O
25. Both legs.	O	O

Checked Sensation: Must ask patient to close eyes for credit

	YES	NO
26. Both arms.	O	O
27. Both legs.	O	O

The SP checklist lists the exact items that should be asked and performed by a student who is competent. This is not the only way to write a checklist; however, many SP educators state that they prefer the first-person POV because it is easier for an SP to remember what he or she said to the student, as opposed to what was asked of him or her. The first-person statements also help each SP portraying the case to use the same wording each time they answer the question.

In the Physical Examination section, basic information is provided for the SP on what will and will not earn credit for a maneuver—this information is covered in more detail during the SP training. It can also be helpful to include these details in the training materials for reference. The SP Guide to Checklist helps the standardized patient know exactly what criteria they are looking for so that they give the correct answer, even if the question is worded differently or asked at an unexpected time.

SP Guide to Checklist—Willow R.

Checklist # *Potential prompts by student*/guidance for responses

HISTORY-TAKING:

1. *How long have you had these headaches?*
   How long has this been going on?

2. *How frequent are they?*
   How often do you get them?

3. *Do you vomit OR have nausea?* (Offer both in response to either query.)

4. *Any flashing lights?*
   Any visual changes you've noticed before the headaches?

5. *Where does it hurt?*
   Can you describe the location on your head?

6. *How long does each headache last?*

7. *Does anything make it feel better?*
   Can add "in a dark room" if sensitivity to light has already been asked.

8. *Have you tried any medications?*
   Do you take anything for them?

9. *Ever had a head injury OR head trauma OR loss of consciousness?*

10. *Any family history of headaches?*
    Does anyone else in your family get these headaches?

11. *Does light bother you when you get them? Any sensitivity to light?* Note: this is different from #4's "visual changes" and "flashing lights"—here you're talking about being bothered by light and preferring a dark room, not visual changes.

12. I haven't had any recent sinus congestion.

PHYSICAL EXAMINATION:

13. Hand washing should take place prior to touching you; use your judgment if student washes at the very beginning and "recontaminates" before touching you (student touches own face, hair, etc.). If answering "No" due to recontamination, make sure to note in comments.

14. Presses front, back and sides of head.

15. Presses forehead and nasal areas.

16. Must use *some* kind of light source—penlight, otoscope, et cetera.—and have you open your mouth (to examine teeth, etc.).

17. Must examine *both* eyes and must use instrument *very close* to your face.

One of the greatest insights an SP can provide is his or her perspective on the student's communication and interpersonal skills. This is extremely valuable simply because once the student graduates, feedback *from the patient* on the practitioner's communication skills will be extremely limited, if not nonexistent. SPs can be trained to provide constructive, subjective feedback on how they felt while working with this student, how well they understood information provided, if they felt the student protected their modesty, and if they would return to see this student again.

A GENERAL CHECKLIST ON INTERPERSONAL/COMMUNICATION SKILLS:

	YES/Likely/ Satisfied	NO/Unlikely/ Unsatisfied
1. The student identified themselves by surname and professional role.	O	O
2. The student treated me with respect.	O	O

3. The student addressed me by my surname.	O	O
4. The student seemed to care about me and my health.	O	O
5. I could easily understand what the student was saying.	O	O
6. The student used smooth, appropriate transitions and seemed organized.	O	O
7. The student listened carefully to me.	O	O
8. The student brought the encounter to a closure.	O	O
9. I understand what this student is planning to do for me.	O	O
10. I trust that this student will help me (confidence in student).	O	O
11. I would do what the student asked me to do (compliance with plan).	O	O
12. I would be willing to return to this student for care in the future.	O	O
13. Overall satisfaction with care.	O	O

A checklist like this will provide you with specific details on the basic history taking and physical examination skills of a graduate nurse.

The Post-Encounter Exercise

Your next step is to consider what information you would like to receive from the student. In most SP encounters, the student is expected to complete a "postencounter exercise" after completing their work with the patient. There are several different types of postencounter exercises, each providing you with different information:

■ *The self-assessment checklist:* This checklist, completed by the student after seeing the patient, is a mirror of the SP checklist. By answering the same questions or you can compare the student answers with the SP answers. Do they both have the same recollection of the encounter? If the student reports asking questions or performing skills that the SP did not give credit for, where is the disparity? Perhaps the student tested sensation but forgot to tell the SP to close his or her eyes. Medical jargon or compound questioning (no fever–chills–rash–cough–nausea? Instead of "Have you had a fever? How about chills? Any rash...") can also cause SPs and students to have different answers. An example of some self-assessment questions are as follows:

I told the student...	**I asked the patient...**
I've been having headaches for 10 years.	*How long have you had these headaches?*
I tried Tylenol but it doesn't help much.	*Have you tried any medicine for these headaches?*

- *The SOAP note:* Teachers find they get a good perspective on a student's progress through a traditional subjective/objective/assessment/plan (SOAP) medical note. Although correct note writing is a skill in itself, having the student complete a patient note after an encounter gives you insight into their thought processes and clinical reasoning. Although electronic medical records are making SOAP notes less common in the clinic or hospital settings, many faculty still feel it is a valuable skill to develop and demonstrate while training.
- *Clinical reasoning exercise:* As graduate nurses advance in their training, their ability to work independently and provide sound clinical reasoning for their decisions becomes more important. Exercises in clinical reasoning can range from the simple (providing a differential diagnosis, justification, or management plan) to the complex (ordering labs, interpreting tests, or imaging results).
- *The clinical consult:* Being able to work within a specific protocol and communicate effectively with fellow health care providers on a patient's behalf is a vital skill. This type of postencounter exercise may have the student advocate for their patient with an attending physician, a social worker, or other provider. "Standardized attendings" (or other coworkers) can be trained to provide data and perspective on the student's performance as well.

The Faculty Evaluation

As students advance, it becomes more difficult to confine a definition of competence to simple tasks. It becomes much more important to know "how" skills were performed rather than simply "if" they were performed. As SP cases become more complex, the issue of what can and cannot be reliably evaluated by an SP also comes into play. Although an SP can be trained to reliably report if they were asked to consent to a surgical procedure—for example, training them to recognize each and every component of giving proper informed consent is both time and cost prohibitive. This is where faculty evaluations of student encounters become a very useful tool.

This is an example of a general faculty evaluation form[*] that can easily be adapted to different types of cases:

	Yes	No	Global Rating		
Professional Behavior					
1. Did the trainee introduce themselves?	☐	☐			
			1	2	3
2. Act with empathy?	☐	☐	☐	☐	☐
History-taking Skills					
3. Obtains the HPI correctly to include symptom nature, quality, duration, severity, and associated symptoms	☐	☐			
4. Asks about Past Med/Surg Hx?	☐	☐			
Notes:					
			1	2	3
5. History *NOT* taken: _____		☐	☐	☐	
Communication Skills					
6. Uses mostly open-ended questions?	☐	☐			
			1	2	3
7. Avoids leading or closed-ended questions? ("You don't have any fevers, do you?" Or "No problems in...?")	☐	☐	☐	☐	☐

[*] Faculty Feedback/Evaluation Form. Joseph O. Lopreiato, MD. Uniformed Services University.

Physical Examination Skills

			1	2	3
8. Focus on areas related to chief complaint?	☐	☐			
9. PE maneuvers done correctly?	☐	☐			
10. PE areas *OMITTED* _____			☐	☐	☐

Case Management

	Yes	No			
12. Did the trainee have a plan for this patient?	☐	☐			

13. Did the trainee explain the plan to the patient?	☐	☐	**Global Rating**		

			1	2	3
14. Avoids using medical jargon; explains DX and plan of action in layman's terms.	☐	☐	☐	☐	☐

Other Notes:

> 1 = Less skill than I expect for a student at this level. Will need some work here. Many omissions.
>
> 2 = Skill level is what I expect for a student at this level. Occasional omissions. Good to go.
>
> 3 = Better than I expect for a student at this level. No errors or omissions.

Review of Patient Note

NOTES:

	Yes	No			
15. Was the Hx recorded adequately? (No novels, contains HPI/PMHx/ pertinent positives and negatives)	☐	☐			
16. Was the PE documented correctly? (appropriate elements recorded for adequate chart review?)	☐	☐			
17. Did the assessment contain a differential?	☐	☐			

18. Was the correct Dx in the assessment or in the differential Dx?	☐	☐	**Global Rating**		

			1	2	3
19. Is the plan reasonable? (Not lots of tests—shotgun approach. Is the plan feasible in their medical setting?)	☐	☐	☐	☐	☐

Overall Rating

☐ Needs to repeat this station (Scores of 1 on two or more global ratings)
☐ Passes the station, but needs lots of feedback (Scores of 1 on only one global rating)
☐ Passes station to my satisfaction, no further feedback (No scores of 1 on any rating)

In the example earlier, note how there are ratings for each individual question and then "global" ratings for the overall performance in each domain. By providing benchmarks for the observer, it makes it easier to ensure that everyone is using the same criteria in evaluating each student.

This next example is of a faculty observation form for an advanced-level case for graduate nurses providing contraception counseling to an SP:

Contraception Case*

Student:_____Date:_____

Standardized Patient: _____**Room:**_____

Key: D—Done satisfactorily; U—Done unsatisfactorily; N—Not done

CIS (Communication and Interpersonal Skills)	2	1	0
Questioning skills			
Introduces him/herself and identifies themselves as an NP			
Gathers information systematically, does not jump around			
Interview/encounter structured with a clear beginning, middle, and end			
Uses transitional statements—sets context for each section of encounter			
Asks one question at a time			
Uses patient verbal and nonverbal clues to progress, listens without interrupting, and appropriate use of silence			
Questions/responses implying judgment—that put patient on the defensive (personal sensitive issues, i.e., smoking, drinking, sexual practice, weight)			
Critical Clinical Questions	**2**	**1**	**0**
LMP			
Menstrual history			
Obstetrical history			
Lactation history			
Gynecologic history			
Current contraceptive use			
Past contraceptive use			
Current sexual history			
Medications used/allergies			
Medical history			
Pertinent family history			
Tobacco/ETOH/drug use			
Desire for another pregnancy			
Impact of an unplanned pregnancy			
Spermicidal agents	**2**	**1**	**0**
Use			
Effectiveness: (Theoretical vs. Actual)			
Risk, benefits, side effects			
Impact on breast feeding			
Combined hormonal contraceptives	**2**	**1**	**0**
Use			
Effectiveness: (Theoretical vs. Actual)			
Risk, benefits, side effects			
Reviewed ACHES			
Impact on breast feeding			

* Contraceptive Counseling Evaluation form. Diane Seibert, PhD, CRNP. Uniformed Services University.

Progestin only contraceptive (POPs)	2	1	0
Use			
Effectiveness: (Theoretical vs. Actual)			
Risk, benefits, side effects			
Impact on breast feeding			
IUD	2	1	0
Use			
Effectiveness: (Theoretical vs. Actual)			
Risk, benefits, side effects			
Impact on breast feeding			

This complex checklist will give a very detailed perspective on the nurse's counseling technique and content. The lack of specific benchmarks on the evaluation form indicates an expectation that an experienced faculty member will be performing the evaluation—expected to judge not only if each item was discussed, but how thoroughly it was explained. Although it may seem like an exhaustive amount of detail, the benefit shows in the collection of data—any weak spots can be easily identified and feedback or remediation can be very individualized.

Putting It All Together

Once you have designed your evaluation tools, SP checklist, student postencounter, and faculty evaluation (if needed), it is time to complete the case. This is where you and your SP trainer will work together to make sure all needed information is contained in one package—that way, when you want to use this case again, you can rest assured that the case will appear just as it was designed to, even if the original case was written a few years prior.

ENCOUNTER INFORMATION

Length of Encounter:

Level of Learner

Case Domains:
   History?
   Physical Examination?
   Patient Counseling?
   Informed Consent?
   Communication Skills?
   Clinical Reasoning?
   Faculty Evaluation?

CASE INFORMATION

Domain: *Acute/Subacute/Chronic*

Diagnosis:

Gender:

Age:

Race:

Incompatible characteristics: *Does the patient have surgical scars that would contra-indicate the complaint, for example?*

Setting: *Clinic? ER? Counseling Center?*

General appearance: *Patient in gown or street clothes? In examination room chair, or on examination table? Is patient well-groomed or disheveled? Are there visible signs of illness or injury?*

Additional characters or confederates: *Is the patient accompanied by a family member? Will the student be expected to work with another provider (attending physician, social worker) during the encounter?*

Chief complaint:

Opening statement:

History of present illness:

Patient emotional affect: *Tense, upset, relaxed, evasive, etc.*

Onset of pain/complaint:

Location of pain/complaint:

Character/quality of pain/complaint:

Severity/pain scale:

Frequency of pain/complaint:

Duration of pain/complaint:

Aggravating factors:

Alleviating factors:

Associated symptoms:

Similar episodes:

Current medications:

PATIENT'S MEDICAL HISTORY

PATIENT'S SOCIAL HISTORY

Occupation:

Lifestyle:

Habits:
Alcohol
Tobacco
Drugs
Diet
Exercise
Sexual History

FAMILY HISTORY

PHYSICAL EXAMINATION RESULTS
Will the standardized patient be expected to show any physical signs of illness or injury (positive rebound tenderness, for example?) Are lab results or x-rays needed?

SCENARIO DEVELOPMENT
SP opening statement: *The first statement you would like the patient to make in response to the student's open-ended question "So what brings you in today?" "How can I help you?"*

Follow-up statement: *Any follow up statement you wish the SP to make if the student gives another open-ended statement: "Can you tell me more about that?"*

Standardized Patient Checklist
Example

Opening statement: *"I have been unusually tired lately."*

HISTORY:

Upon questioning by the student, I responded that:

History Checklist Items

Answer format: *yes/no, always/sometimes/never, done/not done/done incorrectly*

Physical Examination Checklist Items

Answer format: *yes/no, always/sometimes/never, done/not done/done incorrectly*

PATIENT/PHYSICIAN INTERACTION*

Please check appropriate box

The student: Please check appropriate box.

	*Outstanding	Very good	Good	Needs Improvement	Marginal	**Unacceptable
1. Appeared professionally competent—seemed to know what she/he was doing; inspired my confidence; appeared to have my interests at heart.						
2. Effectively gathered information—collected information in a way that seemed organized; began with several open-ended questions and progressed through interview using a balanced ratio of open- to closed-ended questions; summarized periodically.						
3. Listened actively—paid attention to both my verbal and nonverbal cues; used facial expressions/body language to express encouragement; avoided interruptions; asked questions to make sure they understood what I said.						
4. Established personal rapport—introduced self warmly; verbally/nonverbally showed interest in me as a person, not just my condition; avoided technical jargon.						

* Adapted from the East Tennessee State University Rating Form.

5. Appropriately explored my perspective—encouraged me to identify everything that I needed to say.						
6. Addressed my feelings—acknowledged and demonstrated interest in my expressed and unexpressed feelings and experience.						
7. Met my needs—worked toward a plan that addressed both the diagnosis and my concerns about my illness.						

	*Outstanding	Very good	Good	Needs Improvement	Marginal	**Unacceptable
1. As (patient name), rate your overall level of satisfaction with this student encounter.						

* Please provide specific examples of what this student did or said that prompted you to give them an "Outstanding" rating on this section.
** Please provide specific examples of what this student did or said that prompted you to give them a rating of "Unacceptable" on this section. If the student has two or more "unacceptable" ratings on this checklist, please inform the Standardized Patient Educator.

Student Postencounter:
Please use the space below to write your top 3 differential diagnoses:

Defend your #1 diagnosis on your list.

What additional tests/labs would you like to order?

An additional component of the case materials is the Doorway Information (or Student Instructions). This form should contain all information you want the student to know before beginning the encounter as well as any instruction you deem appropriate. An example:

Presenting Situation

PATIENT INFORMATION

Name:

Setting: Clinic

You are working in the Family Medicine Clinic. You have been asked to see *Patient Name*, who has come to the clinic complaining of *Chief Complaint*.

Vital Signs

BP:
Pulse:

Respiration:

Temperature:

Student Instructions

Tasks:
Take a relevant history.
Perform an appropriate physical examination.
Discuss assessment and plan.

Time limit: 15 minutes

Your SP educator is a valuable resource during case creation. Do not hesitate to call upon him or her to help you fill in the details beyond specific medical information. Although the amount of information asked for in the Case Template can appear overwhelming, most faculty report that the actual writing of case details, such as social history, is easier than expected because of their own history of seeing patients with this complaint in the past.

SP CASE EXAMPLES:

Case 1: Pediatric Telephone History/Parent Counseling

Level of learner: End-of-first-year nurse practitioner student

Notes: This case allows faculty to evaluate a student's telephone triage skills and allows standardized patients to report on the communication skills of the student with the added difficulty of a telephone conversation. This case is easily achieved by having the standardized patient in another room—the student's doorway information instructs him/her to call the parent and provides the telephone number. By placing the call on speaker, the faculty can hear and evaluate both sides of the conversation.

SP Training Summary—Helen H.

OPENING STATEMENT
My son Jackie has a fever and a cough. I know Dr. Brown says I call too often, but she said if he gets a fever it would be OK to call. I just want to be sure I'm doing the right things for the baby.

HISTORY OF PRESENT ILLNESS
You are Helen H. You are 22 years old and a first-time mother of 15-month-old Jackie H. (Date of Birth—_____). You have a high school education and no particular medical expertise. Because you were the youngest in your family but do not have any nieces or nephews, you do not have any experience with babies and children. You are not very articulate in volunteering detailed description of the baby's illness but are quite able to give specific answers to concrete questions. You are very open, polite, friendly but clearly very anxious and concerned.

Dr. Brown, a local pediatrician, has been caring for Jackie since his birth. You are very pleased with her services. You did not realize that you were asking for a lot of telephone advice from her and her office until about a week ago, when you called to ask about upcoming shots that would be needed and Dr. Brown told you that you were calling too often and that your questions would in most cases be covered in your regular visits. Jackie has been in good health since his birth with just one previous runny nose or cold when he was 6 months old. Jackie was a full-term, normal baby. He has no other health problems. He has never been in the hospital. He has no allergies that you know of. You only have one child. All three of you have lived together and have been healthy. Neither you nor your husband has any flu or cold symptoms.

---

* "Helen H[...]" (Pediatric Phone Triage). Arthur Jaffe, MD, Oregon Health Sciences University. Adapted from Richard Hawkins, MD, Graceanne Adamo, MA, CMA.

Yesterday morning Jackie seemed to have a cold. He had a cough but did not bring up any mucus or phlegm. He had a runny nose, with clear, colorless, watery drainage. He sneezed a lot. He felt warm all day, but you did not take his temperature until 8 p.m. last night. He was fussy and irritable all day. He had no appetite for food, but he drank his usual four bottles of Enfamil. About 12–14 hours ago, he started having fevers, starting at 8 p.m. yesterday evening with a temperature of 102°F. You took his temperature with a glass thermometer under the armpit. He tossed and turned all night and did not sleep very much at all. Jackie usually sleeps 10–12 hours a night and takes a 2-hour nap from 2 to 4 p.m. This morning, he has just been lying there and almost staring at you, but more like his eyes are not focusing—he "does not seem to be looking at me when I talk to him." He does not want any food or anything to drink at all. His diaper was damp this morning, but not soaked like it usually is in the morning. About 3 hours ago, you gave him a dose (1½ droppers) of children's Tylenol.

You are very worried now and really wanted to call the office a few hours ago but waited hoping that the Tylenol you gave Jackie would finally work. Jackie's temperature was 104 degrees when he woke up this morning and is still 104 degrees.

If asked by the physician on the telephone, you have not noticed any rash on Jackie but will check again now. You are very surprised to find a rash and describe it as about 15–20 tiny, dark red dots on his chest, belly, and back. Let the physician ask further question(s) about the rash and help you to describe it as follows: The dots are flat on the skin and do not fade when you push on them. Jackie is not scratching the rash.

If asked, Jackie does not seem to have any trouble breathing. If you are asked to count Jackie's respirations, you can count 7 to 9 breaths in 15 seconds.

SOCIAL HISTORY

You, your husband (Jackie's father, Jack), and Jackie live in a small apartment. Jack is a carpenter—*medically retired from the military, with lupus*. The place he works just went out of business, so he is unemployed right now, and your family went on public assistance. You, the mother, stay home with Jackie. You used to work as a checker at the local grocery store, but soon after the baby was born you quit. The child care bills were bigger than your paychecks, so now you stay home to take care of the baby.

Both you and your husband graduated high school.

You own a car.

The family has no pets and has not traveled anywhere recently.

FAMILY HISTORY AND SUPPORT SYSTEMS

Your husband is estranged from his family, but your father lives nearby. Your mother died of cervical cancer when you were 12 years old. Your dad has helped you a little financially since your husband lost his job.

SP Checklist—Helen H.

OPENING STATEMENT

My son Jackie has a fever and a cough. I know Dr. Brown says I call too often, but she said if he gets a fever it would be OK to call. I just want to be sure I'm doing the right things for the baby.

	History Checklist	Told Student	Did Not Tell Student
1.	I gave Jackie 1½ droppers of children's Tylenol about 3 hours ago, but it didn't help at all.	O	O
2.	He doesn't take any prescription medications.	O	O
3.	Last night around 8 p.m., his fever was102°, and now it is up to 104°! "Does he have a fever?" Or "What is his temperature?"	O	O
4.	I took his temperature under his arm with an electronic thermometer (from CVS). "How did you take his temperature?"	O	O
5.	He felt warm all day yesterday. "When did the fever start?"	O	O
6.	He's coughing and sneezing. "Any cold symptoms?" *"Is he sneezing?" "Is he coughing?"*	O	O
7.	His nose is running. It's clear stuff.	O	O
8.	His diaper was damp this morning, but not soaked like it usually is.	O	O
9.	When I rubbed his stomach to soothe him, he pulled his legs up like it hurt. "Does his stomach hurt?" Or "Does he have any stomach problems?"	O	O
10.	Yesterday, he only drank his Enfamil, today he won't eat or drink at all!	O	O
11.	I haven't noticed any rash.	O	O
12.	*When asked to check for a rash: Pause as if checking child.* There is a rash! There are 15–20 flat, tiny red spots on his back, stomach, and chest.	O	O
13.	He was fussy and irritable before, but for the past few hours he just lays there quietly. *"What is his mood like?" Or "How is he behaving?"*	O	O
15.	Jackie is 15 months old.		
16.	He has been healthy except for an occasional cold. "Has your child had any significant recent or past medical problems since birth?"		
14.	He seems to be staring straight ahead. I have to touch him or talk really loud to get him to respond to me. "Does he respond to you?" Or "Is he conscious?"	O	O

	Counseling Checklist	Done	Not Done
1.	The student explained that this could be a serious illness.	O	O
2.	The student told me that I did the right thing by calling.	O	O
3.	The student said that I should bring the child in to the clinic or emergency department immediately.	O	O

COMMUNICATION AND INTERPERSONAL SKILL RATING FORM

Please provide and label specific comments on any item for which you assign a *No/Unlikely/Unsatisfied* in the space provided under the *Comments* section below.

	Yes/ Likely/ Satisfied	No/ Unlikely/ Unsatisfied
1. The student identified themselves by surname and professional role.	O	O
2. The student treated me with respect.	O	O
3. The student addressed me by my surname.	O	O
4. The student seemed to care about me and my health.	O	O
5. I could easily understand what the student was saying.	O	O
6. The student used smooth, appropriate transitions and seemed organized.	O	O
7. The student listened carefully to me.	O	O
8. The student brought the encounter to a closure.	O	O
9. I understand what this student is planning to do for me.	O	O
10. I trust that this student will help me (confidence in student).	O	O
11. I would do what the student asked me to do (compliance with plan).	O	O
12. I would be willing to return to this student for care in the future.	O	O
13. Overall satisfaction with care.	O	O

Comments:

_____

_____

_____

_____

_____

Student Instructions

It is a "typical" busy morning in the Family Medicine clinic. Dr. Brown, the Family Medicine attending physician, has been called to another unit for an emergency.

You have been seeing many patients with "influenza-like" illnesses. As you rush out of one examination room to enter another, the clinic nurse stops you. She says that Mrs. H., one of Dr. Brown's patients, is calling about her son, Jackie, who has a fever. You do not know the H. family personally. Your nurse thinks you should call her back now (instead of during your lunch break) because this parent "seems very concerned." You enter the office to call Mrs. H. on your telephone extension.

You have 20 minutes to:

Use the telephone in the examination room.

Press the "Speaker" button on the telephone.

Room 1: Dial xxx-xxx-xxxx

Hang up by pressing "Speaker" again.

Case 2: Burning Urination/Sexual History and STD Counseling

This next case is more complex, appropriate for a second-year nurse practitioner student. Although there is no physical examination component to this case, the student will be expected to take a thorough sexual history, explain the need for specific tests, including invasive exams, and help the patient to feel comfortable disclosing potentially embarrassing information. The SP is asked to comment specifically if he felt that the nurse's attitude toward him changed as the circumstances surrounding his chief complaint become clear.

This case as written does not require the student to perform any invasive exams, but that can be adjusted based on the level of the learner.

The learner is expected to write a SOAP note and complete a self-assessment checklist after seeing the patient.

Standardized Patient Training Summary —Chris W.*

OPENING STATEMENT: "It kind of burns when I urinate."

CURRENT COMPLAINT
You are Christopher (Chris) W., a 40-year-old who has come to the clinic because you are experiencing a burning, stinging sensation when you urinate. This occurs as you initiate stream and urinate. The burning started about a week ago and is getting worse. Initially, the burning was just a minor annoyance, a 4 on a 1–10 scale (1 = no pain at all, 10 = extreme pain), now it is more uncomfortable and much more noticeable, maybe a 6. You also sometimes have a little of a feeling that you need to rush to the bathroom to urinate. This mild urge has only started in the last few days. A few days ago, you also noticed that your underwear briefs seem a little damp, but no discharge or discoloration. (This has happened at least once, but perhaps not only once.)

Your urine is the same color as it always is (yellow) and you are not urinating any more than usual (five to six times a day). You have not seen any blood in your urine. You do not have any pelvic pain, back pain, difficulty starting to urinate, or incontinence. You also do not have any diarrhea, nausea, vomiting, or constipation.

You have never had a problem like this before.

SOCIAL HISTORY
You are a building contractor living in (location). You retired from the Navy 5 years ago as a Lt. Commander.

You eat very healthy since you have always had to stay in shape. You always drink 8–10 glasses of water a day because you know that it is healthy to do so.

You run 5–10 miles a day. You do not smoke or use drugs.

Two weeks ago, you got married to Hannah. You and Hannah have been together for almost 4 years now.

You do not usually drink alcohol now, except once every few years when you are with a group of old Navy buddies.

Two weeks before you got married, your old Navy buddies threw you a crazy bachelor party. You have not seen many of these friends in years. Your buddies kidnapped you and flew you out to Las Vegas for the weekend. That weekend got "pretty wild and out of control." The guys, many of who still lead the swinging single life, arranged for a bunch of strippers on Saturday night. Everyone, including you, drank a lot. You cannot even remember how much you drank. You also cannot remember when you last drank that much. Although your memory of that night is pretty foggy, you do remember that you had sex with one of the strippers. You do not think you used a condom. You passed out in bed, and when you woke up the next morning, the room was a mess and the woman was gone.

Hannah does not know what happened, and you feel terrible about having betrayed her. Although you were very sexually active in your 20s, you have settled down since then. Except for this indiscretion with the stripper, you have been faithful to Hannah ever since you first started dating her 4 years ago.

---

* "Chris W[...]" (Burning Urination). Aileen Zanoni, Richard Hawkins, MD, Graceanne Adamo, MA, CMA, Deb Omori, MD, Eric Marks, MD, Amy Flanagan, MFA, Michelle Lavey, MSN, CRNP.

ADDITIONAL SEXUAL HISTORY

In the past 10 years, you have had three other sexual partners other than Hannah and the woman in Las Vegas (5 partners in 10 years). You have used condoms and were faithful to each of those women and still use condoms with Hannah. This stripper incident is your only incident of high-risk sexual behavior.

Because you are ashamed of what you did in Las Vegas and now because you are concerned about the burning urination, you have been avoiding sexual intimacy with Hannah ever since you returned from your honeymoon. (The burning urination started when you returned from the honeymoon.) Hannah is upset that you have been avoiding making love.

MEDICAL HISTORY

Other than an occasional cold or flu in past years, you have been especially healthy in the past and have no chronic medical problems.

As an active-duty Navy officer, you have a yearly physical. Your last one was about 6 months ago and everything was fine, including the routine HIV test.

FAMILY HISTORY

You are adopted, so you have no knowledge of your biological parents' medical history. Your adoptive parents are both healthy. Your adoptive father was a Navy officer.

TIMELINE:

Today	Came for a walk-in appointment to the ambulatory care clinic
2–3 days ago	Urgency Noticed an instance of damp underwear Pain increases = 6 out of 10
1 week ago	Returned from honeymoon Burning urination started Began avoiding sexual intimacy
2 weeks ago	Wedding Pain = 4 out of 10
4 weeks ago	Bachelor party in Las Vegas
6 months ago	Annual physical, including HIV test. All OK
4 years ago	Started dating Hannah exclusively

SP Checklist*

OPENING STATEMENT: "It kind of burns when I urinate."

HISTORY	YES	NO
Upon questioning by the nurse, I responded that:		
1. (Onset) The burning started about a week ago. *When did it start?*	O	O

* Adapted from Southern Illinois University, Office of Medical Education

2. (Progression) It's been getting worse (burns more).   O   O
   Has it gotten worse?

3. I've never had a problem like this (urinary) before.   O   O

4. My urine is the same color is always is.   O   O

5. I didn't see anything red in my urine.   O   O

6. I'm not urinating any more than usual (5–6 times/day).   O   O
   How often are you urinating?
   Are you urinating more than usual?

7. Well, when I go to the bathroom, I feel like
   I really need to go.   O   O
   Do you ever feel a need to rush to the bathroom?
   Any other symptoms? (Or any open-ended follow-up question)

8. I'm not sure. I did notice my briefs are a little damp.   O   O
   Have you noticed any discharge/pus?

9. My last HIV test at my yearly physical 6 mo. ago was fine.   O   O
   What were the results of your last HIV test?

10. I've never been *tested* for a sexually transmitted disease.   O   O
    Ever tested for sexually transmitted diseases (other than HIV)?

11. (Hx of condom use) I've almost always used condoms.   O   O
    Do you use condoms?
    Do you habitually use condoms?

12. (Recent condom use) I had unprotected sex right before
    I got married, but other than that,
    I've always used condoms.   O   O
    Have you recently had unprotected sex?
    Did you use a condom with the stripper?

13. "Yes, since our wedding." Just before I got married,
    I had sex with a stripper at my bachelor party. Otherwise,
    I've been in a monogamous relationship.   O   O
    Is your wife your only sexual partner?
    Any question about sexual partners

14. No, I'm always so safe. It's so out of character for
    me do something stupid.   O   O
    **Any other question about other high-risk sexual behaviors.
    Have you ever had sex with prostitutes or strippers (other than Las Vegas?)

COUNSELING CHECKLIST   **YES**   **NO**

The student discussed the following with me:

15. It is likely/possible that I have a sexually transmitted infection.   O   O

16. The rationale for testing for hepatitis/HIV.

17. That I should use/continue to use condoms with my wife   O   O
    until all of my test (STD/HIV) results come back.

EXAMINATION CHECKLIST
18. The student advised me that a specimen would need to be collected (either urine or penile swab).

If the student states that an examination is required of the genitalia or rectum, advise the student that results can be found in the drawer.

OPTIONAL QUESTION
Did you ever feel that the attitude of the nurse changed during the course of the encounter? If so, please describe *when* this occurred, *how* the nurse's attitude changed, and *how it made you feel*. Please feel free to mention positive or negative changes in attitude.

_____

_____

_____

_____

COMMENTS:

_____

_____

_____

_____

COMMUNICATION AND INTERPERSONAL SKILL RATING FORM

Please provide and label specific comments on any item for which you assign a *NO/Unlikely/Unsatisfied* in the attached *Comments* sheet as needed.

	YES /Likely /Satisfied	NO /Unlikely /Unsatisfied
1. The student identified his or herself by surname and professional role.	O	O
2. The student treated me with respect.	O	O
3. The student addressed me by my surname. *(Does not indicate confirming pt identity.)*	O	O
4. The student seemed to care about me and my health.	O	O
5. I could easily understand what the student was saying.	O	O
6. The student used smooth and appropriate transitions and seemed organized.	O	O
7. The student listened carefully to me.	O	O
8. The student brought the encounter to a close.	O	O
9. I trust that this student will help me (confidence in student).	O	O
10. I would be willing to return to this Student for care in the future	O	O
11. Overall satisfaction with care.	O	O

PATIENT INFORMATION/STUDENT INSTRUCTIONS
You are asked to see Chris W. who has come to walk-in appointments at the ambulatory care clinic complaining of urination problems.

Vital Signs:

Temperature 99.3°
BP   130/80
HR   86
RR   16

You are to:
Take a focused history.
Perform/discuss physical examination as appropriate.
Educate the patient as needed.
After the encounter, complete your SOAP note and computer checklist.

Student Name_____   Student #_____
Patient Name_____

POSTENCOUNTER FORM

Using the space provided, write a SOAP note for this patient.

SUBJECTIVE

OBJECTIVE

ASSESSMENT

PLAN

Student Self-Assessment Checklist

I asked the patient an open-ended question about why he was here.
"It kind of burns when I urinate."

HISTORY	YES	NO
I asked the patient:		
1. When the burning started (onset—about a week ago).	O	O
2. If it had gotten worse (progression—yes, burns more).	O	O
3. About prior history of current complaint (never had a problem like this before).	O	O
4. About change in color of urine (same as always).	O	O
5. If he'd seen blood or "red" (no).	O	O
6. About frequency of urinating (5–6 times/day).	O	O
7. About urgency—or any follow-up to #6 (do feel like I really need to go).	O	O
8. If he'd noticed any discharge/pus (not sure - noticed briefs a little damp.)	O	O
9. About results of his last HIV test, (at yearly physical 6 mo. ago, was fine).	O	O

10. If ever *tested* for a sexually transmitted disease other than
    HIV (no).   O   O

11. About history of condom use (almost always use condoms).   O   O

12. About recent condom use (had unprotected sex right before
    married, but other than that, always used condoms).   O   O

13. If monogamous/any question about sexual partners (monogamous since   O   O
    wedding, but before, had sex with a stripper at bachelor party).

14. About other high risk sexual behaviors/sex with prostitutes or strippers before.   O   O
    (No, always so safe. So out of character to do something stupid.)

COUNSELING   YES   NO

I told the patient:

15. It is likely/possible that he has a sexually transmitted infection.   O   O

16. Discussed the rationale for testing for Hepatitis/HIV.   O   O

17. He should continue to use condoms with his wife   O   O
    until all of his test (STD/HIV) results come back.

EXAMINATION CHECKLIST

18. I advised the patient that a specimen would need to be collected (either urine or   O   O
    penile swab).

OPTIONAL QUESTION
Did you ever feel that your attitude toward the patient changed during the course of the encounter?
If so, please describe *when* this occurred, *how* your attitude changed, and *if and how you think that
affected the patient's feelings.*

_____
_____
_____
_____

COMMENTS:
_____
_____
_____
_____

COMMUNICATION AND INTERPERSONAL SKILLS*

Place a check beside items that describe your encounter with the patient.

	YES /Likely /Satisfied	NO /Unlikely /Unsatisfied
1. I identified myself by surname and professional role (nursing student).	O	O
2. I treated the patient with respect.	O	O

*Adapted from Southern Illinois University, Office of Medical Education.

3. I addressed the patient by his surname.   O   O

4. I cared about the patient and his health.   O   O

5. I spoke in language easily understandable to the patient.   O   O

6. I used smooth, appropriate transitions, and seemed organized.   O   O

7. I listened carefully to the patient.   O   O

8. I brought the encounter to a close.   O   O

9. I confirmed that the patient understood what I intended to do for him.   O   O

10. I think this patient trusts (has confidence) that I will help him.   O   O

11. I think the patient will do (comply with) what I asked him to do.   O   O

12. I think this patient would be willing to return to me for care in the future.   O   O

13. Overall, I think the patient was satisfied with the care I provided to him.   O   O

Examination Results

Chris W.

Penile Swab—moderate amt yellowish discharge

Rectal Examination—no abnormal findings

Case 3: Nonaccidental Trauma

This is an even more complex case appropriate for graduate nurses nearing the end of their training. The student must interact with two standardized patients portraying a mother and son. He or she is then expected to take a history, to perform an appropriate physical examination, and upon discovery of signs of abuse, to deal with the heightened emotion of the mother and also counsel her on the correct procedure for informing Child Protective Services.

An interesting adjustment to this case would be to add a component where the student is required to present the findings to an attending physician or a Child Protective Services agent.

SP Training Summary —Peg R.*

You are Peg R., a _____-year-old woman with an 8- or 9-year-old son, Evan. Evan is your only child. You discovered that you were pregnant with him shortly after you ended your marriage with Evan's father, Matt; you had no contact with him after telling Matt you were pregnant. When Evan was born, your ex-husband listed Evan as his legal dependent, and so Evan has access to military health care. Other than that, Matt has never tried to have a relationship with Evan or offered you child support. Matt was a Private First Class in the Army when you divorced. You do not know what rank he is now or what he does in the Army, other than he is still active duty. You do not have any idea where he is.

* "Peg and Evan R[...]" (Nonaccidental trauma). Sue Spachimann, Lindsey Lane MD. Adapted from Joseph O. Lopreiato, MD, and Amy Flanagan, MFA. Sue and Lindsey adapted the case from Joseph and Amy.

You work as a florist and own a small floral shop and greenhouse that your parents started years ago. Your parents are now retired and live in Delaware. They love you and Evan and try to see you often, but with school, your work, and everything else, months can go by between visits. You will often take work home and stay up at nights putting together arrangements to make as much money as possible. You do not get a lot of sleep. You try to be home by 4:15 p.m., when Evan arrives home from school, but it is not always possible. You really do not have any kind of support system to help you with Evan: his grandparents are too far away to help with child care; you do not know any other families in the area. You really do not have any kind of a social life and never get a chance to do anything fun on your own. You love Evan completely, but you are really burned out and cannot see anything positive happening.

Evan is in the third grade at (location) Elementary School. He struggled in first and second grade and is now having a really tough time. His favorite subject is science, but all of his grades are poor, especially in reading. The school psychologist has contacted you about Evan's grades and he's been scheduled for a "complete evaluation" in about two weeks. You're not sure what that means or what they'll be evaluating. Evan says that "the other kids don't like me" and although he's never been disciplined for fighting at school, he will come home cut up and bruised sometimes. He broke his arm while climbing trees in the first grade, sprained his ankle last year while riding his bike, and got a large cut on his head once. You really do not remember how he got the cut on his head. He did not have to get stitches for the cut.

Today was a school in-service day, so you have been working from home. Evan has been running in and out of the apartment, playing with friends, generally being loud and messy and demanding. Right after lunch, you noticed that he was being really quiet. You found Evan in the corner of the living room. He looked guilty and when you asked what he was doing, he ran out of the room. You noticed that the edge of the living room rug was charred and smoldering, and you realized that Evan had been playing with matches and set the rug on fire.

In that moment, you lost it. You ran after Evan, grabbed him by the arm, picked up the first thing you saw (the electrical cord on the vacuum cleaner), and whipped him on his torso three times with the cord. He screamed really loudly and you realized that you had really hurt him. Hearing him scream brought you back to your senses. You cried and hugged him for a long time and kept telling him how sorry you were. Evan let you hug and rock him for a while, and in a way, that scared you even more—he's been growing up and not wanting as much physical affection from you as he once did.

After you cooled down you started to get really worried about what you had done. Evan has been really quiet since you hit him, which is not like him at all. You offered him ice cream as an apology and he said he was not hungry. He is always hyper and always active, loud when he's happy and even louder when he's sad or angry. You kept checking the marks on his stomach and back, and as they started to get more bruised, you became more worried and called the pediatric clinic to see if you could bring him in "because he has a cold." They had a free appointment space and so you bundled Evan into the car and brought him right here.

Evan did have a cough and runny nose a few days ago, but it did not seem to bother him much and it's been getting progressively better. You could not think of anything else to tell the receptionist on the telephone, so you said his cold has been getting worse. As you're sitting in the office right now, you really do not know what to say, so you keep insisting that you're worried because his cold is worse, he does not want to eat, and "he's not himself."

You do not mention anything about the whipping unless the physician lifts Evans shirt for the physical examination and discovers the welts. When the doctor asks you about the whip marks, you break down and begin telling the doctor everything: "I just lost control...he was playing with matches and scorched the rug...I didn't even realize what I was doing until it was too late..."

You are ashamed, but you answer all the doctor's questions truthfully. When the doctor mentions the need to contact Social Services, you become panicked and try to bargain with him or her: "Please don't call anybody...I swear, I have never done anything like this before and I will never again...that's why I brought him here, because I love him and want him to be okay...if you call them, they will take him away from me!"

The Family Nurse Practitioner student should:

Stand firm and not back down from the decision to call Social Services.

Explain to you why there is a need to call Social Services, and that he or she has a legal obligation to call;

Give you details about the process and let you know what to expect;

Discuss the need for you to have help and a support system for yourself.

Child: Moulage, three whip marks on back, do not use child's real mother so it is clear that this is an acting, child should have a handheld game or cell phone game that he plays with while he tries to ignore the interaction between the mother and student.

Standardized Patient Checklist		
History (Hx)		

"Evan started a cold a few days ago, but he seems much worse today."

Upon questioning by the FNP, we responded that:
COMMUNICATION AND INTERPERSONAL SKILL RATING FORM

1. He started with a runny nose about 3 days ago.	[ ] Yes	[ ] No
2. He does have a cough, and it sounds a lot worse today.	[ ] Yes	[ ] No
*3. The resident asked Peg about the whip marks. (Peg: I just can't take him anymore...)	[ ] Yes	[ ] No
4. I just lost it...he was playing with matches, he knows that's not allowed ever, and he scorched the rug.	[ ] Yes	[ ] No
5. It was the vacuum cleaner cord. I just grabbed it without thinking.	[ ] Yes	[ ] No
6. No, I've never even spanked him before. I'm not that kind of mom!	[ ] Yes	[ ] No
7. Evan's really hyper and he's tough to control. I'm the only one at home and it's really hard.	[ ] Yes	[ ] No
In response to the FNP asking if you have stresses in your life.		
8. He's always bringing home bad report cards and notes from teachers.	[ ] Yes	[ ] No
9. They scheduled him for an evaluation with the school psychologist. It's not for another two weeks.	[ ] Yes	[ ] No
*10. He's a kid... broke his arm climbing a tree in first grade, sprained his ankle riding bikes, cut his head once doing I don't know what.... Evan, honey, how did you cut your head that time? Evan: Don't know.	[ ] Yes	[ ] No
11. No, I've never done any drugs! I would never do anything like that!	[ ] Yes	[ ] No
12. My husband and I divorced before Evan was born. I don't know where he is. He's never wanted to help with Evan.	[ ] Yes	[ ] No
13. Comments on the checklist above: (NS)		
Physical Examination (Px)		
The Nurse:		
14. Washed his or her hands before beginning the physical examination or putting on gloves.	[ ] Yes	[ ] No
*15. Undressed Evan, or lifted up his shirt to examine his chest.	[ ] Yes	[ ] No
16. Inspected skin on upper extremities.	[ ] Yes	[ ] No
17. Inspected skin on lower extremities.	[ ] Yes	[ ] No
18. Palpated Evan's rib cage.	[ ] Yes	[ ] No

19. Palpated upper extremities.	[ ] Yes	[ ] No
20. Palpated lower extremities.	[ ] Yes	[ ] No
21. Comments on physical examination: (NS)		
Counseling (Cx)		
The FNP student:		
Involved Evan in the history taking at least twice.	[ ] Yes	[ ] No
Asked Peg about social support (I'm the only one at home…I don't know where his father is…school planning an evaluation)	[ ] Yes	[ ] No
*The FNP explained to me (Peg) about the need and obligation to involve social services.	[ ] Yes	[ ] No
The FNP gave details about the social services process and what we should expect to happen.	[ ] Yes	[ ] No
*The FNP responded FIRMLY in the negative when I challenged him or her not to report the abuse.	[ ] Yes	[ ] No
The FNP discussed with me the need for me to have support with Evan.	[ ] Yes	[ ] No
Comments: (NS)		

Please provide and label specific comments on any item for which you assign an *Unsatisfactory* in the space provided under the *Comments* section below.

COMMENTS:

	Satisfactory	Unsatisfactory
The learner identified himself/herself by surname and professional role.		
The learner treated me/my child with respect.		
The learner addressed me by my surname.		
The learner seemed to care about my child and my child's health.		
I could easily understand what the learner was saying.		
The learner used smooth, appropriate transitions and seemed organized.		
The learner listened carefully to me and my child.		
The learner brought the encounter to a close.		
I understand what this learner is planning to do for me and my child.		
I trust that this learner will help my child (confidence in learner).		
I would do what the learner asked us to do (compliance with plan).		
I would be willing to return to this learner for care in the future.		
Total		

Adapted from the Office of Medical Education, Southern Illinois University

PATIENT INFORMATION

You are asked to see 7-year-old Evan R., who presents with his mother, Peg R. Mrs. R. says that Evan has had a runny nose and cough for the past few days but that the symptoms worsened today and she became worried. Mrs. R. has noticed that Evan is quieter, has lost his appetite, and "just doesn't seem like himself."

Vital Signs:

Temperature: 99.0°F
Pulse: 100
RR: 18
BP: 115/70

YOU ARE TO:

Take a focused history.
Perform an appropriate physical examination.
Answer Mrs. R.'s questions and provide appropriate counseling.

SUGGESTED READINGS

Barrows, H. (1993). An overview of the uses of standardized patients for teaching and evaluating clinical skills. *Academic Medicine, 68*(6), 443–453.

Cohen, D. S., Colliver, J. A., Marcy, M. S., Fried, E. D., & Swartz, M. H. (1996). Psychometric properties of a standardized-patient checklist and rating-scale form used to assess interpersonal and communication skills. *Academic Medicine, 71*(Suppl. 1), S87–S89.

Eaton, J.A. & Cappiello, J.D. (1998). *A day in the office: Case studies in primary care.* St. Louis, MO: Mosby.

Ebbert, D. W., & Connors, H. (2004). Standardized patient experiences: evaluation of clinical performance and nurse practitioner student satisfaction. *Nursing Education Perspectives, 25*(1), 12–155.

Kaiser, S., & Bauer, J. J. (1995). Checklist self-evaluation in a standardized patient exercise. *American Journal of Surgery, 169*(4), 418–420.

O'Connor, F., Albert, M., & Thomas, M. D. (1999). Incorporating standardized patients into a psychosocial nurse practitioner program. *Archives of Psychiatric Nursing, 13*(5), 240–247.

Yoo, M. S., & Yoo, I. L. (2003). The effectiveness of standardized patients as a teaching method for nursing fundamentals. *Journal of Nursing Education, 42*(10), 444–448.

CHAPTER 17

Human Simulation for Nurse Anesthesia

Lewis Bennett and Ferne Cohen

A Certified Registered Nurse Anesthetist (CRNA) is a registered professional nurse who is educated at the master's, postmaster's, or doctoral level in the advanced nursing specialty of nurse anesthesia. According to the Annual Report from the Council on Accreditation (2010), of the 108 nurse anesthesia programs currently in the United States, 96% offer a master's degree and 3% of the programs are at the doctoral level. Fifty-seven percent are within a nursing department and 12% fall within health sciences (Council on Accreditation, Annual Report 2010). All programs are accredited by the Council on Accreditation of Nurse Anesthesia Educational Programs, which provides quality assurance of the educational process and compliance with the standards for accreditation. To be eligible to practice, graduates must pass the national certification examination and are then certified as a CRNA. CRNAs have been administering high-quality anesthesia care in the United States since the middle of the 19th century. As the first professional group to administer anesthesia care, nurse anesthetists practice in a variety of clinical settings including hospitals, ambulatory surgery centers, pain clinics, and physicians' offices. CRNAs are the largest provider of anesthesia care for U.S. military personnel and deliver most of the anesthesia care in rural hospitals as solo practitioners (American Association of Nurse Anesthetists, n.d.). In the United States, approximately 40,000 CRNAs practice in collaboration with anesthesiologists, surgeons, and other health care providers to administer more than 30 million anesthetics each year (American Association of Nurse Anesthetists, n.d.). A recent study by Dulisse and Cromwell (2010) confirmed that "CRNAs provide safe, high-quality" cost-effective anesthesia care. "The analysis of Medicare data for 1999 to 2005, encompassing more than 481,000 hospitalizations, found that allowing CRNAs to work independently without oversight by an anesthesiologist or surgeon had little or no effect on mortality and morbidity rates" (Dulisse & Cromwell, 2010, p. 1469). Although "CRNAs practice according to their expertise, state statutes and regulations, and institutional policy" (American Association of Nurse Anesthetists, 2010, p. 2), the scope of practice can be delineated into four general areas. These include (1) preanesthesia assessment and formulation of anesthesia plan of care, (2) intraoperative or procedural anesthetic management, (3) postanesthesia care, and (4) perianesthesia (anesthesia related) clinical support services outside the operating room (Jordan, 1994; http://www.aana.com/qualifications.aspx). In addition to providing high-quality anesthesia care as clinicians, nurse anesthetists pursue other roles in education, research, administration, and business (Waugaman, 1994, p. 17).

SIMULATION

Since the early 1960s, the military, nuclear engineering, and aviation industries have used simulation. The military uses simulation to mimic war situations, which aids in training, critical thinking, and decision-making and improved technical skills. Simulation in nuclear engineering is used to simulate a nuclear power plant reactor accident, promoting the development of risk analysis awareness (Galloway, 2009; Glasstone, 1994; Macedonia, Gherman, & Satin, 2003). Aviation's use of simulation exposes pilots to flight maneuvers involved in air combat and provides the opportunity to react to in-flight emergencies; this improves critical thinking skills and has been used to help avoid air disasters (Brown, 1976).

The literature includes multiple studies validating the use of simulation to teach concepts in a realistic environment (Beaubien & Baker, 2004; Durham & Alden, 2008; Farnsworth, Egan, & Johnson, 2000; Feingold, Calaluce, & Kallen, 2004; Fort, 2010; Gaba & DeAnda, 1988), which "enhances both acquisition and retention of knowledge, sharpens critical thinking and psychomotor skills, and is more enjoyable" (Raven, 2004, p. 50). As such, there have been movements to integrate these experiences into the health care program's curriculum because it provides "risk-free practice (for students)...and to teach, practice, and/or evaluate critical thinking skills" (Raven, 2004, p. 47). The literature identifies two broad types of simulation that flow on a continuum from low-to high-fidelity simulation (see Figure 17.1). Beaubien and Baker (2004) note that learning

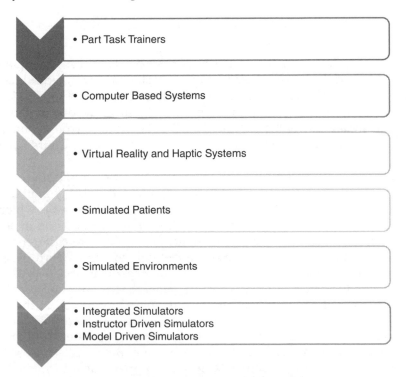

Figure 17.1 *Classification of simulators.*
Source: Adapted from Maran and Glavin (2003).

outcomes are not always correlated to the level of simulation but are more related to the execution of the simulated experience.

According to Beaubien and Baker (2004, p. 52), fidelity simulation consists of three components, which can be manipulated to achieve the desired competencies of the controlled learning experience.

1. Environment fidelity is measured by how similar the audio, visual, and olfactory components of the simulated environment models the replicated clinical setting.
2. Equipment fidelity is evaluated by how authentic the simulated equipment is when matched against the actual equipment.
3. Psychological fidelity inculcates the belief that the simulated experience is genuine when compared with the clinical setting.

The use of simulation has several advantages for the learner, as the experience provides the ability to (a) perform tasks in a real environment without the risk of patient harm caused by inexperience, indecision, or insecurity; (b) learn from an error and immediately repeat the task utilizing the correct methodology; (c) gain experience in emergency scenarios that are critical but infrequent; and (d) teach teamwork among professionals engaged in critical fields so roles are identified and communication skills are enhanced (Beaubien & Baker, 2004; Durham & Alden, 2008; Maran & Glavin, 2003). Durham and Alden (2008, p. 12) note that simulation also benefits the faculty member, as it promotes student–faculty interaction in a dynamic and mutually beneficial learning environment that increases job satisfaction.

USE OF SIMULATION IN NURSE ANESTHESIA

The use of simulation in the field of nurse anesthesia has grown exponentially over the past several years as it provides "opportunities for standardized, reproducible critical events in a realistic and safe environment" (Gaba & DeAnda, 1988, pp. 387). Although the use of simulation as a learning tool is growing in the field of nurse anesthesia and an increasing number of lectures on the topic are noted at professional anesthesia conferences, the number of publications related to simulation in nurse anesthesia is sparse.

The incorporation of both low- and moderate-fidelity simulation into the nurse anesthesia curriculum at Drexel University began in 2005. Newly matriculated students are enrolled in a 10-week course titled Overview of Anesthesia, which includes a 20-hour didactic lecture component followed by weekly hands-on experiences in the simulation laboratory. Each week, students are exposed to different features of anesthesia in a controlled learning environment, which begins with the perioperative overview and includes the intraoperative management of aspects such as airway management, induction, maintenance, emergence, and neuraxial insertion techniques. Most of the student's experience in simulation involves the use of task trainers, which provide repetitive "hands-on" experience to increase proficiency in a particular skill set. Task trainers are considered low-tech trainers and are designed to assist in teaching basic training skills (Beaubien & Baker, 2004). Most task trainers are used to simulate a particular body part or anatomical location. The Nurse Anesthesia program utilizes an airway mannequin and a regional mannequin as adjuncts to the didactic lectures. These task trainers provide first-year students with the opportunity to practice the skills of airway management, such as mask ventilation, intubation, and laryngeal mask airway insertion. In the second year, central line mannequins are utilized to teach ultrasound-guided central vascular access techniques to students before the open heart clinical experience. Although task trainers do not promote proficiency in these tasks, they introduce the student to the skill before entering the clinical practicum. For the novice student, the experience gained from the repetitive performance of the task, such as managing an airway, performing a regional technique, or inserting a central line catheter, increases confidence and technical skills and decreases anxiety when these newly acquired tasks are attempted in the clinical environment (Henrichs, Rule, Grady, & Ellis, 2002).

The Nurse Anesthesia program also incorporates high-fidelity simulation, utilizing Laerdal's SimMan. SimMan's capabilities include cardiopulmonary functions and voice interaction. This provides the student with the ability to respond to the simulated scenario by implementing various interventions and examining the effects of these decisions or indecisions in a controlled environment. The realism of the simulated experience may aid in decreasing students' fears, stress, and anxiety when experiencing a similar patient scenario in the clinical area. SimMan is utilized to simulate the induction, maintenance, and emergence phases of anesthesia and also introduces students to basic complications, such as hemodynamic lability or respiratory compromise. In 2011, a simulated monitored anesthesia care (MAC) case scenario will be added to the curriculum because these are the typical cases that first-year students are exposed to when beginning the clinical practicum. A MAC simulation experience will expose students to the challenges of titrating sedatives, analgesics, and hypnotics to avoid undesirable effects, such as airway obstruction, apnea, or hypotension and achieve the desired effect of a relaxed, sedated patient who minimally responds to surgical stimulation yet is easily arousable.

The varied critical scenarios that can be programmed using SimMan or Medical Education Technologies, Inc. (METI) provides the anesthesia trainee with the ability to practice specific anesthesia skills in a safe, simulated environment; however, the remainder of this chapter will focus on the standardized patient (SP) experience during the preoperative anesthetic evaluation and includes experience design, administrator's concerns, challenges, and evaluation feedback.

THE SP EXPERIENCE

SPs were first introduced by Barrows and Abrahamson in 1964. The SPs are usually paid actors; however, some institutions use students, faculty, or former patients. Typically, the SPs are not trained in health care and have no previous medical knowledge (Levine & Swartz, 2008). The SP provides students with the opportunity to interview and assess a live actor in an environment that simulates the preoperative anesthesia period. This experience can help decrease stress, increase confidence, and enhance communication skills before performing a preoperative assessment on an actual patient in the clinical area. May, Park, and Lee (2009, p. 490) performed a review of the literature over a 10-year period from 1996 to 2005 and determined that the "educational use of SPs was indeed valuable, from both self-reported scores as well as more objective data such as higher scores on performance examinations." They recommended that "future research should focus on the impact of using SPs on change in behavior or change in patient outcomes or change in health systems. More rigorous designs with randomized control or comparison groups, multicenter studies, and triangulation through use of both qualitative and quantitative studies could overcome the weakness or intrinsic bias."

In 2010, the Nurse Anesthesia program incorporated the SP experience into the curriculum to expose novice students to the preoperative interview before beginning the clinical practicum. The SP experience was designed to build on the student's didactic knowledge and provide students with a real-life patient to interview in a simulated environment with the goal of enhancing communication skills and self-confidence and creating comfort with the patient assessment.

Before the implementation of this experience into the curriculum, the faculty began planning in 2009 and considered the following issues to evaluate the feasibility as well as the cost–benefit of the added experience:

a. Scheduling of the simulation laboratory—the availability of the laboratory and actors—was a concern because of the extremely heavy use of the laboratory. Approximately 6 months before the proposed scheduled time frame, the anesthesia faculty met with the director of the Center for Interdisciplinary Clinical Simulation and Practice to discuss the details of the experience for the nurse anesthesia students. It was determined that a cohort of 20 students would require 5 SP actors and that 30 minutes per encounter would be needed to complete 1 full session of the SP experience (a session is defined as 15 minutes for the student to perform a preoperative assessment with the patient actor, 5 minutes for the actor to complete a 10-question evaluation (Appendix 17.A) of the student's performance, 5 minutes for the actors to provide feedback to the student and a 5-minute break for the actors between sessions).

b. Schedule of the SP encounter—the faculty formulated a schedule to accommodate 20 students that were divided into 5 groups (Appendix 17.B). Each group interviewed an SP actor who was simulating a patient from 1 of 5 different scenarios. For example, group 1 interviewed a 56-year-old woman undergoing a right total knee replacement, whereas group 2 interviewed a 29-year-old man scheduled for a right knee arthroscopy (Appendix 17.C).

c. Expense of actors—the actors are compensated at a rate of $20.00 per hour, which is incorporated into the student's simulation fee. During training sessions, the actors are paid for the actual number of hours associated with the training; however, the actors are paid a minimum of 4 hours per SP encounter. The actors were scheduled for training from 8:00 to 9:00 a.m., with the SP experience scheduled from 9:30 to 11:30 a.m. The 5 actors were each paid $100 for the entire SP encounter.

d. Time constraints—because of the amount of content in the current curriculum, integrating additional experiences is quite challenging. However, the faculty felt that the experience would prove to be quite beneficial, so after review of the curriculum, it was determined that the SP experience would be integrated into the ninth week of the first 10-week quarter. This would provide the students the time to obtain the didactic lectures on preoperative patient assessment, imparting the theory needed before the SP experience.

e. SP scenarios—the patient scenarios, which included past medical, surgical, and anesthesia history and current medications, were distributed to the SP actors for review approximately one week before the scheduled experience. The scenarios were developed based on the didactic lecture material and given that students had never interviewed patients from an anesthetic perspective, the surgical procedures included in the scenario were "bread and butter" type cases and the comorbid disease processes were not complex. To expose the students to the three different types of anesthetic techniques (general, regional, and MAC), each patient scenario included a different surgical procedure. The information gathered by the student during the SP interview would provide the foundation required to develop a patient-specific anesthesia care plan.

The first set of SP experiences was scheduled to begin at 9:30 a.m. Faculty met with the patient actors at 8:00 a.m. to review the scenarios, clarify their roles, and answer any questions. At 8:45 a.m. the faculty met with the students during the prebriefing to review the expectations for the SP experience. The students were provided with a template of questions to guide the preoperative interview, and the importance of maintaining eye contact and establishing a rapport was also emphasized. Finally, students were informed that the SP experience would be videotaped and they would have access to the recording the following day. All students received an e-mail from the Center for Interdisciplinary Clinical Simulation and Practice the day after the encounter, which included an individual ID, password, and web-link to the recording. All students previously signed a photo consent form, which included the use of videotape recording.

At 9:25 a.m., the actors were situated in the examination room while the students waited outside for the announcement to begin the experience. At 9:30 a.m., an overhead announcement was made and the students entered the room. Upon entering the room, students were expected to wash their hands and introduce themselves as a student registered nurse anesthetist from the anesthesia department. The students then proceeded to interview the patient to assess past medical, surgical, and anesthesia history and inquire about current medication therapy. A physical assessment was also performed to auscultate heart and lung sounds. The students reviewed the informed surgical consent with the patient to ensure that it listed the correct procedure, identified their surgeon, and that it was signed by the patient. Once the assessment was complete, the student briefly discussed the various anesthetic options appropriate for the patient's history and surgical procedure and answered any questions asked by the patient actors. The student also educated the patient on the importance of not eating or drinking anything after midnight the night before the scheduled procedure. Upon completion of the interview, the students were instructed to wash their hands and exit the room. Two nurse anesthesia faculty members observed the students during the 15-minute preanesthesia assessment patient interview from the control room. Faculty had both audio and video access during the student interview, with the ability to toggle between each of the 5 examination rooms (Figure 17.2).

At the completion of the interview, the actors had five minutes to complete an online evaluation of the student's performance. Once the evaluation was complete, the students re-entered the room to obtain feedback from the SP actor regarding their performance. Upon conclusion of the experience, each group of five students met with the anesthesia faculty for a short debriefing to review the overall group performance, with comments that included the following:

1. A few students needed to establish more eye contact.
2. Two students did not wash their hands at the end of the experience.

3. One student was unable to answer questions about the type of anesthesia, which did not instill confidence in the patient. Establishing a rapport is an important component of the patient interview process.
4. Three students did not introduce themselves to the SP actor as a student registered nurse anesthetist.

The 15-minute interview, as well as the 5-minute period allotted for the actors to complete the evaluation, was videotaped. The recorded session was made available online for a 2-week period for the students to review, which they accessed with their individual ID and password.

After the SP experience, the students had one week to research the disease process, the surgical procedure and anesthetic implications and develop an anesthetic care plan to present to their classmates. The following week, the students were placed in groups based on the patient scenario. Each student discussed his or her plan under the guidance of the anesthesia faculty who provided feedback related to the care plans and discussed other anesthetic options the students may not have considered. It was interesting to hear the various anesthesia techniques that students selected to administer to the same patient. For example, some students selected a regional technique to administer for the total knee scenario whereas others chose general anesthesia. It was

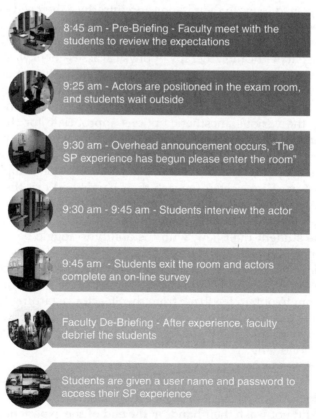

8:45 am - Pre-Briefing - Faculty meet with the students to review the expectations

9:25 am - Actors are positioned in the exam room, and students wait outside

9:30 am - Overhead announcement occurs, "The SP experience has begun please enter the room"

9:30 am - 9:45 am - Students interview the actor

9:45 am - Students exit the room and actors complete an on-line survey

Faculty De-Briefing - After experience, faculty debrief the students

Students are given a user name and password to access their SP experience

Figure 17.2 *SP timeline.*

an excellent student learning experience as they witnessed that practitioners may opt to manage the same patient scenario differently, which is a challenging concept for a novice student to grasp. Having this experience before entering the clinical practicum is invaluable.

STUDENT FEEDBACK

The review of the student evaluations of the SP experience indicated that all students found the experience to be extremely beneficial and that they were more comfortable when having to perform a preoperative assessment in the clinical practicum. A few student comments included the following:

- "Great experience," "very realistic"
- "I was extremely nervous, not knowing what to expect"
- "It was so realistic that it didn't seem like I was in a simulated experience"
- "The SP experience really helped to combine theory to application"
- "The SP experience offered a great opportunity for the students to learn"
- "The SP experience was a great introduction to what we will do in clinical"
- "Having the day with the SP actors was a good way to learn how to do an anesthesia preoperative interview"
- "I really liked the day with the SP actors and I think the tradition should continue for next year"

Most students also indicated that they reviewed their recorded session online, which provided additional feedback related to their interaction with the SP actor.

LESSONS LEARNED

Upon review of the student and faculty evaluations of the SP experience, the future recommendations include the following:

1. The need for the students to wear scrubs and white laboratory coats to simulate appropriate operating room attire. When planning for the SP experience, the faculty did not consider the students' attire and the students wore street clothes, which could have decreased the "realistic feeling" of the experience. Environmental and psychological fidelity are key components that add to the realism of the experience, increasing skills, knowledge, and self-confidence, which can carry over into the student's clinical performance.
2. The need to video record the feedback period when the actors meet with the students to discuss the student's performance. This part of the session was not recorded, which was an oversight and will be incorporated for the 2011 experience. The faculty and director of the SP laboratory believe that having the ability to review the evaluation online provides the opportunity to analyze the SP interaction and gain further insight regarding their performance, which will enhance the student's overall experience.

3. The need for a more detailed and personalized debriefing after the SP encounter. For 2011, the Nurse Anesthesia faculty will review the videotaped interview with each student and provide individual feedback on their performance. According to Stafford (2005, p. 1083), "Debriefing allows for discharge of emotion and capturing the learning." Reviewing the videotape session with the student may help them see how they "actually" performed during the interview session, as opposed to how they "imagine" they performed. This debriefing period would also provide time for the faculty to obtain feedback from the students regarding their perception as to the realism of the SP experience.

CONCLUSIONS

Simulation in anesthesia can be a valuable learning tool that enables the student to learn and practice newly acquired tasks before the actual performance in the clinical environment. Although various types of simulators have been used in anesthesia training programs, the literature addressing the advantages of SP actor encounters for nurse anesthesia students to perform a preoperative patient assessment is limited. The SP experience, in conjunction with didactic lectures and classroom discussion and collaboration, can increase the student's confidence, decrease anxiety, and enhance student–patient communication skills, easing the transition into the clinical practicum.

REFERENCES

American Association of Nurse Anesthetists. (n.d.). *Certified registered nurse anesthetists (CRNAs) at a glance*. Retrieved from http://www.aana.com/ataglance.aspx

American Association of Nurse Anesthetists. (2010). Scope and standards for nurse anesthesia practice. Retrieved from http://www.aana.com/qualifications.aspx

Beaubien, J., & Baker, D. (2004). The use of simulation for training teamwork skills in health care: How low can you go? *Quality and Safety in Health Care, 13*(1), 51–56.

Brown, J. L. (1976). Visual elements in flight simulation. *Aviation, Space, and Environmental Medicine, 47*, 913–914.

Dulisse, B., & Cromwell, J. (2010). No harm found when nurse anesthestists work without supervision by physicians. *Health Affairs, 29*(8), 1569–1575.

Durham, C., & Alden, K. (2008). Enhancing patient safety in nursing education through patient simulation. In R. G. Hughes (Ed.), *Patient safety and quality. An evidence-based handbook for nurses* (pp. 1–26). Rockville, VA: Agency for Healthcare Research and Quality.

Farnsworth, S. T., Egan, T. D., & Johnson, S. E. (2000). Teaching sedation and analgesia with simulation. *Journal of Clinical Monitoring and Computing, 16*(4), 273–285.

Feingold, C. E., Calaluce, M., & Kallen, M. A. (2004). Computerized patient model and simulated clinical experiences: Evaluation with baccalaureate nursing students. *Journal of Nursing Education, 43*(4), 156–163.

Fort, C. (2010). So good it's unreal: The value of simulation education. *Nursing Management, 41*(2), 22–25.

Gaba, D. M., & DeAnda, A. A. (1988). Comprehensive anesthesia simulation environment: Re-creating the operating for research and training. *Anesthesiology, 69*, 387–394.

Galloway, S. J. (2009). Simulation techniques to bridge the gap between novice and competent healthcare professionals. *Online Journal of Issues in Nursing, 14*(2), Manuscript 3.

Glasstone, S. (1994). *Nuclear reactor engineering* (4th ed., p. 488). New York: Chapman & Hall.

Henrichs, B., Rule, A., Grady, M., & Ellis, W. (2002). Nurse anesthesia students' perceptions of the anesthesia patient simulator: A qualitative study. *AANA Journal, 70*(3), 219–225.

Levine, A. I., & Swartz, M. H. (2008). Standardized patients: The "other" simulation. *Journal of Critical Care Issue, 23*(2), 179–184.

Macedonia, C. R., Gherman, R. B., & Satin, A. J. (2003). Simulation laboratories for training in obstetrics and gynecology. *Obstetrics & Gynecology, 102*(2), 388–392.

Maran, N. J., & Glavin, R. J. (2003). Low- to high-fidelity simulation—A continuum of medical education? *Medical Education, 37*, 22–28.

May, W., Park, J. H., & Lee, J. P. (2009). A ten-year review of the literature on the use of standardized patients in teaching and learning: 1996–2005. *Medical Teacher, 31*(6), 487–492.

Raven, C. A. (2004). Simulation as a teaching strategy for nursing education and orientation in cardiac surgery. *Critical Care Nurse, 2*, 46–51.

Stafford, F. (2005). The significance of de-rolling and debriefing in training medical students using simulation to train medical students. *Medical Education, 39*, 1083–1085.

Waugaman, W. R. (1994). Professional roles of the certified registered nurse anesthetist. In S. Foster & L. Jordan (Eds.), *Professional aspects of nurse anesthesia practice* (pp. 347–367). Philadelphia, PA: F. A. Davis Company.

APPENDIX 17.A

SP Checklist

Institute Name   Drexel

Case Name   Nu Anes Interview I

Q. No.   Question Text

Category:- Communication

1. Introduces Self (name and title)

    ○ Done   ○ Not Done

2. Good eye contact (50% or greater of the time)

    ○ Done   ○ Not Done

3. Speaks clearly in terms the patient can understand (three strikes rule)

    ○ Done   ○ Not Done

4. Active Listener

    ○ Done   ○ Not Done

5. Asks patient's age or date of birth

    ○ Done   ○ Not Done

6. Checked identification by checking ID band.

    ○ Done   ○ Not Done

7. Asks about allergies

    ○ Done   ○ Not Done

8. Asks about current medications I am taking

    ○ Done   ○ Not Done

9. Asks about smoking history

    ○ Done   ○ Not Done

10. The student instructed me to not have anything to eat or drink after midnight

    ○ Done   ○ Not Done

Source: Adapted from Education Management Solutions. © 2008.

APPENDIX 17.B

Drexel University
College of Nursing and Health Professions
Nurse Anesthesia Program

PRE-ANESTHESIA ASSESSMENT SCHEDULE

Time	Room 1 Scenario 1 *Female*	Room 2 Scenario 2 *Male*	Room 3 Scenario 3 *Male*	Room 4 Scenario 4 *Female*	Room 5 Scenario 5 *Female*
9:30 am–10:00 am	Student 1	Student 2	Student 3	Student 4	Student 5
10:00 am–10:30 am	Student 6	Student 7	Student 8	Student 9	Student 10
10:30 am–11:00 am	Student 11	Student 12	Student 13	Student 14	Student 15
11:00 am–11:30 am	Student 16	Student 17	Student 18	Student 19	Student 20

Source: Drexel University, College of Nursing and Health Professions, Nurse Anesthesia Program.

APPENDIX 17.C

SCENARIO I

56-year-old woman

Procedure: Right total knee replacement

Height/weight: 5'8" 225 lbs   **Airway assessment:** MP II good CROM

PMH: HTN, GERD, migraine headaches, smoker 1ppd, no ETOH

Meds: Lisinopril, prevacid   NKDA

PSH: 1995: Breast reduction under GA with PONV

Labs: H/H: 13.6/40.6 plts: 140K

Lytes:

140	104	16	
4.2	30	109	0.9

SCENARIO II

29-year-old woman

Procedure: Right knee arthroscopy

Height/weight: 6'1" 260 lbs   **Airway assessment:** MP II-III good CROM

PMH: anxiety disorder, sleep apnea, NIDDM, nonsmoker no ETOH

Meds: ativan, elavil, buspar, glucophage

Allergies: PCN

PSH: none

Labs: H/H: 15.6/43.7 plts: 258K

Lytes:

140	101		
3.9	31	127	

CHAPTER 18

Human Simulation with Critically Ill Patients

Pilar Hernández Pinto and Alejandro Martínez Arce

INTRODUCTION

A critically ill patient can be found in different places, such as operating rooms, inten-sive care units, emergency rooms, delivery rooms, different wards, or mobile inten-sive care units, and poses different problems to health care professionals.

Recognizing that a patient has become or is becoming critically ill is a major chal-lenge because early intervention may significantly reduce morbidity and mortality. Assessment and initial treatment should be carried out by a multidisciplinary team, and the time and coordination in decision making is essential as it may affect the results (Sinz, 2004).

These patients are usually presented with complex clinical problems, both in acute and in severe form, which require immediate attention. Typically, they do not occur often enough to allow time for training, and when they do occur, the provider often lacks the necessary experience to carry out an efficient approach. This usually generates a high level of stress and therefore the increase of possible errors arises.

In the case of nurses who are required to have extensive clinical skills that are com-plex and rapidly changing, they must also decide when to call the physician. Nurses require ongoing education to confront challenges related to increased complexity of both patient status and increased complexity of technology (Cato & Murray, 2010).

Health care professionals need to be trained to solve these rare problems by practic-ing different skills and teamwork training, thereby improving patient safety.

In this way, simulation helps to train health care professionals in critically ill patient care. Simulation allows the experience to be repeated as often as required, and their development takes place without risk to the patient. It provides a safe, support-ive educational environment (Bradley, 2006). It encourages the acquisition of skills through experiential learning, ideally in a realistic situation or setting, and will allow reflection on performance.

A variety of simulation modalities has been used for teaching critical care skills, including partial-task trainers, mannequins, computer screen–based simulation, standardized patients (SPs), hybrid patients (HPs), animals, human cadaver, video-tapes, and full-scale human–patient simulators (HPSs). When regarding simulation in the critically ill patient compared with other specialties, HPSs have been widely used because critically ill patients frequently require invasive procedures. They are highly monitored and often unable to move about, speak, or even communicate. These systems make it possible to simulate different situations that require the application of action protocols or the management of new drugs in the clinical practice. That in turn promotes teamwork and the rational use of resources in urgent care of the critical and multiple-injured patients (Quesada Suescun et al., 2007; Rall & Dieckmann, 2005). In comparison, the use of human actors trained as SPs or HPs are used in Advanced Trauma Life Support courses and Advanced Cardiac Life Support courses and during Objective Structured Clinical Examinations. These models are limited by their inability to simulate high-risk scenarios such as difficult airway management or tension pneumothorax. In our experience, training with SPs allows for greater involvement of the participants. It is possible to simulate high-risk scenarios using SPs and partial-task trainers together, provided that participants in the simulation are well-informed of it, resulting in a doubly enriching simulation experience. Throughout the chapter, we will discuss our experience in using simulation for training critically ill patient care.

WHY USE SIMULATION FOR TRAINING CRITICAL PATIENT CARE?

The health care profession, in its many facets, makes extensive use of the three major learning domains: cognitive, affective, and psychomotor. Teaching engages all aspects of the learners' and practitioners' capabilities.

Health care professionals draw upon the three domains in the following ways:

- Cognitive (knowing) domain: focusing on knowledge acquisition and intellectual skills and abilities (e.g., the diagnosis of disease, strategizing treatment options). According to Bloom's (1956) taxonomy, cognitive domain has six major categories ranging from the simplest behavior to the most complex. The categories can be thought of as degrees of difficulty. That is, the first one must be mastered before the next one can take place: knowledge, comprehension, application, analysis, synthesis, and evaluation.
- Psychomotor (doing) domain: relating to skills that require varying levels of well-coordinated physical activity and precise manipulative procedures (e.g., simple suturing of an open wound, performing an endoscopic examination, or performing sophisticated surgical procedures).
- Affective (feeling) domain: dealing with feelings, emotions, mindsets, and values, including the nurturing of desirable attitudes for personal and professional development (e.g., allaying the concerns and fears of patients, displaying empathy for the relatives of a patient who has just died, displaying mutual trust and respect in working with members of the health care team, or upholding high ethical standards in practice).

To optimize care of critically ill patients, it is necessary to train health care professionals. Specific educational strategies should be used to improve knowledge, skills, attitudes, and relationships with the team. Adult educational methodology requires careful preparation of the talks and conferences, practical sessions for skills development, and analysis and discussion working with small groups. Professional learning is enhanced when the content is relevant to their own practice, the objectives are clearly defined, and a supportive environment is provided. Then participants engage in the learning process, allowing for broad discussion of the issues, establishing an information exchange between teacher and student, reflecting on the new lessons learned, and allowing them to identify what was done well and those weaker or erroneous aspects of their performance.

Simulation-based training in health care can be applied when teaching different areas of knowledge, skills, and behaviors. High-fidelity simulation helps to integrate knowledge acquired from classes, readings, psychomotor skills, and clinical practice. Furthermore, simulation develops critical thinking and clinical judgment skills by submersion of the participant in a critical clinical environment. The opportunity to debrief and carry out constructive feedback of a crisis scenario increases participant reflection and understanding of event outcomes. Simulation can reproduce these critical care clinical situations in a controlled environment so that they are readily understood and managed and provides opportunities for repeated exposure to identify and correct deficiencies noted in knowledge or skill (Cato & Murray, 2010). Simulation also supports lifelong learning for health care clinicians in relation to achieving specific levels of competency (Cannon-Diebl, 2009).

WHICH AREAS ARE MORE IMPORTANT TO TRAIN?

Critically ill patients are a challenge for every team: complex patient, complex environment, decision making in a limited time setting, high stakes situation, and different professionals working together with a common goal. We can improve safety in critically ill patient care by way of training technical, clinical, and behavior skills, as well as teamwork by using simulation. The decision about the type of simulator required must be based on the objectives and needs of the application.

Technical Skills

Among those specialty-specific domains lies procedural competency, an area where there is an ever present risk for patient discomfort and harm. Acquiring skill at procedural tasks is of great importance for early learners—students or interns and residents—but it is also important for experienced personnel who need practice at new procedures as they are being introduced or with existing tasks and procedures that do not frequently occur in clinical practice.

In clinical training, simulation has become accepted as a safe alternative to practicing procedural skills on patients. Simulation offers an opportunity for focused, deliberate practice in a safe, controlled learning environment, thus allowing learners to practice skills repeatedly until mastery is achieved (Del Moral et al., 2001).

Different sorts of tasks and skills can be simulated in the critically ill patient using different kinds of immersive and simulation models:

Part-task trainer models reproduce the key portions of a procedure. Part-task trainers in plastic or other forms cannot fully replicate performing the task on real patients, but they do allow learners to acquire the basic steps of the procedures and some of the basic skills needed to then be later taught the fine art of doing the procedures under supervision on actual human beings.

Some examples of part-task trainers in critically ill patients may include the following:

1. Plastic **"intravenous arm"** containing soft plastic skin with plastic "veins" underneath. These can be stuck with standard intravenous or blood-drawing needles in just the way this is done for real veins in real patients.
2. **Airway management head.** These replicate the face, the head, and the "airways" (mouth, nose, throat, and windpipe) of patients. These can allow ventilation via a face mask with or without mechanical ventilation devices like a breathing bag, direct and indirect intubation, as with video laryngoscopes, or insertion of special breathing tubes such as an endotracheal tube (in the windpipe) or laryngeal mask airway (sitting just above the windpipe).
3. **Urinary catheter trainer.** This replicates the genital structures containing the urethra. Students can physically learn the process of inserting a urine collecting tube (a "Foley catheter") in either male or female patients.
4. **Central venous catheterization (CVC) trainer.** This consists of a pad of a special soft plastic material with a special surface that can be stuck with a standard CVC system. CVC is associated with patient risks known to be inversely related to clinician experience. Recent studies have demonstrated that simulation-based training can improve the CVC insertion skill and reduce associated complications (Smith et al., 2010; Barsuk et al., 2009).
5. **Lumbar puncture part-task trainer.** Lumbar puncture procedure is important because it is commonly performed for a wide array of diagnostic and therapeutic reasons. These include diagnosis of subarachnoid hemorrhage, meningitis, elevated intracranial pressure, and the performance of spinal or epidural anesthesia (Conroy et al., 2010).
6. **Pelvic examination trainer.** Various sorts of plastic models replicate the pelvic structures of female patients and allow practice of examination without causing any discomfort to real patients. The most advanced of these part-task pelvic trainers contain electronic force sensors to let the student know exactly what portions of the anatomy they felt and how hard they or their instruments pressed on various areas. This kind of feedback may be highly beneficial.
7. **Diagnostic ultrasound trainer.** It is a kind of box with gelatin and other materials to simulate catheterization or puncture guided by ultrasound.

Animals. Parts of animals, such as a dissected trachea, can be used to practice, for example, tracheotomy or cricothyroidotomy. Full animals may be used to train chest tube placement, intravenous lines catheterization, or peritoneal puncture lavage.

Virtual reality simulators. Advantages include skill training and assessment of surgical and invasive procedures, extended training time, no risk to patient, repeatable difficulty level, reliable feedback, and avoidance of ethical issues with animal-based training (Aggarwal & Darzi, 2006).

Examples of virtual reality simulators in a critically ill patient:

1. Fibrobronchoscopy, for the airway management
2. Diagnosis by ultrasound
3. Endoscopic and laparoscopic surgery

Mannequins. They are widely used to train a variety of technical skills, such as basic or advanced life support or airway management.

Table 18.1 *Technical Skills*

Airway management
Bronchoscopy
Central venous catheter insertion
Chest tube placement
Defibrillation
Hemofiltration
Intraosseous puncture
Intravenous pumps, monitors, and other equipment
Invasive monitors
Lumbar puncture
Peritoneal puncture lavage
Urinary catheter insertion
Ventilator management

Table 18.1 shows a list of technical skills that can be trained with simulation.

Clinical Skills

In daily practice, health care professionals face clinical situations that require not only knowledge or the application of specific techniques, but also clinical decision making, referred to as *clinical reasoning, clinical judgment, clinical inference,* and *diagnostic reasoning.* Different models can be used to train these aspects in simulation with the critically ill patient.

SPs are actors trained to act out the story and symptoms of specific diseases. In the critically ill patient, SPs can put on makeup to simulate, for example, cyanosis, jugular engorgement, wounds, burns, abrasions, or bumps, and the actors can simulate different aspects such as the Glasgow Coma Scale, seizures, dyspnea, or pain.

HPS is the most widely used model in simulation with critically ill patients. It can be used in the case of those participants needing to perform invasive procedures. For example, in case of pneumothorax, the abolition of breath sounds on auscultation is more realistically reflected.

The use of an appropriate mix of these devices can optimize learning and mainte-nance of skill for providers at all levels of experience.

HPs are a combination of a part-task physical trainer with a living, breathing SP: for instance, CVC using the specific part-task model and the SP actor. Such a pad can be strapped on the neck of an SP actor and then draped with appropriate clinical material. The student not only has to perform the elements of CVC, but also has to do so as in real life while attending to the patient's needs and conversing with the patient and family.

In simulation in the critically ill patient, we choose the type of simulator that bet-ter helps to achieve the objectives. For example, in our center, to train the protocol of analgesia and sedation for critically ill patient protocol, we use SP because they express feelings and emotions, interact with the participants, and engage them better. If a respi-ratory depression due to opiate overdose needs to be replicated, and the use of invasive techniques, such as ventilation or intubation, is required, we usually use HPS. Another option is to use hybrids. For example, a part-task trainer can be placed adjacent to the neck of an SP to insert a central line in a patient with a Glasgow Coma Scale of 12. This option is cheaper and easier to use than HPS, and the learning objectives can be per-fectly achieved.

Table 18.2 *Examples of Clinical Skills: Protocols*

General Competencies	Critical Care	Anesthesia	Obstetrics
Hypovolemic, cardiogenic, distributive, and obstructive shock Advanced cardiac life support (neonatal, pediatric, and adult) Sepsis	Analgesia and sedation for the critically ill patient Trauma care	Anaphylaxis Malignant hyperthermia Difficult airway Poisoning by local anesthetics Management of critical events in surgical patients	Massive postpartum hemorrhage Eclampsia Amniotic liquid embolism

Simulation scenarios covered during courses on management of critically ill patient at one simulation center.

Other examples of clinical skills are shown in the Table 18.2. Sepsis and postpartum hemorrhage will be more widely discussed at the end of the chapter as example scenarios.

Teamwork and Behavioral Skills

Errors in health care are most frequently due to an interaction of human factors like poor teamwork and poor communication, rather than individual mistakes (Kohn et al., 1999). Patients in critical care settings are at particularly high risk because of complex medical problems, incomplete or conflicting information, dynamic situations, and intense time pressure. Training team and communication competencies have been considered an effective tool for the provision of safe and effective health care (Table 18.3).

Human patient simulation has been widely advocated to evaluate, test, and practice team communication and interaction under challenging situations (Gaba, 2000). Models such as SP, HPS, or HP can be used to effectively train these skills. However, it is difficult to assess the knowledge and skills acquired after training, mainly due to the difficulty in finding instruments for measurement and rating scales (Gaba et al., 1998).

Teamwork skills can be elicited in a number of ways. Role clarity can be challenged by placing the team in an unfamiliar or unexpected environment, by creating scenarios where plans must substantially change with time, by having confederate players to create leadership conflict, and by distracting or task overloading single members of the team. Communication skills can be assessed by introducing particular data into the scenario from various sources to individual members and by seeing how such data are transferred to the team. Keeping some team members apart from the simulation scenario at the outset and introducing them as the case develops can aid the evaluation of support issues. Injecting equipment failures, incompatibilities, and unfamiliar models of devices can highlight resource issues. Finally, global assessment skills can be brought out by making the etiology of the problem unclear and by placing several suggestive data throughout the scenario (Table 18.4).

The learning environment affects behavior. Realism provided within simulation is an important factor.

THE ROLE OF SIMULATION IN CRITICALLY ILL PATIENT SAFETY

One method to get the utmost out of simulation as a learning tool is by using it to train multidisciplinary teams in behaviors, cognitions, and attitude to facilitate coordinated

Table 18.3 *Teamwork*

Communication, organization, and coordination in and among medical teams
Role clarity
Optimize support
Resource utilization
Global assessment

Source: Adapted from Raemer, D. B. (2004).

Table 18.4 *Behavioral Skills*

Social or interpersonal skills (easily observable)	Cognitive or mental skills (partially observable)
Leadership	Situation awareness
Teamwork	Decision making
Communication	Task Management and Planning

Source: Adapted from Fletcher et al. (2002).

adaptive performance in a contextual environment. Simulation can facilitate these teams to improve their performance by exposing them to an experiential and contextual learning. Several researchers reveal that certain skills and attitudes are blocked with relative ease when conditions change routine of our work. Workload, fatigue, stress, time pressure, or lack of resources quietly leads professionals to make mistakes (Alonso-Felpete et al., 2004).

LIMITATIONS OF SIMULATION-BASED TRAINING

Although it is true that simulation as a training tool has gained importance and has been expanding in the health care field in recent years, there are still some barriers to its full implementation.

One of the main difficulties to integrate simulation into the daily clinical activity is the production pressure in combination with the still incipient patient safety culture among health care providers.

Another major barrier is the availability of qualified instructor–clinicians who can provide excellent hands-on teaching in selecting objectives, designing scenarios, and using the analysis for the reflection of the performance. Designing a realistic clinical critical care simulation course requires the contribution of educators specialized in adult learning and clinicians that have extensive knowledge of the environment and patient population attempting to be replicated (Summers & Kingsland, 2009).

The final barrier is resources, including the time to train instructors and the time spent by instructors and participants during the courses, the purchase and maintenance of the equipment and facilities, and the cost of administration and development of the program.

EXAMPLES OF SCENARIOS IN CRITICALLY ILL PATIENTS IN THE VALDECILLA VIRTUAL HOSPITAL

Example 1

Case title: Postpartum hemorrhage

SIMULATION PERFORMANCE OBJECTIVES

Clinical objectives:

Review the 4T causes of postpartum hemorrhage + 1: "tone" (uterine atony), "trauma" (laceration or hematoma), "tissue" (retained placental tissue), "thrombosis" (clotting disorder), and "traction" (uterine inversion), and the predisposing factors and potential etiology.

Therapeutic approach: Primary interventions common to all hemorrhage with examination focus on airway, breathing, and circulation, including oxygen supplementation, intravenous fluid, insertion of a second large-bore intravenous, monitoring, Foley catheter, laboratory studies, preparation for a possible blood transfusion; and secondary interventions, for example, in case of uterine atony, vigorous fundal uterine massaging, imaging studies (ultrasonography), vaginal examination, Bakri probe, uterotonic medication as oxytocin, methylergonovine (Methergin), carboprost (Hemabate), and misoprostol (Cytotec).

Behavioral objectives (team work):

Call for help early: ask for senior obstetrician-gynecologist, anesthesiologist, and intensive care specialist.

Communication and coordination between midwife, obstetrician-gynecologist, and anesthesiologist and intensive care staff. Also consult blood bank.

PARTICIPANTS AND ACTORS

Participants: midwife, resident and faculty in obstetrics and gynecology, resident and faculty in anesthesiology.

Actors: one plays SP, a second actor plays a relative of the patient with the baby, and a third actor plays nursing assistant.

CASE STEM TO BE READ TO PARTICIPANTS

You will be called by a nursing assistant to assist a 30-year-old female patient who has just delivered a baby, noninstrumental vaginal delivery, after 8 hours of induction because of prolonged pregnancy. The placenta is out. Her past medical history is negative for any systemic illness. She does not take medication or have any known drug allergies.

SCENARIO SETUP

Room: delivery room.

Hybrid female patient (standardized female patient and pelvic examination trainer) is lying supine on delivery room table with legs. An HPS dressed as a female patient with a wig can also be used.

Props

Delivery room table with legs.

Hybrid female patient with large-bore peripheral intravenous access and epidural catheter connected to a PCA pump.

Standard monitors (electrocardiogram, noninvasive blood pressure [BP], and pulse oximetry) are available but are not in place until the participant asks for it.

Anesthesia machine, additional crystalloid and colloid fluids, previously mentioned medications to treat uterine atony and other anesthesia medications, and Foley catheter and Bakri probe are available.

Face mask and equipment for endotracheal intubation are available too.

In our center, we simulate vaginal bleeding by pressing a system, consisting of a plastic bottle with dyed red softener, connected through tubes to the vagina of the pelvic examiner trainer. The uterus is simulated with a balloon.

The relative of the female patient is in the delivery room with the baby in his or her arms. He or she is instructed to push the plastic bottle containing the simulated blood (which is hidden under the delivery room table) with his or her foot. The baby's crying is simulated with a recording.

The nursing assistant will be present throughout the scenario to help the participants.

A table prepared with tweezers, scissors, several gauzes dyed red, valves for review, rings, holders, sutures, and a placenta with intact membranes (we make the placenta with gelatinous material).

Medical record

Personal history: Unknown drug allergies, primigravida.

Anesthesia record of the epidural anesthesia without complications.

Physical examination

Weight and height: 160 cm and 67 kg.

Vital signs: temperature, 36°C; heart rate, 90 bpm; and BP 110/60 mm Hg.

Laboratory and other relevant studies

Normal electrocardiograph record: weight of fetus, 3800 g; Apgar score, 9/9.

Chest x-ray: unavailable.

Electrocardiogram: sinus rhythm.

Hematocrit: 35%.

Prothrombin activity: 100%.

Platelets: 250,000/mm^3.

INSTRUCTIONS FOR SIMULATOR TECHNICIAN

Baseline: Patient is initially awake, alert, and breathing spontaneously, becomes dizzy and anxious with cold sweaty skin, and is hemodynamically stable.

Vital signs evolution: temperature, 36°C; heart rate, 90–140 bpm; systolic BP, 120–60 mm Hg; respiratory rate, 18 breaths/minute to apnea; and oxygen saturation, 97%–80%.

SCENARIO SCRIPT

After the midwife participant has taken care of the patient, profuse vaginal bleeding is presented. At this time, midwife is expected to call the obstetrician-gynecologist resident, to monitor the patient, and to start diagnosis and treatment—fundal uterine massage, oxygen, and intravenous fluid. Initially, the patient will be hemodynamically stable.

Three minutes after the obstetrician-gynecologist resident participant has arrived, the patient becomes dizzy and anxious, and vaginal bleeding continues profusely. Vital signs deteriorate: BP, 60/30; heart rate, 140 bpm; and oxygen saturation, 80%. At this time, the obstetrician-gynecologist resident is expected to call the obstetrician-gynecologist and anesthesiology staff and reevaluate the steps that have been made by the midwife and continue or initiate basic and specific treatment (and differential diagnosis).

The obstetrician-gynecologist and anesthesiologist faculty are expected to communicate adequately, to retrieve information from the team, to reevaluate the current situation, and to continue diagnosis or treatment if they have not been made.

The scenario ends when an accurate differential diagnosis, basic and specific treatment, and good communication between the professionals involved are made.

DEBRIEFING GUIDE

Usually, we prepare some questions to help us explore the trainee's perspective on scenario events. We use the theory and method for debriefing with good judgment described by Rudolph et al. (2006).

Example 2

Case title: postoperative sepsis

SIMULATION PERFORMANCE OBJECTIVES

Clinical objectives

Early detection of sepsis.

Initial steps of treatment.

Nonclinical objectives

Detect organizational barriers and their negative clinical impact.

Effective communication between team members.

PARTICIPANTS AND ACTORS

Actors: SP, one family member, and a nursing assistant.

Participants: two nurses and two physicians (resident and faculty).

CASE STEM TO BE READ TO PARTICIPANTS

Nurse participants are informed they will be the team responsible for the general surgery ward. It is the beginning of the afternoon shift. Faculty are on call.

A nurse will be called by a nursing assistant to evaluate a 76-year-old male patient operated by laparoscopy 5 days ago because of a rectal neoplasm. The family finds the patient confused and nervous. During the morning nurse shift, laboratory orders have been extracted and are pending evaluation by the surgeon in charge, who has been all morning in the operating room.

SCENARIO SETUP

Room: general surgery ward

A standardized male patient wears a nightgown and has a suprapubic scar and four small dressings: navel, pit right iliac, and left and right vacuum.

Props:

Bed and bedside table with a bottle of water, glass, and magazines.

Manual sphygmomanometer and pulse oximeter in the room. Other monitors, such as electrocardiogram or defibrillator, are available but are not in place.

The relative of the patient is in the room and will be able to provide information if required.

Medical record
Medical history: 76-year-old male patient, atrial fibrillation, hypertension, and depression (his wife died 3 months ago). In treatment with 5 mg of anhydrous amiloride HCl and 50 mg/day of hydrochlorothiazide, 325 mg/day of aspirin, and 0.125 mg/day of digoxin. No known drug allergies.
Surgical record
Surgical intervention: neoplasm in the recto sigmoid junction, laparoscopic resection performed with end-to-end anastomosis 5 days ago by Dr. R.
Postoperative Day 1: stable constants, afebrile, limited serous and bloody drainage (<20 mL), 1200 mL of urine, and depressible and slightly painful abdomen to deep palpation. Signature: Dr. R.
Postoperative Day 2: No changes. Signature: Dr. B.
Postoperative Day 3: Afebrile and without changes. Urinary catheter is removed and diet to be initiated orally. Signature: Dr. R.
Postoperative Day 4: Drainage is removed. Oral diet well-tolerated. Signature Dr. R.

Postoperative Day 5: Patient reports that he is restless, does not know what is happening, and does not feel well. Exploration of the abdomen seems normal. New laboratory orders are requested. Signature: Dr. J.

Nursing record

Days 1 to 4: Normal evolution.

Day 4, night: Patient is anxious and is constantly calling. Temperature, 37.8°C.

Day 5, morning: Dr. J. ordered new analysis early in the morning. I phoned him when the results came, but he was in the operating room. He will come to see them when he finishes.

INSTRUCTIONS FOR SIMULATOR AND ACTORS

Patient baseline: disoriented, complains of abdominal pain, and asks urgently for painkillers; oxygen saturation, 94%; heart rate, 110 bpm; and BP, 90/50 mm Hg.

The patient's relative should remain nervous during the scenario.

The nursing assistant must have a passive attitude and help the nurses with the material and keep them oriented.

SCENARIO SCRIPT

Beginning of the scenario:

A nurse is called to the room by the nursing assistant because the patient refers general discomfort and intense pain in the abdomen.

The patient appears anxious; temperature, 38.5°C; heart rate, 110 bpm; oxygen saturation, 95%; and BP, 90/50 mm Hg.

The nurse is expected to assess the patient, to review the medical record, and to call for help.

Another participant nurse arrives to the scenario:

Exchange of information between the nurses is expected; they should reassess the patient, call for help, and begin to perform initial treatment.

The patient feels more pain and begins to become more disoriented and confused, the family gets very nervous; heart rate, 125 bpm; oxygen saturation, 92%; and BP, 85/45 mm Hg.

Doctor called by telephone:

The assistant nurse may suggest so in case there is a delay in calling for help.

The nurse is expected to transmit all the possible information about the patient's condition.

Ideally, sepsis criteria should be noted.

Doctor (participant) comes:

Communication and exchange of information between team members are expected.

Depending on the treatment previously initiated, the patient may deteriorate and becomes unconscious; heart rate, 130 bpm; oxygen saturation, 91%; and BP, 80/40 mm Hg.

Scenario ends when the presence of sepsis diagnostic criteria is highlighted, differential diagnosis is discussed, and sepsis laboratory profile, hemoculture, and x-ray examinations are ordered. Also, treatment with fluids and antibiotics should be initiated, and contact with the critical care unit should be made.

If it is necessary to help the participants, the nursing assistant may suggest calling the critical care physician who will come and take care of the patient.

DEBRIEFING GUIDE

Usually, we prepare some questions to help us explore the trainee's perspective on scenario events. We use the theory and method for debriefing with good judgment described by Rudolph et al. (2006).

ACKNOWLEDGMENT

The authors would like to thank Valdecilla Virtual Hospital, IFIMAV (Instituto de Formación e Investigación "Marqués de Valdecilla") and Fundación Marqués de Valdecilla for assistance they provided during the writing of this chapter.

REFERENCES

Aggarwal, R., & Darzi, A. (2006). Technical-skills training in the 21st century. *New England Journal of Medicine, 355,* 2695–2696.

Alonso-Felpete, A., Abajas, R., De la Horra, I., Hoz, V., Llata, G., López, L. M., et al. (2004). Simuladores de escala real en el entrenamiento de enfermería. *Revista Rol de Enfermeria, 27*(7–8), 510–518.

Barsuk, J. H., McGaghie, W. C., Cohen, E. R., Balachandran, J. S., & Wayne, D. B. (2009). Use of simulation-based mastery learning to improve the quality of central venous catheter placement in a medical intensive care unit. *Journal of Hospital Medicine, 4,* 397–403.

Bloom, B. S. (Ed.). (1956). *Taxonomy of educational objectives: The classification of educational goals: Handbook I. Cognitive domain.* New York: Longmans, Green.

Bradley, P. (2006). The history of simulation in medical education and possible future directions. *Medical Education, 40,* 254–262.

Cannon-Diebl, M. R. (2009). Simulation in healthcare and nursing state of the science. *Critical Care Nursing Quarterly, 32*(2), 128–136.

Cato, D. L., & Murray, M. (2010). Use of simulation training in the intensive care unit. *Critical Care Nursing Quarterly, 33*(1), 44–51.

Conroy, S. M., Bond, W. F., Pheasant, K. S., & Ceccacci, N. (2010). Competence and retention in performance of the lumbar puncture procedure in a task trainer model. *Simulation in Healthcare, 5,* 133–138.

Del Moral, I., Rabanal, J. M., & Díaz de Terán, J. C. (2001). Simuladores en anestesia. *Revista Española de Anestesiología y Reanimación, 48,* 423–433.

Fletcher, G.C. L., McGeorge, P., Flin, R.H., Glavin, R.J., & Maran, N.J. (2002) The role of non-technical skills in anaesthesia: a review of current literature. *Br J Anaesth* 2002; 88: 418–29.

Gaba, D. M. (2000). Simulation-based crisis resource management training for trauma care. *American Journal of Anesthesiology, 27,* 199–200.

Gaba, D. M., Howard, S. K., Flanagan, B., Smith, B. E, Fish, K. J., Botney, R. (1998). Assessment of clinical performance during simulated crises using both technical and behavioral ratings. *Anesthesiology, 89,* 8–18.

Hammond, J. (2004). Simulation in critical care and trauma education and training. *Current Opinion in Critical Care, 10,* 325–329.

Kohn, L. T., Corrigan, J. M., & Donaldson, M. S. (Eds.). (1999). *To err is human: Building a safer health system.* Committee on Health Care in America, Institute of Medicine. Washington, DC: National Academy Press.

Mitchell, L., & Flin, R. (2008). Non-technical skills of the operating theatre scrub nurse: Literature review. *Journal of Advanced Nursing, 63*(1), 15–24.

Quesada Suescun, A., Burón, F. J., Castellanos, A., Del Moral, I., González Fernández, C., Olalla Antolín, J. J., et al. (2007). Formación en la asistencia al paciente crítico y politraumatizado: Papel de la simulación clínica. *Medicina Intensiva, 31*(4), 187–193.

Raemer, D. B. (2004). Team-oriented medical simulation. In W. F. Dunn (Ed.), *Simulators in critical care and beyond* (pp. 42–46). Des Plaines, IL: Society of Critical Care Medicine.

Rall, M., & Dieckmann, P. (2005). *Crisis resource management to improve patient safety.* Euroanaesthesia 2005: Annual Meeting of the European Society of Anaesthesiology Vienna, Austria, May 28–31.

Rudolph, J. W., Simon, R., Dufresne, R. L., & Raemer, D. B. (2006). There's no such thing as "non-judgmental" debriefing: A theory and method for debriefing with good judgment. *Simulation in Healthcare, 1,* 49–55.

Sinz, E. H. (2004). Partial-task-trainers and simulation in critical care medicine. In W. F. Dunn (Ed.), *Simulators in critical care and beyond* (pp. 33–41). Des Plaines, IL: Society of Critical Care Medicine.

Smith, C., Huang, G. C., Newman, L. R., Clardy, P. F., Feller-Kopman, D., & Ennacheril, T. (2010). Simulation training and its effect on long-term resident performance in central venous catheterization. *Simulation in Healthcare, 5,* 146–151.

Summers, K., & Kingsland, K. (2009). Simulation: Issues and challenges. *Paediatric Nursing, 21*(3), 33.

CHAPTER 19

Human Simulation with Perioperative Patients

Jorge L. Gomez-Diaz, Mary Ellen Bednar,
Fabien Pampaloni, and Linda Wilson

INTRODUCTION

*T*he world of the perioperative nurse changes frequently. As technically skilled as they are, they also utilize critical thinking in every surgical case. As such, ongoing education is provided for them throughout their surgical career, from assembly and troubleshooting of equipment to new surgical procedures. When in the surgical arena, of course, perioperative nurses work with the surgical team as skilled communicators to ensure safe patient outcomes.

To work in the operating room as a circulating nurse or a scrub nurse, special education is required. Most hospitals and health care systems recommend that the nurse experience 1 year of medical surgical nursing to develop organizational skills. However, some hospitals have programs that admit new nursing graduates. The Periop 101 program from the Association of periOperative Registered Nurses (AORN) is highly recognized by most hospitals for providing initial perioperative education. However, some hospitals provide their own homegrown perioperative programs with clinical orientations lasting from 1 to 2 years. At the same time, most hospitals encourage certification for perioperative nurses through AORN (as a Certified Nurse of the Operating Room).

In the past, operating room nurses were generally viewed as the hospital intraoperative care providers. Since the late 1980s, however, the role has evolved into what we now know as the perioperative nurse. Because of technological advances and new minimally invasive procedures, many surgical procedures are now performed in outpatient surgi-centers, radiology departments, and even office-based surgery. It is very common to see a perioperative nurse in charge of the preadmission and testing office, working in same-day surgery or even providing care in the postanesthesia care unit. Here, as elsewhere, the nursing process is used to assess, plan, and implement patient care. When assessing patients, the nurse must carefully review the patient's current and past health history in a holistic manner to ensure the best postoperative outcomes. Care plans are revised as necessary throughout the surgical experience and typically address patient safety, which is crucial, as well as psychological and physiological changes that can provoke negative patient outcomes if not monitored.

Another kind of opportunity for preoperative nursing exists at hospitals, outpatient surgical centers, invasive departments, and office-based surgery. They may be allowed to work with selected surgical populations, depending on the volume of patients undergoing surgery. It is very common for perioperative nurses to choose to work within a surgical specialty, such as open heart, organ transplants, neurosurgery, orthopedic, and others.

PERIOPERATIVE ROLES

Although there are two traditional roles in perioperative nursing—the circulating nurse and scrub nurse—today, new roles have evolved, such as certified registered nurse first assistant (RNFA), perioperative nurse specialist, perioperative educator, and so on.

CIRCULATING NURSE

The circulating nurse is responsible for managing the nursing care of all patients assigned within the operating room and coordinates the needs of the entire surgical team with other care providers. The nurse makes certain that the procedure runs smoothly throughout the surgical experience: the necessary equipment is setup and functional; properly positions, preps, and drapes the patient; assures that proper aseptic or sterile techniques are used; and observes for any break in sterile techniques during the procedure. The nurse is accountable for the count of all instruments, needles, and sponges used during the procedure. Simply, the circulating nurse is an expert who manages the operating room environment throughout the duration of the entire surgical experience, including but not limited to troubleshooting problems with equipment, providing critical information about the patient, and making sure that all specimens are properly prepared and labeled for analysis. The circulating nurse becomes the patient advocate to ensure patient safety protocols are followed while measuring outcomes against recommended AORN Practices and other regulatory agencies, such as the Joint Commission.

SCRUB NURSE

The scrub nurse works directly with the surgeon within the sterile field, passing instruments, sponges, and other necessary items needed during surgery. The nurses who work within the sterile field have scrubbed their hands and arms with special disinfecting soap or alcohol-based solutions to ensure reduction of skin bacteria. The scrub nurse also works hand in hand with the circulating nurse to ensure all instruments, needles, sponges, and so forth, are accounted for at the end of the surgical procedure.

CERTIFIED RNFA

The RNFA holds a national certification as Certified Nurse of the Operating Room and has gone through additional, extensive education and training to deliver surgical care following the AORN RNFA curriculum. The RNFA will work with a clinical preceptor who evaluates competency and has a minimum of 120 clinical hours. The RNFA assists the operating surgeon by controlling bleeding, using surgical instruments or medical devices, handling tissue, and suturing during the procedures. To be eligible for certification as an RNFA, the candidate must possess a bachelor's degree in any field and have a minimum of 2,000 hours as a first assistant.

PERIOPERATIVE NURSE SPECIALIST

The role of a clinical nurse specialist has not been completely defined. Scientific advances can be attributed to the evolution of specialist roles within nursing, however, increasing the knowledge base, in this instance, within the perioperative field. Many perioperative nurses have a master's degree in nursing or science of nursing with four primary components; clinical expert, consultant, educator, and researcher.

Given the very specialized area of practice for the perioperative nurse, she or he is a fundamental member of the surgical team, working in collaboration with other health care professionals to decrease an ever-growing number of cases of preventable deaths and to provide a protected and safe environment for the surgical patient.

The following universal protocol illustrates a simulation for perioperative nursing and includes nurse, physician, and team grading questionnaires.

PERIOPERATIVE SIMULATION—UNIVERSAL PROTOCOL

NAME: Mr./Mrs. Fran K.

SETTING: Operating room

SESSION DETAILS:
> 20-minute encounter
> 5 minutes for checklist completion in the computer
> 10 minutes for feedback
> 5-minute turnaround time

SCENARIO: The patient is in the operating room and scheduled for an open reduction internal fixation of the left hip. Patient is slightly sedated. Patient is prepped for surgery on the right hip. The universal protocol is performed and the error is identified.

INSTRUCTIONS/DOOR SIGN: Mr./Mrs. Fran K. came to the emergency room with a fractured left hip and is now scheduled to have an open reduction internal fixation of the left hip. You have 20 minutes to finish preparing the patient for surgery start. Please refer to the patient chart for any specific patient orders, consents, and surgical paperwork.

TRAINING QUESTIONS:

What is your age? Use your own

Are you married? Use your own

Occupation? Use your own

Do you have any chronic illnesses? Use your own

Health history

>   Neurological (none)
>   Cardiovascular (none)
>   Respiratory (none)
>   Gastrointestinal (none)
>   Genitourinary (none)
>   Gynecological (none)
>   Obstetrical (use your own)

Have you ever been hospitalized before? No.

Have you ever had surgery? Not before this.

Have you ever been pregnant? Use your own

How is your father? Use your own

How is your mother? Use your own

How is/are your sibling(s)? Use your own

Immunizations up to date? All immunizations are up to date.

Diet: I try to eat healthy.

Activity/exercise: I do a lot of walking.

How did you injure your hip? I fell off a ladder taking down decorations.

Medications: None.

Psychosocial history

>   Smoking history (use your own)
>   Alcohol history (use your own)
>   Sexual history (use your own)
>   Recreational drug use (none)

You should be in a hospital gown, bra, and underwear, lying down on the table.

Graded items should have options for—done/not done/N/A

Nurse Grading

COMMUNICATION
__ Introduced self (name and title)
__ Good eye contact (50% or greater of the time)
__ Spoke clearly in terms the patient can understand (three strikes rule)
__ Active listener
__ Created an atmosphere that put the patient at ease
__ Asked about what surgery you are having done today
__ Asked about allergies
__ Asked about activity/exercise
__ Asked about current medications
__ Asked about smoking history
__ Asked about alcohol history
__ Verified patient's identity using two identifiers
__ Checked if surgical consent form is on the chart
__ Checked if anesthesia consent form is on the chart
__ Checked if blood transfusion consent form is on the chart
__ Verified surgical site
__ Completed universal protocol

PHYSICAL EXAMINATION

— Washed hands before examination
— Explained to me what she/he was doing with each step of exam
— Helped to position me
— Was professional in manner

Physician Grading

COMMUNICATION

— Introduced self (name and title)
— Good eye contact (50% or greater of the time)
— Spoke clearly in terms the patient can understand (three strikes rule)
— Active listener
— Created an atmosphere that put the patient at ease
— Asked about what surgery you are having done today
— Asked about allergies
— Asked about activity/exercise
— Asked about current medications
— Asked about smoking history
— Asked about alcohol history
— Verified patient's identity using two identifiers
— Checked if surgical consent form is on the chart
— Checked if anesthesia consent form is on the chart
— Checked if blood transfusion consent form is on the chart
— Verified surgical site
— Completed universal protocol

PHYSICAL EXAMINATION

— Washed hands before examination
— Explained to me what she/he was doing with each step of exam
— Helped to position me
— Was professional in manner

Team Grading

Did the perioperative team work well together?

Did the perioperative team demonstrate mutual respect for each other?

Did the perioperative team have good eye contact with each other?

■ **SP will also provide feedback**

Feedback to nurse(s)/feedback to physician/feedback on team function.

CHAPTER 20

Human Simulation with Perianesthesia Patients

Linda Wilson, H. Lynn Kane, and Linda Webb

This chapter provides an overview of perianesthesia nursing and some examples of perianesthesia human simulation cases for standardized patient simulation. Perianesthesia nursing practice involves caring for individuals in all phases of the perianesthesia continuum. In these settings, perianesthesia patients are either preanesthesia or postanesthesia.

The perianesthesia continuum includes the following phases: (1) preanesthesia preadmission, (2) preanesthesia day of procedure, (3) postanesthesia phase I, (4) postanesthesia phase II, and (5) extended observation. These settings can be located in hospitals, free-standing surgical centers, specialized physician offices, and specialty departments such as radiology and endoscopy.

In the preanesthesia preadmission phase, the focus of nursing care is on holistic preparation of the patient for the procedure as well as identifying actual or potential problems (ASPAN, 2010). Preoperative teaching by the professional nurse is initiated in this phase, and includes what to expect during the process: pain and comfort goals, patient's expectations, and discharge instructions.

In the preanesthesia day of procedure phase, the perianesthesia nurse focuses on validating information, reinforcing preoperative teaching, reviewing discharge instructions, and completion of preparation for the procedure (ASPAN, 2010, p. 6). The perianesthesia nurse will (1) complete a patient history; (2) complete a patient assessment, including current and accurate height and weight; (3) examine the presence and completion of multiple informed consents on the patient's chart; (4) review all laboratory and diagnostic test results and ensure any abnormal results are communicated to the appropriate physician or licensed independent practitioner with appropriate documentation; and (5) reinforce preoperative patient teaching and discharge instructions.

In postanesthesia phase I, nursing care focuses on immediate postanesthesia and postoperative care based on the type of anesthesia and surgery the patient received (ASPAN, 2010). The perianesthesia nurse monitors the patient for any signs of complications from the anesthesia or surgery, including patient pain and comfort management, and patient safety as priorities. In this setting, the perianesthesia nurse potentially cares for a variety of patients in all age ranges and varying acuity, which can include elective surgery patients, postprocedural patients, critical care patients, and trauma patients. In addition, the postanesthesia phase I nurse focuses on the transition of the patient to the next patient care setting, such as postanesthesia care phase II, the inpatient setting, or a critical care setting (ASPAN, 2010, p. 7).

In postanesthesia phase II, nursing care is focused on preparing the patient for discharge to home or transfer to a rehabilitation facility or extended care facility (ASPAN, 2010, p. 7). In this phase, the patient is assessed for readiness for discharge in a variety of areas including (1) respiratory function, (2) stability of vital signs, (3) level of consciousness, (4) mobility, (5) appropriate reflexes, (6) hydration and elimination, (7) anesthesia recovery, (8) nausea and vomiting, and (9) pain and comfort management.

In the extended observation phase, nursing care is focused on the specific care needed by patients who have already been discharged from postanesthesia phase I or postanesthesia phase II (ASPAN, 2010, p. 7). Examples of types of patients that may be cared for in this setting include patients waiting for a ride home and patients requiring extended recovery time.

There are many opportunities for using human simulation with standardized patients to train perianesthesia nurses. Some examples of simulation scenarios include (1) preanesthesia assessment, (2) preoperative teaching, (3) postanesthesia assessment, (4) malignant hyperthermia, (5) laryngospasm, (6) bronchospasm, (7) chest pain, (8) postanesthesia assessment after regional anesthesia, (9) respiratory arrest, (10) cardiac arrest, (11) discharge teaching, and many others. Several examples of human simulation cases for use with standardized patients are provided below.

PERIANESTHESIA SIMULATION—PREOPERATIVE/PREANESTHESIA ASSESSMENT

NAME: Mrs. Fran H.

SETTING: Preanesthesia day surgery unit

SESSION DETAILS:

> 20-minute encounter
> 5 minutes for checklist completion in the computer
> 10 minutes for feedback
> 5-minute turnaround time

SCENARIO: The patient is in the preanesthesia day surgery unit being prepared for a left breast biopsy under monitored anesthesia care. She is scheduled to go home after surgery.

INSTRUCTIONS/DOOR SIGN: Mrs. Fran H. came to the preanesthesia day surgery unit to be prepared for a left breast biopsy under monitored anesthesia care. She is scheduled to go home after surgery. You have 20 minutes to complete the preoperative/preanesthesia assessment. Please refer to patient chart for any specific patient orders, consents, laboratory results, x-ray results, and so forth.

TRAINING QUESTIONS:

What is your age? Use your own

Are you married? Use your own

Occupation? Use your own

Do you have any chronic illnesses? None.

Do you have any allergies to food(s) or medication(s)? None.

Health history:

> Neurological (none)
> Cardiovascular (none)
> Respiratory (none)

> Gastrointestinal (none)
> Genitourinary (none)
> Gynecological (none)
> Obstetrical (use your own)

Have you ever been hospitalized before? No.

Have you ever had surgery? Not before this.

Have you ever been pregnant? Use your own

How is your father's health? Use your own

How is your mother's health? Use your own

How is/are your sibling's health? Use your own

Immunizations up to date? All immunizations are up to date.

Diet—I try to eat healthy.

Activity/exercise: I go to the gym at least three times a week.

When did you find the lump in your left breast? I found it 2 weeks ago while doing my self-breast examination.

Has anyone discussed resources for support with you? No.

Would you like some information on support groups that are available? Yes.

Would you like to speak to someone from our pastoral care department? Sure.

How are you feeling about this experience? I am very concerned about the biopsy outcome, and I am very stressed.

Medications: None.

Psychosocial history

> Smoking history (none)
> Alcohol history (social)
> Sexual history (use your own)
> Recreational drug use (none)

You should be in a hospital gown, bra, and underwear, sitting on the table.

Graded items should have options for—Done/Not Done/N/A

Nurse Grading

COMMUNICATION
__ Introduced self (name and title)
__ Good eye contact (50% or greater of the time)
__ Spoke clearly in terms the patient can understand (three strikes rule)
__ Active listener
__ Created an atmosphere that put the patient at ease
__ Asked about what surgery you are having done today
__ Asked about allergies
__ Asked about activity/exercise
__ Asked about current medications
__ Asked about smoking history
__ Asked about alcohol history
__ Verified patient's identity using two identifiers
__ Checked if surgical consent form is on the chart
__ Checked if anesthesia consent form is on the chart
__ Checked if blood transfusion consent form is on the chart

— Verified surgical site as per policy and procedure
— Asked about a responsible adult to drive me home after surgery
— Asked if anyone discussed resources for support with me
— Asked if I would like some information on support groups that are available
— Asked if I would like to speak to someone from the pastoral care department
— Asked how I am feeling about this experience

PHYSICAL EXAMINATION

— Washed hands before examination
— Explained to me what she/he was doing with each step of examination
— Helped to position me
— Was professional in manner
— Maintained modesty during examination (if applicable)
— Listened to my heart in at least four places anterior on skin
— Listened to my lungs in at least four places (two pairs) bilateral anterior on skin
— Listened to my lungs in at least four places (two pairs) bilateral posterior on skin

PATIENT TEACHING

— Discussed the importance of deep breathing and coughing exercises after surgery
— Discussed the importance of taking pain medications as prescribed
— Discussed resources that are available for support
— Discussed the importance of not driving for 24 hours after surgery
— Discussed the importance of not operating any heavy machinery for 24 hours after surgery
— Discussed the importance of not signing any important papers for 24 hours after surgery

   ▮ **SP will also provide feedback**

PERIANESTHESIA SIMULATION—MALIGNANT HYPERTHERMIA

NAME: Mr./Mrs. Adrian L.

SETTING: Postanesthesia care unit (PACU)

SESSION DETAILS:
   20-minute encounter
   5 minutes for checklist completion in the computer
   10 minutes for feedback
   5-minute turnaround time

SCENARIO: The patient is in the PACU after an appendectomy under general anesthesia. While in the PACU, it is noted that the patient is hyperthermic and the patient's temperature is rising very quickly. The PACU nurse notifies the anesthesia department and prepares to treat the patient for a malignant hyperthermia crisis.

INSTRUCTIONS/DOOR SIGN: Mr./Mrs. Adrian L. is in the PACU after an appendectomy under general anesthesia. While in the PACU, it is noted that the patient is hyperthermic and the patient's temperature is rising very quickly. The PACU prepares to treat the patient for a malignant hyperthermia crisis. You have 20 minutes for the encounter. Please refer to patient chart for any specific patient orders, consents, and surgical paperwork.

TRAINING QUESTIONS:

What is your age? Use your own

Are you married? Use your own

Occupation? Use your own

Do you have any chronic illnesses? None

Health history

> Neurological (none)
> Cardiovascular (none)
> Respiratory (none)
> Gastrointestinal (none)
> Genitourinary (none)
> Gynecological (none)
> Obstetrical (use your own)

Have you ever been hospitalized before? No.

Have you ever had surgery? Not before this.

Have you ever been pregnant? Use your own

How is your father's health? Use your own

How is your mother's health? Use your own

How is/are your sibling's health? Use your own

Immunizations up to date? All immunizations are up to date.

Diet—I try to eat healthy.

Activity/exercise: I do a lot of walking.

How did you injure your hip? I fell off a ladder taking down decorations.

Medications: None.

Psychosocial history

> Smoking history (none)
> Alcohol history (social)
> Sexual history (use your own)
> Recreational drug use (none)

You should be in a hospital gown, bra, and underwear, lying down on the table.

Graded items should have options for—Done/Not Done/N/A

Nurse Grading

COMMUNICATION

__ Introduced self (name and title)
__ Good eye contact (50% or greater of the time)
__ Spoke clearly in terms the patient can understand (three strikes rule)
__ Active listener
__ Created an atmosphere that put the patient at ease
__ Provided emotional support and reassurance
__ Asked about allergies
__ Asked about current medications
__ Contacted anesthesia department to come and evaluate the patient

PHYSICAL EXAMINATION

__ Washed hands
__ Explained to me what she/he was doing with each step
__ Helped to position me
__ Was professional in manner
__ Intravenous access confirmed
__ Intravenous fluids administered as per physicians orders
__ Dantrolene prepared and mixed with preservative-free sterile water for Intravenous injection stat

___ Patient-cooling measures initiated (ice packs, cool IV saline, cooling blanket, and so forth)
___ Labs obtained as per physician orders
___ ABGs obtained as per physician orders

PATIENT TEACHING AFTER STABILIZATION

___ Discussed what malignant hyperthermia is
___ Discussed the importance of having a caffeine halothane contracture test completed as part of follow-up for the patient's safety for future surgical procedures
___ Discussed the importance of having other family members have a caffeine halothane contracture test completed
___ Discussed resources available from the Malignant Hyperthermia Association of the United States
___ Discussed the importance of wearing a medical alert bracelet identifying malignant hyperthermia susceptibility

■ **SP will also provide feedback**

Feedback to nurse(s)/feedback to physician/feedback on team function.

REFERENCE

ASPAN. (2010). *Perianesthesia nursing standards and practice recommendations 2010–2012.* Cherry Hill, NJ: ASPAN.

CHAPTER 21

Human Simulation for Women's Health

Amy K. Nakajima and Glenn D. Posner

INTRODUCTION

*H*istorically, medical education has followed a master–apprenticeship model of "see one, do one, teach one," whereby novice doctors learn on the job while doing progressively more complex and central tasks under the supervision of a master (Patel, Glaiberman, & Gould, 2007; Pugsley & McCrorie, 2007). However, advances in educational theory, societal trends of litigation, and increasing awareness of patient safety (Institute of Medicine, 2001)—along with changing patterns in health care, emphasis on operating room efficiency, and increasing morbidity of patients with more clinically complex problems that result in diminished teaching time—suggest that the master–apprenticeship model is no longer sufficient (Bradley, 2006; Higham, 2006; Reznick and MacRae, 2006). Simulation is a logical solution to address these various needs and pressures. By providing a risk-free environment where learners can successfully master skills needed to become capable clinicians through "deliberate practice" (Ericsson, 2004), simulation has come into its own. In the specialty of obstetrics and gynecology, simulation has been incorporated into teaching, training, assessment of performance of technical and nontechnical skills, and assessment of performance of individuals and of teams (Bonin & Posner, 2004). A wide spectrum of technologies has been implemented in this regard, from the technologically very simple to the very complex (Cooper and Tacqueti, 2004; Gaba, 2004).

OVERVIEW OF SIMULATION AND SIMULATORS IN OBSTETRICS

Obstetrics is a high-risk specialty, and the availability of skilled attendants to prevent, to detect, and to manage obstetric complications is important to prevent maternal and fetal morbidity and mortality. Education, training, and clinical experience is necessary for the various members of the multidisciplinary team to acquire the knowledge, skills, and attitudes to become safe practitioners and function well together, from the obstetrician and pediatrician to the anesthesiologist and nursing personnel (Birch et al., 2007).

Macedonia, Gherman, and Satin (2003) indicated that simulations can be used to "teach, test or prepare for rare life-threatening scenarios," and that one of the advantages of simulation is its ability to expose learners to rare but critical events. They point out that teaching can become "awkward and counterproductive" when an "unpredictable life-threatening emergency [occurs with an] awake patient...a unique aspect of obstetrics." Ziv, Wolpe, Small, and Glick (2006) made a compelling argument for simulation-based medical education to "enhance patient safety, and decrease reliance on vulnerable patients for training."

Gardner (2007) defined the term *obstetric simulation* as "the reenactment of routine or critical clinical events involving a woman who is pregnant or recently delivered, and her fetus or newborn, for procedural or behavioral skills training, practice, evaluation, or research. The overall goal of obstetric simulation is to improve the quality and safety of care for women and newborns."

An excellent overview of simulation in obstetrics and gynecology by Gardner and Raemer (2008) also includes a fascinating account of the history of obstetric simulators. Obstetric simulators, known as "phantoms," were developed in the 1600s to demonstrate the birthing process and to teach midwives how to manage deliveries. Later, in the 1800s to the mid-1900s, pelvic models were developed to teach anatomy of the female pelvis and obstetric maneuvers. Other part-task trainers have been developed to teach and train skills, such as assessment of cervical dilation, episiotomy repair, and operative deliveries.

In contrast to part-task trainers, life-size, high-fidelity birthing simulators are now commercially available, which contain motor-driven mechanics that push a fetal mannequin down through the pelvis of the birthing simulator (Noelle; Gaumard Scientific Inc., Miami, FL). The most technologically sophisticated models have wireless, computer-based software.

Obstetric hybrid simulation can be performed with a live person holding a birthing pelvis and draped to achieve the appearance of seamlessness (Gardner & Raemer, 2008). The addition of a live person to a simulation scenario imparts increased realism to the scenario and the need for the participant to perform in a contextualized environment, not only to perform an individual task but also to respond and to relate to the "patient" while doing so (Ellaway, Kneebone, Lachapelle, & Topps, 2009).

OVERVIEW OF SIMULATION AND SIMULATORS IN GYNECOLOGY

Nowhere else in health science is the application of simulation, standardized patients (SP), and part-task trainers more useful than in gynecology, and these tools have revolutionized the manner in which skills are learned and assessed. Although peers can examine all other parts of each other's bodies during the learning process, the sensitive parts of the anatomy remain areas that are not routinely appropriate for these types of reciprocal teaching exercises. Teaching the speculum examination and bimanual pelvic examination remains a challenge in modern medical and nursing education.

Gynecologic Teaching Associates

To fill this need, gynecologic teaching associates (GTAs) have emerged as a way of filling that gap in skill acquisition. GTAs are women who are hired to act as SPs for medical or nursing students who are learning to perform speculum examination and bimanual pelvic examination of the female genitalia. Descriptions of GTA programs for the instruction of medical and nursing students in North America began to emerge in the literature in the mid-1980s (Beckmann, Spellacy, Yonke, Barzansky, & Cunningham, 1985; Muggah & Staseson, 1988; Plauché & Baugniet-Nebrija, 1985). By the mid-1990s, this practice was adopted at medical schools as far away as Australia (Robertson, Hegarty, O'Connor, & Gunn, 2003). In 1986, Beckmann, Sharf, Barzansky, and Spellacy studied students' experiences with this form of instruction and found that their students "emphasized the importance of the ability of the teaching associates to provide immediate informative feedback and to reduce anxiety during the teaching sessions." Women who offer themselves as GTAs are usually motivated by a desire to teach health professionals the proper way to examine women in a sensitive and respectful manner. In a study of nurse practitioner students taught using GTAs or volunteer peers, Theroux and Pearce (2006) found that the students who were taught by GTAs "rated their learning experiences [on a Likert scale] more positively and reported a better understanding of examination techniques than students who learned to perform examinations by voluntary examination of classmates." They also found that all students felt anxious, both during the educational activity and during their first clinical experiences. Theroux and Pearce also echoed the earlier findings of Beckmann et al. (1986) and reported that the advantage of the GTAs was that they "provided immediate feedback to students, decreased their feelings of anxiety, and increased their confidence in performing examinations." In general, the advantages of the GTA program are clear: Enthusiastic, altruistic, patient advocates are allowing our trainees to practice on their intimate anatomy. These women are typically very comfortable with their anatomy and can even direct trainees to their own ovaries. When organized properly into small groups of learners with discrete objectives, the GTAs can be an invaluable resource. In a randomized controlled trial, Pickard, Baraitser, Rymer, and Piper (2003) demonstrated that 44 medical students taught by GTAs had significantly better physical examination skills than 48 of their peers trained using traditional methods. In a study of Swedish medical students, Siwe, Wijma, Stjernquist, and Wijma (2003) found that students trained by GTAs "were more skilful in palpating the uterus and ovaries and performed more physical examinations during the clinical clerkship" than students trained on clinical patients.

The disadvantages of the GTA programs are cost, accessibility, potential political motivation, and trainee discomfort. GTAs provide teaching and put their own discomfort after students' needs, and as such, they expect compensation for their educational activities. This cost can often be significant when teaching budgets are tight. Accessibility can be an obstacle, as programs such as this do not exist in proximity to every nursing school. This can lead to a further increase in cost when schools choose to pay the GTAs' travel expenses to transport them from another city. In 1992, Beckmann, Lipscomb, Williford, Bryant, and Ling reviewed the source of funding for GTA programs for medical students in the United States and Canada and found that although medical schools were footing most of the bill, department chairs were being asked to use discretionary funds to pay for an increasing proportion of the cost. They worried that economic constraints would lead to the cancellation of GTA programs as "expendable luxuries."

Although the mission of the average GTA is to educate health care professionals, there are often political messages about patient empowerment associated with the teaching session. Of course, patient empowerment is also a primary goal of nursing, so this is not meant as a criticism; however, sometimes it can be felt that the political message being disseminated is more important than the clinical education that is being provided. The potential political agenda is mentioned only to sensitize schools to the notion of ensuring that their objectives match those of the GTAs. During the early years of the GTA programs, Beckmann et al. (1985) outlined the type of training that should be received by these educators. Interestingly, it has been found that students trained by laywomen had better interpersonal skills (as assessed by SPs) than students trained by physicians, although both groups demonstrated the same technical skills (Kleinman et al., 1996).

Trainee discomfort as a disadvantage of the GTA program is meant as a comparison with pelvic part-task trainers; when trainees examine GTAs, regardless of the fact that they are being paid to let them examine them, some trainees feel intimidated and rush through the examination without wanting to cause undue discomfort to the GTA. In contrast, trainees learning on a part-task trainer can spend as much time as they need feeling for the pelvic organs without causing anyone harm.

Part-Task Trainers

Where GTAs are not available or cost is a concern, models of the pelvic anatomy can be purchased and curricula developed involving their use. As it pertains to gynecology, part-task trainers are available for the female pelvis that feature normal anatomy or can include different ovarian and uterine pathology for trainees to encounter. One can perform a speculum examination on these models, allowing the teaching of Pap tests and cervical cultures for sexually transmitted infections. Numerous types of part-task trainers are available for teaching the breast examination that include interchangeable pathology or the option of strapping the model onto an individual's chest. The fidelity of these models varies and should be chosen to suit the learning objectives. For example, a model that will be used to teach the speculum examination needs to have a vaginal canal that reasonably simulates real flesh and a cervix that is properly positioned, but does not need a palpable uterus.

The advantages of part-task trainers in teaching the examination of the female genitalia relate to their inanimate nature and their reusability. First, students can feel uninhibited when practicing on these models and palpate anatomy with impunity. A sensitive approach to the examination can still be reinforced, but the students can experiment with how to manipulate the speculum inside the vagina or how to position their hands to assess the uterus without worrying about patient discomfort. Second, once the cost of these models is borne, there is very little ongoing maintenance required. Depending on the number of students palpating each model, they can be used for three or four years before they start to lose their integrity and require replacement. One benefit of owning the models is that they can be used for training and then be reused for assessment at a later time, as opposed to the GTAs where this practice would be prohibitively expensive and perhaps more difficult to gauge student performance. However, despite the potential financial constraints, GTAs have been successfully used in the evaluation of medical students' communication and examination skills (Hillard & Fang, 1986).

Conversely, the major disadvantage of part-task trainers also relates to their inanimate nature; nothing can truly replace an actual human when learning the physical examination. Whether it is the amount of pressure required to find an ovary or the correct way to part the labia when inserting a speculum, there is no substitute for practicing on a real patient. However, if trainees attempt their first few examinations on a model, they will be further along the learning curve when they have their first opportunity to practice on live patients and will gain more from that experience while causing less discomfort. Other disadvantages of the part-task trainer include the initial outlay of money to purchase an adequate number of models and the need for sufficient storage space.

As of the publication of this text, there is no randomized controlled trial comparing competence of students trained by GTAs to those trained by part-task trainers.

Standardized Patients

The use of SP has evolved into an established teaching and assessment tool since Dr. Howard Barrows (1968) suggested using SPs in a test format to assess medical students. Feedback from the SP may also be included as an additional means to assess a learner's performance of both technical and nontechnical skills (Nestel, Kneebone, & Black, 2006). Richardson, Resnick, Leonardo, and Pearsall (2009) described the design and implementation of the use of undergraduate nursing students as SPs in objective structured clinical examination stations to assess the history-taking, physical examination, and diagnostic and communication skills of advanced practice nursing students. Nestel and Kneebone (2010) described a process of incorporating the patient into the simulation by interviewing real patients about their experiences of undergoing procedures and surgeries. These interviews were taped and used to construct SP roles and scenarios. They feel that this approach of integrating actual patient experiences into the simulations enables them to place the "authentic patient voice at the center of the learning experience."

Because of the issues related to the sensitive anatomy that have been previously explored, the classic SP in gynecology is relegated to the teaching and assessment of history-taking skills. However, the specialty of gynecology involves not only sensitive anatomy but also awkward topics of conversation that are best practiced on SPs before exposure to actual patients. For example, nursing students learning to elicit a sexual history could practice this potentially uncomfortable conversation on an SP before confronting a patient. This particular use is well-described by Boendermaker, Faber, and Weijmar Schultz (2008). The SPs are widely used in objective structured clinical examinations, where trainees are required to provide contraceptive counseling, to discuss the results of an abnormal Pap test, or to provide education about sexually transmitted infections.

Hybrid Simulation

Hybrid simulation, whereby benchtop task trainers are combined with an SP, was explored as a new conceptual model for integrated skills teaching of a clinical procedure by Kneebone et al. (2002). They indicated that performing a clinical procedure required integration of the acquisition of a technical clinical skill with effective communication skills. In this pilot study, they explored the feasibility of this new model and the subjective responses of their participants who were second- and third-year medical students. The students undertook two scenarios: The first was a urinary catheterization scenario consisting of a standard catheterization model, placed adjacent to an SP, with the joint covered so that there was an appearance of seamlessness. The second was a wound closure scenario, with an SP who had a simulated tissue skin pad mounted on the arm and again draped to give the appearance of seamlessness. The students' performances were video recorded. The students provided their feedback and in turn received feedback from the SP and tutors and then, subsequently, had the opportunity to review their videotape. On the basis of tutor observation and group interviews, which took place immediately after the simulation sessions, the students felt that the opportunity to integrate communication and technical skills on an SP was a valuable and challenging learning experience. Key points and findings included the realism of the scenarios, the difficulties that the students encountered in integrating skills from different domains, and the value of immediate feedback in technical and communication skills. The group had developed a teaching method to support integrated learning of technical and communication skills within a safe and supportive learning environment that encouraged reflection.

In a later study, Higham, Nestel, Lupton, and Kneebone (2007) developed a hybrid simulation model with which to facilitate teaching and learning how to perform a gynecologic examination. Three scenarios, developed for fifth-year medical students, were structured into an initial verbal consult with an SP followed by a physical examination, for which a pelvic simulator was placed adjacent to the SP, and using pillows and a sheet, made to look seamless.

Kneebone et al. (2006) described their approach of patient-focused simulation (PFS) as a combination of a live person with high-fidelity-simulated environments. The authors describe application of PFS in low-, medium-, and high-complexity settings. They emphasize that participants are better able to suspend disbelief and to "buy" into the experience with the presence of a real "patient" and allows the tapping into "a complex web of conscious and unconscious professional responses...[which] include empathy, communication, clinical judgment, and decision-making." They suggest that the use of PFS may act as a mirror of actual practice and, as such, may facilitate assessment of practice. In a thought-provoking article, Kneebone (2009) argued that, in fact, a "decontextualized approach [might] have a counterproductive effect, fostering misleading expectations of real-world care." Furthermore, he makes the case that simulation should reflect "the messy realities and challenges of clinical practice."

Hybrid simulation has also taken the form of pairing simulators with other simulators. For example, in obstetrics and gynecology, a low-fidelity birthing pelvis can be paired with a high-fidelity mannequin to enhance capability and to augment realism in an obstetric scenario (Gardner & Raemer, 2008). Girzadas et al. (2009) also performed a study in which an endovaginal ultrasound trainer was combined with a high-fidelity mannequin (SimMan, Laerdal, Wappingers Falls, New York) to assess emergency residents' performance and interpretation of endovaginal ultrasound in a scenario wherein the patient has an ectopic pregnancy.

PATIENT SAFETY AND SIMULATION IN OBSTETRICS

The Harvard Medical Practice Study found that 1.5% of obstetric patients admitted to a hospital suffered an adverse event and that 38.3% of these outcomes were related to negligent care (Brennan et al., 1991). A retrospective analysis of 90 consecutive obstetrics and gynecology-related internal review files, opened by a center's risk managers between 1995 and 2001, was performed by White, Pichert, Bledsoe, Irwin, and Entman (2005). The group found that half of the cases were associated with inpatient obstetrics and aimed to identify potentially avoidable contributing factors. They found at least one such factor in 78% of cases.

The Joint Commission on Accreditation on Healthcare Organizations (JCAHO, 2004) published an alert on preventing infant death and injury during delivery. This alert included a summary of the identified root causes associated with 47 cases of perinatal death or permanent disability that had been reported to the JCAHO for review under the Sentinel Event Policy. On the basis of these root causes, the institution of emergency obstetric training drills was identified as a risk-reduction strategy, in addition to team training. Other strategies incorporated education (physician edu- cation and counseling), training approaches (orientation and training processes to be revised), competency assessment, and medical staff credentialing and privileging processes.

The JCAHO (2010) recently published an alert that addresses maternal mortality rates, which may, in fact, be increasing in the United States. Since 1996, a total of 84 cases of maternal death have been reported to JCAHO's sentinel event database, with the largest numbers of events reported in 2004, 2005, and 2006. According to the National Center for Health Statistics of the Centers for Disease Control and Prevention, in 2006, the national maternal mortality rate was 13.3 deaths per 100,000 live births (Heron et al., 2009). Embolism, hemorrhage, and pregnancy-induced hypertension complications were the leading causes of pregnancy-related deaths during 1991–1999 (Chang et al., 2003).

The JCAHO (2010) alert, "Preventing Maternal Death," outlined suggested actions that could be undertaken by hospitals and by providers to prevent maternal deaths, including adoption of the use of simulation in the form of protocols and drills for "responding to changes, such as hemorrhage and preeclampsia. Use the drills to train staff in the protocols, to refine local protocols, and to identify and fix systems problems that would prevent optimal care."

EDUCATIONAL PROGRAMS AND OBSTETRIC SKILL DRILLS

There are a number of educational and training programs for obstetric providers to teach and to assess both technical and nontechnical skills necessary for effective and appropriate management of obstetric emergencies. These programs or courses tend to be held over a few days, covering a number of topics, often combining didactic lectures with practical hands-on exercises. The targeted audience may be unidisciplinary, mul- tidisciplinary, or transdisciplinary in nature. The Managing Obstetric Risk Efficiently (MORE[OB]), the Advanced Life Support in Obstetrics (ALSO), the Managing Obstetric Emergencies and Trauma (MOET), and the Multidisciplinary Obstetric Simulated Emergency Scenarios (MOSES) courses are all examples of this approach.

Another training approach involves the use of skill drills, also known as "emer- gency drills" or "fire drills." In contrast to the abovementioned programs, these exer- cises tend to have more narrowly focused learning objectives, often held in situ on the labor floor (or other clinical units), and often with a team approach with care providers that normally work together. Deering, Rosen, Salas, and King (2009) outlined the advan- tages of these drills:

1. Less staff time is required to implement.
2. No travel time to an external facility is required.
3. Less scheduling difficulties are encountered, allowing more frequent training.
4. On-the-job training is facilitated.
5. System problems may be identified (Osman, Campbell, & Nassar, 2009).

Disadvantages of holding training programs or skill drills in the clinical setting include the need to ensure that patient care is adequately covered. If the unit becomes too busy, the session may need to be cancelled. There may also be concerns on how the patients perceive the training exercises. For instance, patients may become alarmed if they mistakenly believe that there is a genuine obstetric emergency occurring on the unit.

Specific Obstetric Programs

Gardner, Walzer, Simon, and Raemer (2008) described the rationale, the design, the implementation, and the evaluation of an obstetric simulation-based team training course on the basis of crisis resource management (CRM) principles. The Harvard medical community's medical malpractice closed captive insurer, the Controlled Risk Insurance Company (CRICO), Risk Management Foundation (RMF) of the Harvard Medical Institutions, had reviewed 149 perinatal closed claims and identified poor communication and poor team interactions in 43% of those cases and concluded that formal training in teamwork and communication for care providers in labor and delivery units would lead to improved perinatal outcomes. The pilot course was based on a 4-hour format, which included covering the CRM principles and 2 scenarios for the pilot course. The course participants included obstetricians, anesthesiologists, and nurses. Immediate postcourse evaluations were completed by participants, and feedback was very positive. On the basis of the experiences from the pilot, the faculty further developed the course curriculum, and the course was lengthened to 7 hours with 3 scenarios. The course participants were requested to complete immediate postcourse questionnaires to evaluate how well participants felt that the course fulfilled the stated objectives and also to document participation for continuing education credits, as the curriculum had been approved for continuing education credits for physicians, midwives, and nurses. Overall, the participants rated the course very highly. A second follow-up questionnaire was sent out to participants by mail, the "One Year or Longer Ob CRM Follow-up Survey." The overall response rate was 33%. The survey included questions asking about the participants' experience with a difficult or critical event since taking the course and the participant's perceptions of the team performance during that critical event in terms of teamwork and communication. Most survey respondents were senior clinicians, and most respondents indicated having experienced such an event since having attended the course. Most felt that their team's performance in managing a difficult case had improved since having attended the course. Most respondents who had experienced a difficult event felt that CRM principles were useful for obstetric faculty and that what they had learned during the course had been useful in their practice. CRICO/RMF has endorsed obstetric simulation-based team training as one of the risk reduction activities in their "Obstetrical Incentive Pilot Program," a voluntary program that awards a 10% malpractice insurance premium credit to obstetricians completing a series of perinatal risk reduction and team training activities.

The MORE[OB] program is a proprietary program developed by the Society of Obstetricians and Gynecologists of Canada and is now being offered through the Salus Global Corporation (2010). The MORE[OB] program is an educational program for caregivers and administrators in hospital obstetric units and emphasizes improving communication and collaboration between team members, encouraging effective teamwork, and learning through reflective practice. The program also supports the development of a culture of patient safety and system improvements.

The MORE[OB] program is structured into three modules. The first module, Learning Together, presents core clinical content, skill drills, and workshops to ensure that team members have the same background knowledge. The second module, Working Together, contains more clinical content and skill drills and introduces communication and teamwork tools. The third module, Changing Culture, introduces methods to assess and to evaluate clinical cases and reviews the program's impact to identify areas for improvement. Currently, the MORE^OB program does not incorporate the use of high-fidelity simulation.

The ALSO program is a proprietary educational program for obstetric care providers to acquire knowledge and skills necessary in the management of urgent and emergent conditions that occur during pregnancy, labor, and delivery. A number of variations exist, but the most common program structure consists of weeklong series of courses using a train-the-trainer model. A syllabus and slide set are available. A case-based approach and the use of mannequins are utilized in the acquisition of knowledge and skills.

The ALSO program was developed in the United States through a group of family physicians in Wisconsin; the course grew rapidly and is currently managed by the American Academy of Family Physicians. The program has been introduced into Canada, the United Kingdom, Europe, Asia/Pacific, South America, Central America, the Middle East, and Africa. The program is structured to encourage promulgation of the course within the host country. Host-country clinicians that attend ALSO instructor courses are evaluated and assisted as they, in turn, teach a new group of host-country clinicians. Factors for successful self-sustainability of the ALSO program include a local champion, infrastructure (a local professional organization to administer the program), finances (for the instructional materials, translation, travel, etc.), and program materials that fit the host country's stage of medical development (Deutchman, Dresang, & Winslow, 2007). Outcomes include participants' increased confidence in their skills and knowledge (Bower, Wolkomir, & Shubot, 1997).

The Royal College of Obstetricians and Gynaecologists (RCOG) and the Royal College of Midwives issued recommendations on labor ward management, which included the importance of rehearsing the management of emergencies using scenarios and models. The RCOG recognized the need for a course aimed at teaching advanced skills to specialist registrars and updating other senior clinicians, and in 1998, the RCOG's Implementation Committee commissioned the development of the MOET course. Literature on obstetric emergencies had been reviewed and collated into evidence-based guidelines, which became the core of the MOET manual. Separately commissioned reviews on trauma in pregnancy and nationally available guidance on adult life support comprised the general components of the theoretical teaching. The MOET project aims to improve professional performance, encouraging effective and efficient care, and through risk management, ultimately improve the clinical outcome for patients (Johanson et al., 1999).

Faculty for the MOET course had backgrounds in resuscitation courses, including leading members of the Battlefield Advanced Trauma Life Support, ALSO, and others with experience from Advanced Trauma Life Support, Advanced Cardiac Life Support, and Advanced Paediatric Life Support. Participants were mainly registrars from the West Midlands Region. Baseline knowledge of the participants was assessed with multiple choice questions (MCQs) completed before the first session. The original course was conducted for more than 3 days, with the first day covering adult life support and the management of trauma and the second day covering obstetric emergencies. A variety of teaching methods was used. Each topic was introduced by a short summary lecture followed by hands-on practice on the basis of real-life scenarios and using five different types of models: animal cadaver, "Resusci Annie," purpose-made assisted delivery model, symphysiotomy model, and moulage (simulated casualties) with actors.

The third morning was used for an assessment of the candidates who managed one obstetric emergency and one adult life-support scenario and completed a set of post-training MCQs. Participants received individual feedback. The first two courses were run in 1998. Because of the feedback from the first course, an extra cardiopulmonary resuscitation module was included in the second course. The original project recorded participants' feedback and evaluations, which were largely positive. A follow-up postal survey was sent to the participants 10 months after the first and 4 months after the second course. Sixty-three percent responded to the postal survey, and the results suggest that the participants felt that the course was useful clinically and should be incorporated into residency training.

The adoption of the MOET course in the United Kingdom seems to have been quite successful, with increasing numbers of courses being held each year and continued positive feedback from attendees. In November 2000, UNICEF sponsored a MOET course in Bangladesh, the format of which was similar to the UK-based courses. It ran for more than two days, covering adult life support and the management of burns and trauma, obstetric, neonatal, and anesthetic emergencies, using a variety of teaching methods. On the third morning, attendees underwent an obstetric emergency simulation, and their performances were assessed by a pair of instructors; they also underwent a post-test identical to the pretest. The participants received individual feedback and were requested to assess the course. Overall scores demonstrate improvement in the posttest. The participants rated the course highly (Johanson, Akhtar, et al., 2002).

The MOET course has been run in Armenia with a similar format as the course in Bangladesh. Findings were also similar in that all candidates showed improvement in postcourse scores (Johanson, Menon, et al., 2002).

The MOSES course was developed by clinician-educators at Barts and the London Medical Simulation Centre, London, to address the need for better interprofessional teamwork in obstetric care (Freeth et al., 2009). The emphasis of this course, unlike other programs, is not on the clinical aspects of patient management during obstetric emergencies, but rather on the nontechnical aspects of care and their impact on patient safety. The targeted participants of this one-day simulation-based continuing education course consist of experienced midwives, obstetricians, and obstetric anesthetists held in a simulation center.

MOSES courses promote key principles to support patient safety on the basis of the key points of anesthesia CRM.

1. Share clear goals and objectives.
2. Anticipate and plan together.
3. Communicate effectively.
4. Share information freely.
5. Develop a climate of support and trust.
6. Work through conflict.
7. Have leadership appropriate to the members and situation.
8. Distribute workload appropriately.
9. Develop the team members.
10. Review progress regularly.

The interprofessional scenarios were video recorded and were followed by facilitated debriefing sessions. The participants were later interviewed by telephone or by e-mail.

The results of the interviews were then coded and analyzed. One of the themes that emerged was that the course was appreciated as an educational opportunity to learn together as peers. The course appeared to facilitate relationship building between the group members and allowed participants to explore the roles within the group. The second theme that emerged was that the participants appeared to have learned about the role of communication and leadership in crisis situations. The third theme that emerged was that a number of the participants appeared to have taken what they had learned during the course and integrated that learning into their daily clinical practice. The authors suggest that there has been transfer of learning, but this is based on the participants' self-report and not on observed objective performance assessment (Gardner et al., 2008).

Deering et al. (2009) described the development and implementation of the Mobile Obstetric Emergencies Simulator (MOES) system. MOES is a package of simulation technology, scenario-based training curriculum, and performance measurement and debriefing tools designed to build and maintain preparedness for obstetric emergencies. The development of the MOES system was prompted by four overarching goals of improving patient safety, improving teamwork and technical performance, identifying and correcting systems issues unique to each labor and delivery unit, and meeting JCAHO recommendations.

Teamwork skills are incorporated into the MOES curriculum through alignment with another training program, Team Strategies and Tools to Enhance Performance and Patient Safety (TeamSTEPPS). MOES incorporates the following features:

1. Mobility so that simulations can be run on the actual L&D unit.
2. A standardized curriculum.
3. The ability to evaluate both teamwork and technical competency.
4. Incorporation of best practices in debriefing to maximize learning outcomes.
5. Capacity to track performance over time.
6. Realization of the preceding goals in a cost-effective manner.

Obstetric Skill Drills

Skill drills and systematic, organized, sometimes proprietary obstetric courses have been developed for training and assessment of knowledge and skills needed to manage obstetric emergencies. Some initiatives emphasize knowledge and technical skills, and others may highlight nontechnical skills of the individual practitioners. Practitioners involved in training may range in experience from the novice to the expert (Deering, Brown, Hodor, & Satin, 2006; Deering, Poggi, Macedonia, Gherman, & Satin, 2004; Goffman, Heo, Pardanani, Merkatz, & Bernstein, 2008). Other initiatives may focus on the team aspects of the obstetric team, such as teamwork, team communication, and its multidisciplinary nature. Rall and Dieckman (2005) suggested that simulation may be used "to train and safely experiment on subsystems like the operating room or the intensive care unit with effects on patient safety in the larger system." Maslovitz, Barkai, Lessing, Ziv, and Many (2007) identified recurrent errors by trainees, consisting of residents and midwives grouped into teams participating in obstetric simulation scenarios held in a simulation center. The scenarios were eclamptic seizure, postpartum hemorrhage, shoulder dystocia, and breech extraction. The most common management errors were identified as follows: delay in transporting the bleeding patient to the operating room (82%), unfamiliarity with prostaglandin administration to reverse uterine atony (82%), poor cardiopulmonary resuscitation techniques (80%), inadequate documentation of shoulder dystocia (80%), delayed administration of blood products to reverse consumption coagulopathy (66%), and inappropriate avoidance of episiotomy in shoulder dystocia and breech extraction (32%).

Osman et al. (2009) conducted a prospective trial at three hospitals in Beirut, Lebanon. This study aimed to assess the feasibility and usefulness of conducting in situ obstetric skill drills that tested the hospital system. Two different emergency drills were held at two points in time between January and May 2006. Problems affecting patient care were identified and categorized. Unsurprisingly, inappropriate management was noted as a factor; for example, magnesium sulfate was not given during the eclampsia drill. Interestingly, the study highlighted other categories that contributed to suboptimal care, such as "lack of correct equipment/drugs in the correct place," "lack of medications or inadequate quantities of medications in the ER," "problems in communication," and "problems with policies for emergencies." The study identified hospital policies and systems that needed to be clarified or changed.

Crofts et al. (2006) assessed the effectiveness of simulation training for shoulder dystocia management and also compared two methods of training: training with low-fidelity mannequins compared with training with high-fidelity mannequins with force monitoring. In a later study, Crofts, Bartlett, et al. (2007) studied skill retention in management of shoulder dystocia 6 and 12 months after initial training. More recently, Draycott et al. (2008) performed a retrospective observational study comparing the management of shoulder dystocia and associated neonatal injury before and after the introduction of shoulder dystocia training for all staff in a single maternity unit in the United Kingdom. Intrapartum and postpartum records of term cephalic singleton vaginal deliveries were reviewed, with 15,908 and 13,117 eligible births pretraining and posttraining, respectively. Rates of shoulder dystocia in the two groups were similar: 324 (2.04%) for pretraining and 262 (2.00%) for posttraining. Training was performed using the PROMPT Birthing Trainer (Limbs and Things Ltd., Bristol) and included risk factors, diagnosis and demonstration of the maneuvers to resolve shoulder dystocia, and appropriate documentation in addition to a simulation of a delivery complicated by shoulder dystocia. They found that clinical management, as measured by performance of the maneuvers to resolve shoulder dystocia, improved after training was introduced. Moreover, there appeared to be an effect on clinical neonatal outcomes, as there was a reduction in the rate of brachial plexus injury at birth after the introduction of training.

In addition to drills created for shoulder dystocia training (Crofts et al., 2006; Crofts, Bartlett, et al. 2007; Deering et al., 2004; Goffman et al., 2008), drills have also been created for training management of eclampsia (Ellis et al., 2008; Maslovitz et al., 2007; Osman et al., 2009; Thompson, Neal, & Clark, 2004), vaginal breech delivery (Deering et al., 2006; Maslovitz et al., 2007), and postpartum hemorrhage (Birch et al., 2007; Maslovitz et al., 2007).

SIMULATION AND TEAMWORK TRAINING IN OBSTETRICS

In their article, Birnbach and Salas (2008) described the rationale for the use of simulation and team training to reduce medical errors in the labor and delivery unit. Crew resource management training and the prerequisites for successful implementation of training are outlined. In addition, they discuss how miscommunication and unprofessional behaviors contribute to adverse patient outcomes and that simulation may be used to improve team behaviors.

Nielsen and Mann (2008) described the application of crew resource management from aviation to medicine. In this article, they discuss error theory, the importance of leadership in culture change, and the development of a teamwork training program, TeamSTEPPS, which comprises four competencies:

■ Team leadership, which includes the skills of role clarity, resource management, teamwork behaviors, and conflict resolution
■ Situation monitoring, which includes situation awareness and shared mental models
■ Mutual support, which includes the skills of task assistance, advocacy, and feedback
■ Communication, which includes the practices of call-out and check back, the concept of the two-challenge rule, and the techniques of SBAR and DESC

Mann and Pratt (2008) described a curriculum on the basis of TeamSTEPPS with a detailed discussion of the teamwork concepts, tools and skills, and helpful examples of both.

Very recently, Merien, van de Ven, Mol, Houterman, and Oei (2010) published a systematic review of the literature on the effectiveness of multidisciplinary teamwork training in a simulation setting to improve patients, outcomes by preventing errors in acute obstetric emergencies. They searched MEDLINE, Embase, and the Cochrane database from inception to June 2009, identifying 97 studies. They searched only for articles that reported on objective measures in the management of obstetric emergencies by teamwork training of staff on the labor ward using simulation models, and found eight articles fitting their criteria. Four of the eight were randomized controlled trials (Crofts et al., 2006; Crofts, Ellis, et al., 2007; Crofts et al., 2008; Ellis et al., 2008), and the other four were studies that incorporated pretraining versus posttraining comparisons without a control group (Birch et al., 2007; Draycott et al., 2006; Maslovitz et al., 2007; Robertson et al., 2009). Outcomes in these studies included patient outcomes, knowledge, technical skills, communication, team performance, and the effect of teamwork in obstetric emergencies.

Planning and Designing an Obstetric Simulation

Flanagan, Nestel, and Joseph (2004) emphasized the need to couple effective curriculum and assessment of performance in using the simulator, which they remind us is only a teaching tool, regardless of the modality. Similarly, Salas and Burke (2002) emphasized that simulation is a tool, and for simulation to be effective for training, certain conditions need to be fulfilled:

1. Instructional features are embedded within the simulation.
2. Carefully crafted scenarios are embedded within the simulation.
3. Simulation contains opportunities for assessing and diagnosing individual or team performance.
4. Learning experience is guided.
5. Simulation fidelity is matched to training requirements.
6. There is a reciprocal partnership between subject matter experts and learning/training specialists.

Fahey and Mighty (2008) provided an elegant and stepwise approach to create and implement shoulder dystocia training. They begin by providing background and current literature review of the topic, which clearly explains the relevance of developing and implementing training and the potential benefit of improved patient outcomes. Next, they describe the need for establishing clear goals and objectives. With goals and objectives in place, they walk the reader through the process of designing a training session and pose key questions:

1. Where and by whom will the training be conducted?
2. When and how often will the training be conducted?
3. What sort of model/trainer/mannequin/simulator will be needed?
    a. A very helpful discussion is included, which discusses how to choose a simulator on the basis of needs, budget, and proposed usage.
4. What management approach is going to be taught?
    a. Select an appropriate management protocol/guideline to standardize the content of the training session and to help in creating an assessment tool. Protocols should be in alignment with current literature.
    b. Incorporation of teamwork principles, training both on documentation and on disclosure, and discussion of adverse events with patients are discussed.
5. Should force monitoring be used in the training?
6. What sort of evaluation/debriefing tools will be used?

Apart from the fifth question on the use of force monitoring, which may be most relevant to shoulder dystocia training, the other questions can be used to guide the development and implementation of training sessions of other types of obstetric emergencies, such as eclampsia or postpartum hemorrhage.

Assessment of Performance and Evaluation of Programs

In addition to planning and developing a single scenario, a training program, or a curriculum on a larger scale, the inclusion of assessment is as important as the establishment of goals and objectives and the design of the educational session (Flanagan et al., 2004; Salas & Burke, 2002). Feedback is often requested from participants in the form of questionnaires or surveys, immediately after the completion of the learning activity. Participants may be asked for their perceptions of course quality, quality of debriefing, realism of the scenarios, value of the didactic sessions, and recommended course frequency (Gardner et al., 2008). Other outcome measures include participants' increased confidence in their skills and knowledge (Bower et al., 1997). Follow-up surveys have also been used (Gardner et al., 2008; Johanson et al., 1999). Feedback may also be obtained through the use of interviews and focus groups (Freeth et al., 2009).

Assessment can be made on the performance within the simulation of technical and nontechnical skills and also on the performance of the individual participant and the team (Morgan, Pittini, Regehr, Marrs, & Haley, 2007; Nielsen et al., 2007). Learning may be assessed through the use of prescenario and postscenario testing in the form of MCQs or written tests. Retention of learned skills may be studied with repeated scenarios over an interval of time (Crofts, Bartlett, et al., 2007).

The effectiveness of a drill or program may be reflected in system or organizational change, including the adoption of evidence-based protocols and guidelines, the simplification and standardization of requisitions, and the physical changes in the layout of the workplace (such as organizing all the cupboards on the labor and delivery unit in a standard fashion). A positive change in staff attitude and organizational culture may be reflected in measures such as decreased staff sick leave (Sorensen et al., 2009) and improved safety climate of the ward or hospital (Pettker et al., 2009).

The most important parameter is the one most difficult to measure: the true impact that a drill or training program has on actual patient outcomes because the aim of these training programs and drills incorporating simulation is to reduce the occurrence of adverse events and to optimize patient safety (Draycott et al., 2008).

REFERENCES

Association of Professors of Gynecology and Obstetrics. (2004). *Association of Professors of Gynecology and Obstetrics (APGO) Medical Student Educational Objectives* (8th ed.). Crofton, MD: Author.

Barrows, H. S. (1968). Simulated patients in medical teaching. *Canadian Medical Association Journal, 98*, 674–676.

Beckmann, C. R., Lipscomb, G. H., Williford, L., Bryant, E., & Ling, F. W. (1992). Gynaecological teaching associates in the 1990s. *Medical Education, 26*, 105–109.

Beckmann, C. R., Sharf, B. F., Barzansky, B. M., & Spellacy, W. N. (1986). Student response to gynecologic teaching associates. *American Journal of Obstetrics and Gynecology, 155*, 301–306.

Beckmann, C. R., Spellacy, W. N., Yonke, A., Barzansky, B., & Cunningham, R. P. (1985). Initial instruction in the pelvic examination in the United States and Canada, 1983. *American Journal of Obstetrics and Gynecology, 151*, 58–60.

Birch, L., Jones, N., Doyle, P. M., Green, P., McLaughlin, A., Champney, C., et al. (2007). Obstetric skills drills: Evaluation of teaching methods. *Nurse Education Today, 27*, 915–922.

Birnbach, D. J., & Salas, E. (2008). Can medical simulation and team training reduce errors in labor and delivery? *Anesthesiology Clinics, 26*, 159–168.

Boendermaker, P. M., Faber, V., & Weijmar Schultz, W. C. (2008). Dealing with difficult sexual questions during consultations: A new training program. *Journal of Psychosomatic Obstetrics and Gynaecology, 29*, 79–82.

Bonin, B., & Posner, G. D. (2004). Simulation in obstetrics and gynecology. In G. E. Loyd, C. L. Lake, & R. Greenberg (Eds.), *Practical healthcare simulations*. Philadelphia, PA: Mosby.

Bower, D., Wolkomir, M., & Shubot, D. (1997). The effects of the ALSO® course as an educational intervention for residents. *Family Medicine, 29*(3), 187–193.

Bradley, P. (2006). The history of simulation in medical education and possible future directions. *Medical Education, 40*, 254–262.

Brennan, T., Leape, L., Laird, N., Hebert, L., Localio, A., Lawthers A., et al. (1991). Incidence of adverse events and negligence in hospitalized patients: Results of the Harvard Medical Practice Study. *New England Journal of Medicine, 324*, 370–376.

Chang, J., Elam-Evans, L. D., Berg, C. J., Herndon, J., Flowers, L., Seed, K. A., et al. (2003). Pregnancy-related mortality surveillance—United States, 1991–1999. *MMWR Surveillance Summaries, 52*(SS02), 1–8.

Cooper, J. B., & Tacqueti, V. R. (2004). A brief history of the development of mannequin simulators for clinical education and training. *Quality and Safety in Health Care, 13*(Suppl. 1), i11–i18.

Crofts, J. F., Bartlett, C., Ellis, D., Hunt, L. P., Fox, R., & Draycott, T. J. (2006). Training for shoulder dystocia: A trial of simulation using low-fidelity and high-fidelity mannequins. *Obstetrics and Gynecology, 108*, 1477–1485.

Crofts, J. F., Bartlett, C., Ellis, D., Hunt, L. P., Fox, R., & Draycott, T. J. (2007). Management of shoulder dystocia: Skill retention 6 and 12 months after training. *Obstetrics and Gynecology, 110*, 1069–1074.

Crofts, J. F., Bartlett, C., Ellis, D., Winter, C., Donald, F., Hunt, L. P., & Draycott, T. J. (2008). Patient–actor perception of care: A comparison of obstetric emergency training using manikins and patient-actors. *Quality and Safety in Health Care, 17,* 20–24.

Crofts, J. F., Ellis, D., Draycott, T. J., Winter, C., Hunt, L. P., & Akande, V. A. (2007). Change in knowledge of midwives and obstetric emergency training: A randomized controlled trial of local hospital, simulation centre and teamwork training. *British Journal of Obstetrics and Gynaecology, 114,* 1534–1541.

Deering, S., Brown, J., Hodor, J., & Satin, A. J. (2006). Simulation training and resident performance of singleton vaginal breech delivery. *Obstetrics and Gynecology, 107,* 86–89.

Deering, S., Poggi, S., Macedonia, C., Gherman, R., & Satin, A. J. (2004). Improving resident competency in the management of shoulder dystocia with simulation training. *Obstetrics and Gynecology, 103,* 1224–1228.

Deering, S., Rosen, M. A., Salas, E., & King, H. B. (2009). Building team and technical competency for obstetric emergencies: The Mobile Obstetric Emergencies Simulator (MOES) system. *Simulation in Healthcare, 4,* 166–173.

Deutchman, M., Dresang, L., & Winslow, D. (2007). Advanced Life Support in Obstetrics (ALSO®) International Development. *Family Medicine, 39*(9), 618–622.

Draycott, T. J., Crofts, J. F., Ash, J. P., Wilson, L. V., Yard, E., Sibanda, T., et al. (2008). Improving neonatal outcome through practical shoulder dystocia training. *Obstetrics and Gynecology, 112,* 14–20.

Draycott, T. J., Sibanda, T., Owen, L., Akande, V., Winter, C., Reading, S., et al. (2006). Does training in obstetric emergencies improve neonatal outcome? *British Journal of Obstetrics and Gynaecology, 113,* 177–182.

Ellaway, R. H., Kneebone, R., Lachapelle, K., & Topps, D. (2009). Practica continua: Connecting and combining simulation modalities for integrated teaching, learning and assessment. *Medical Teacher, 31,* 725–731.

Ellis, D., Crofts, J. F., Hunt, L. P., Read, M., Fox, R., & James, M. (2008). Hospital, simulation center, and teamwork training for eclampsia management: A randomized controlled trial. *Obstetrics and Gynecology, 111,* 723–731.

Ericsson, K. A. (2004). Deliberate practice and the acquisition and maintenance of expert performance in medicine and related domains. *Academic Medicine, 79,* S70–S81.

Fahey, J. O., & Mighty, H. E. (2008). Shoulder dystocia: Using simulation to train providers and teams. *Journal of Perinatal and Neonatal Nursing, 22,* 114–122.

Flanagan, B., Nestel, D., & Joseph, M. (2004). Making patient safety the focus: Crisis resource management in the undergraduate curriculum. *Medical Education, 38,* 56–66.

Freeth, D., Ayida, G., Berridge, E. J., Mackintosh, N., Norris, B., Sadler, C., et al. (2009). Multidisciplinary Obstetric Simulated Emergency Scenarios (MOSES): Promoting patient safety in obstetrics with teamwork-focused interprofessional simulations. *Journal of Continuing Education in the Health Professions, 29*(2), 98–104.

Gaba, D. M. (2004). The future vision of simulation in health care. *Quality and Safety in Health Care, 13*(Suppl. 1), i2–i10.

Gardner, R. (2007). Simulation and simulator technology in obstetrics: Past, present and future. *Expert Review in Obstetrics and Gynecology, 2*(6), 775–790.

Gardner, R., & Raemer, D. B. (2008). Simulation in obstetrics and gynecology. *Obstetrics and Gynecology Clinics of North America, 35,* 97–127.

Gardner, R., Walzer, T. B., Simon, R., & Raemer, D. B. (2008). Obstetric simulation as a risk control strategy: Course design and evaluation. *Simulation in Healthcare, 3,* 119–127.

Girzadas, D. V., Antonis, M. S., Zerth, H., Lambert, M., Clay, L., Bose, S., et al. (2009). Hybrid simulation combining a high fidelity scenario with a pelvic ultrasound trainer enhances the training and evaluation of endovaginal ultrasound skills. *Academic Emergency Medicine, 16,* 429–435.

Goffman, D., Heo, H., Pardanani, S., Merkatz, I. R., & Bernstein, P. S. (2008). Improving shoulder dystocia management among resident and attending physicians using simulations. *American Journal of Obstetrics and Gynecology, 199,* 294.e1–294.e5.

Heron, M., Hoyert, D. L., Murphy, S. L., Xu, J., Kochanek, K. D., & Tejada-Vera, B. (2009). Deaths: Final data for 2006. National Center for Health Statistics. *National Vital Statistics Reports, 57*(14), 1–117.

Higham, J. (2006). Current themes in the teaching of obstetrics and gynaecology in the United Kingdom. *Medical Teacher, 28*, 495–496.

Higham, J., Nestel, D., Lupton, M., & Kneebone, R. (2007). Teaching and learning gynaecology examination with hybrid simulation. *Clinical Teacher, 4*, 238–243.

Higham, J., & Steer, P. J. (2004). Gender gap in undergraduate experience and performance in obstetrics and gynaecology: Analysis of clinical experience logs. *British Medical Journal, 328*, 142–143.

Hillard, P. J., & Fang, W. L. (1986). Medical students' gynecologic examination skills. Evaluation by gynecology teaching associates. *Journal of Reproductive Medicine, 31*(6), 491–496.

Institute of Medicine. (2001). *To err is human: Building a safer health system*. Washington, DC: National Academy Press.

Johanson, R., Akhtar, S., Edwards, C., Dewan, F., Haque, Y., & Jones, P. (2002). MOET: Bangladesh—An initial experience. *Journal of Obstetrics and Gynaecologic Research, 28*(4), 217–223.

Johanson, R. B., Cox, C., O'Donnell, E., Grady, K., Howell, C. J., & Jones, P. W. (1999). Managing obstetric emergencies and trauma (MOET). Structured skills training using models and reality based scenarios. *Obstetrics and Gynecology, 1*(2), 46–52.

Johanson, R. B., Menon, V., Burns, E., Kargramanya, E., Osipov, V., Israelyan, M., et al. (2002). Managing Obstetric Emergencies and Trauma (MOET) structured skills training in Armenia, utilising models and reality based scenarios. *BMC Medical Education, 2*(5), 1–7.

Joint Commission on Accreditation on Healthcare Organizations. (2004). Preventing infant death and injury during delivery. *Sentinel Event Alert, 30*.

Joint Commission on Accreditation on Healthcare Organizations. (2010). Preventing maternal death. *Sentinel Event Alert, 44*.

Kneebone, R. (2009). Simulation and transformational change: The paradox of expertise. *Academic Medicine, 84*, 954–957.

Kneebone, R., Kidd, J., Nestel, D., Asvall, S., Paraskeva, P., & Darzi, A. (2002). An innovative model for teaching and learning clinical procedures. *Medical Education, 36*, 628–634.

Kneebone, R., Nestel, D., Wetzel, C., Black, S., Jacklin, R., Aggarwal, R., et al. (2006). The human face of simulation: Patient-focused simulation training. *Academic Medicine, 81*, 919–924.

Macedonia, C. R., Gherman, R. B., & Satin, A. J. (2003). Simulation laboratories for training in obstetrics and gynecology. *Obstetrics and Gynecology, 102*, 388–392.

Mann, S., & Pratt, S. D. (2008). Team approach to care in labor and delivery. *Clinical Obstetrics and Gynecology, 51*, 666–679.

Maslovitz, S., Barkai, G., Lessing, J. B., Ziv, A., & Many, A. (2007). Recurrent obstetric management mistakes identified by simulation. *Obstetrics and Gynecology, 109*, 1295–1300.

Merien, A. E. R., van de Ven, J., Mol, B. W., Houterman, S., & Oei, S. G. (2010). Multidisciplinary team training in a simulation setting for acute obstetric emergences. *Obstetrics and Gynecology, 115*, 1021–1031.

Morgan, P. J., Rittini, R., Regehr, G., Marrs, C., & Haley, M. F. (2007). Evaluating teamwork in a simulated obstetric environment. *Anesthesiology, 106*, 907–915.

Muggah, H. F., & Staseson, S. (1988). The Gynecological Teaching Associates Program. *Canadian Nurse, 84*(2), 28–30.

Nestel, D., & Kneebone, R. (2010). Authentic patient perspectives in simulations for procedural and surgical skills. *Academic Medicine, 85*, 889–893.

Nestel, D., Kneebone, R., & Black, S. (2006). Simulated patients and the development of procedural and operative skills. *Medical Teacher, 28*, 390–391.

Nielsen, P., & Mann, S. (2008). Team function in obstetrics to reduce errors and improve outcomes. *Obstetrics and Gynecology Clinics of North America, 35*, 81–95.

Nielsen, P. E., Goldman, M. B., Mann, S., Shapiro, D. E., Marcus, R. G., Pratt, S. D., et al. (2007). Effects of teamwork training on adverse outcomes and process of care in labor and delivery: A randomized controlled trial. *Obstetrics and Gynecology, 109*, 48–55.

Osman, H., Campbell, O. M. R., & Nassar, A. H. (2009). Using emergency obstetric drills in maternity units as a performance improvement tool. *Birth, 36*(1), 43–50.

Patel, A. A., Glaiberman, C., & Gould, D. A. (2007). Procedural simulation. *Anesthesiology Clinics, 25*, 349–359.

Pettker, C. M., Thung, S. F., Norwitz, E. R., Buhimschi, C. S., Raab, C. A., Copel, J. A., et al. (2009). The impact of a comprehensive patient safety strategy on obstetric adverse events. *American Journal of Obstetrics and Gynecology, 200,* 492.e1–492.e8.

Pickard, S., Baraitser, P., Rymer, J., & Piper J. (2003). Can gynaecology teaching associates provide high quality effective training for medical students in the United Kingdom? Comparative study. *British Medical Journal, 327,* 1389–1392.

Plauché, W. C., & Baugniet-Nebrija, W. (1985). Students' and physicians' evaluations of gynecologic teaching associate program. *Journal of Medical Education, 60(11),* 870–875.

Posner, G., & Nakajima, A. (2010). Development of an undergraduate curriculum in obstetrical simulation. *Medical Education, 44,* 520–521.

Pugsley, L., & McCrorie, P. (2007). Improving medical education: Improving patient care. *Teaching and Teacher Education, 23,* 314–322.

Rall, M., & Dieckmann, P. (2005). Simulation and patient safety: The use of simulation to enhance patient safety on a systems level. *Current Anaesthesia and Critical Care, 16,* 273–281.

Reznick, R. K., & MacRae, H. (2006). Teaching surgical skills—Changes in the wind. *New England Journal of Medicine, 355,* 2664–2669.

Richardson, L., Resnick, L., Leonardo, M., & Pearsall, C. (2009). Undergraduate students as standardized patients to assess advanced practice nursing student competencies. *Nurse Educator, 34,* 12–16.

Robertson, B., Schumacher, L., Gosman, G., Kanfer, R., Kelley, M., & De Vita, M. (2009). Simulation-based crisis team training for multidisciplinary obstetric providers. *Simulation in Healthcare, 4,* 77–83.

Robertson, K., Hegarty, K., O'Connor, V., & Gunn, J. (2003). Women teaching women's health: Issues in the establishment of a clinical teaching associate program for the well woman check. *Women's Health, 34,* 49–65.

Salas, E., & Burke, C. S. (2002). Simulation for training is effective when... *Quality and Safety in Health Care, 11,* 119–120.

Salus Global Corporation. (2010). MORE[OB] brochure. Retrieved from http://salusgc.com/moreob_overview.html

Siwe, K., Wijma, K., Stjernquist, M., & Wijma, B. (2007). Medical students learning the pelvic examination: Comparison of outcome in terms of skills between a professional patient and a clinical patient model. *Patient Education and Counseling, 68(3),* 211–217.

Sorensen, J. L., Lokkegaard, E., Johansen, M., Ringsted, C., Kreiner, S., & McAleer, S. (2009). The implementation and evaluation of a mandatory multi-professional obstetric skills training program. *Acta Obstetricia et Gynecologica Scandinavica, 88,* 1107–1117.

Theroux, R., & Pearce, C. (2006). Graduate students' experiences with standardized patients as adjuncts for teaching pelvic examinations. *Journal of the American Academy of Nurse Practitioners, 18(9),* 429–435.

Thompson, S., Neal, S., & Clark, V. (2004). Clinical risk management in obstetrics: Eclampsia drills. *British Medical Journal, 328,* 269–271.

White, A. A., Pichert, J. W., Bledsoe, S. H., Irwin, C., & Entman, S. S. (2005). Cause and effect analysis of closed claims in obstetrics and gynecology. *Obstetrics and Gynecology, 105,* 1031–1038.

Ziv, A., Wolpe, P. R., Small, S. D., & Glick, S. (2006). Simulation-based medical education: An ethical imperative. *Simulation in Healthcare, 1,* 252–256.

APPENDIX 21.A

OBSTETRICS SIMULATION FOR UNDERGRADUATE MEDICAL STUDENTS

Drs. Glenn Posner and Amy Nakajima
The Ottawa Hospital, The University of Ottawa

Background and Rationale

We developed an undergraduate simulation curriculum in obstetrics in 2008 at the University of Ottawa, Ottawa, Canada (Posner & Nakajima, 2010). We found that the medical students had varied experiences on the clinical rotation in obstetrics and often felt that they were not part of the team, and in fact were a burden to the residents, nursing staff, and attending physicians. The opportunities for students to become involved in routine physical examinations (speculum, digital examinations), routine procedures (artificial rupture of membranes), and uncomplicated vaginal deliveries also varied, depending on the site of the rotation, the assertiveness of the student, the individual attending, the dynamics of the nursing staff, and the gender of the student. We developed a short interactive obstetric curriculum, using an obstetric simulator, for groups of 10 students at a time, to address the potential unevenness of the clinical experience and to act as an introduction to the rotation. The curriculum consists of a single obstetric patient whose clinical course the students follow and assess, starting at a triage visit, through her admission, to the eventual delivery.

The development of this curriculum was in response to the students' feedback of the shortcomings of the current didactic lectures and the feeling of not being integrated into the health care team when on their clinical rotation. In addition, published literature regarding undergraduate experiences of obstetric rotations suggested that with medicolegal concerns, students are experiencing less hands-on learning opportunities (Higham, 2006). We hoped that this curriculum would address the existence of a gender bias (Higham & Steer, 2004); male students appear to have additional challenges in obtaining good clinical exposure, given that the patients were all women, and some clearly preferred female students; also that the nurses were, again, all women and may have had reservations against male learners.

We had debated on the structure of our simulation curriculum and had decided that it would be useful for it to take the form of case-based learning. The students will cover the following items in "chronologic" sequence, as if faced with a single patient. That is, when meeting a patient in triage, a student would start with taking a history, then progress to performing a physical examination to make a diagnosis of labor, decide when to admit the patient, and then consider elements of management of labor, including pain control.

Our curriculum was originally designed for undergraduate medical students on their obstetrics rotation, but could easily be modified for students in advanced practice nursing and midwifery programs.

Introduction

Because of the sensitive and often emergency nature of obstetrics, students are often placed in an observational role rather than functioning as a full member of the medical team. Students rarely have the opportunity to think through a problem and manage an obstetric case from start to finish without the intervention of residents or attending physicians. It is our belief that hands-on experience with Noelle (Gaumard Scientific Company, Inc., Miami, FL), the high-fidelity birthing simulator, in conjunction with small-group learning will facilitate student learning of bread and butter obstetrics.

Through the use of Noelle, medical students will be introduced to the course of normal labor and delivery and be coached how to assist and perform a vaginal delivery in a safe, supportive environment, which allows time for rehearsal of newly learned skills. The curriculum will also include an introduction to patient safety and CRM. The content of the curriculum will incorporate those educational objectives outlined in the *Association of Professors of Gynecology and Obstetrics (APGO) Medical Student Educational Objectives*, eighth edition (APGO, 2004). The simulator curriculum will be integrated into the existing structure of the undergraduate curriculum, consisting of didactic lectures and clinical clerkship. We hope that this curriculum will aid the medical students to acquire the knowledge, skills, and attitudes outlined in the APGO Educational Objectives and to spark enthusiasm and engagement during their clinical rotation.

Overall Goals of the Curriculum

The ultimate goal of the program is to expose the new clerkship students to the fundamentals of obstetrics in an interactive and hands-on manner to maximize interest, knowledge retention, and skill development.

Goals and Objectives

Students participating in this simulation session will be able to

a. Take a focused history from an obstetric patient presenting in the triage unit.
b. Perform a focused physical examination on an obstetric patient in labor.
c. Synthesize the findings on history and physical, to confirm a diagnosis of labor.
d. Define labor and all of its stages.
e. Decide whether or not to admit an obstetric patient to the labor and delivery unit.
f. Take a focused history from an obstetric patient with hypertension, related to the diagnosis of preeclampsia.
g. Perform a focused physical examination on an obstetric patient with suspected preeclampsia.
h. Order appropriate investigations for a patient with preeclampsia.
i. Describe the options available to augment labor, such as amniotomy and oxytocin infusion.
j. Describe the pain control options available to patients in labor and when they are appropriate—that is, narcotics, nitrous oxide, epidural, massage, Jacuzzi, birthing ball, and so forth.
k. Demonstrate the techniques of amniotomy and placement of an internal fetal monitor.
l. Interpret the fetal heart rate monitor tracing, including baseline, variability, accelerations, and decelerations.
m. Discuss the management of the second stage of labor.
n. Demonstrate the proper technique of spontaneous vaginal delivery and management of the third stage of labor.
o. Describe the indications and criteria for operative vaginal delivery and observe a demonstration of the technique of forceps or vacuum delivery on a mannequin.
p. Demonstrate the management of a delivery complicated by shoulder dystocia and review the maneuvers required to resolve the shoulder dystocia.
q. Describe the indications for cesarean section.
r. Describe the first steps of basic neonatal resuscitation.

Teaching Methods

The session will begin with introductory remarks about the goal and objectives of the session. The students will be oriented to Noelle and the simulation room and take their seats around Noelle. Noelle will be preloaded with a baby and dilated to 2–3 cm. The case will then be presented:

"A 25-year-old woman presents to the OAU stating that she thinks she is in labor."

The students will be gently challenged to make a decision. The process of decision making includes the taking of a focused history from this patient and performing a focused physical examination.

The students will ask questions in a round-table format and will be answered by the mannequin. The relevance of each question will be discussed, and clinical ramifications will be explored.

History

This is the patient's first pregnancy, gravida 1, at 40 weeks and 3 days of gestation. She is healthy, with no ongoing medical problems. She has no allergies and takes no medications other than prenatal vitamins. She does not smoke or use alcohol or street drugs. She has had good prenatal care and has had an uneventful pregnancy, with no evidence of either gestational diabetes or hypertension. Fetal movement continues to be good, with no per vagina (PV) bleeding and no suggestion of ruptured membranes. She has been contracting every 4 to 5 minutes, lasting 30 seconds over the last 2 hours. She has good social supports and lives 15 minutes from the hospital. She was examined in Dr. Posner's office yesterday and was found to be 1 cm dilated.

Physical Examination

She is initially 2 cm dilated, and students examine her and decide on dilatation. Students are asked if she should be admitted, and discussion ensues.

Fetal Heart Rate

The patient demonstrates a normal tracing. Fetal heart rate interpretation is reviewed, samples of abnormal tracings demonstrated.

Admission

Patient is sent walking and returns for examination in 2 hours. Students examine her again, now 3–4 cm and contracting every 3–4 minutes, lasting 45–60 seconds. Patient should be admitted.

Nurse comments that her BP is 130/90. The students are asked if this is due to preeclampsia or anxiety.

Discussion of Preeclampsia

The students review the symptoms of preeclampsia. The patient denies having headache, scotoma, or epigastric or RUQ pain. Physical examination demonstrates normal reflexes, and urine dip is negative for protein. Blood work is requested, and results are all normal.

Discussion of Analgesia and Frequency of Examinations

The students are asked, "When should we examine the patient again?" And Noelle asks, "What can you give me for the pain?"

Discussion of Augmentation of Labor If There Is No Progress After Epidural

Students are shown technique of amniotomy and have the opportunity to practice hand movements on balloon in pelvis. The students examine the fetal scalp electrode as it is passed around; the technique of internal monitor placement is then demonstrated.

Discussion of Management of Second Stage of Labor and Indications for Operative Vaginal Delivery

"Noelle is fully dilated, when should she start pushing?" leads to a discussion of the management of second stage, and when to start pushing, depending on whether the patient is a primipara or multipara, with or without epidural.

"After 2 hours of pushing, you are called to the delivery" leads to a review of the technique of spontaneous vaginal delivery. The students are shown how to perform a spontaneous vaginal delivery—from start to finish, including an introduction to the delivery tray and instruments.

1. Put on gloves.
2. Set up tray, check instruments.
3. +/– support perineum.
4. Control the head.
5. Watch for restitution.
6. Check for cord.
7. Deliver anterior shoulder.
8. Deliver posterior shoulder.
9. Place baby onto bed or onto patient.
10. Clamp cord and offer scissors to partner to cut cord.
11. Take cord gases and blood.
12. Place green towel on patient.
13. Support uterus and give gentle traction on cord.
14. Deliver placenta.
15. Administer oxytocin (or with anterior shoulder).
16. Check placenta.
17. Check for genital tract injuries.
18. Repair lacerations (+/– local anesthetic).
19. Check uterine fundus one last time.
20. Clean up, including reminder to place used needles into sharps container.

All students have a chance to practice a delivery. They are then shown the vacuum and forceps and given a demonstration of application. If time permits, students may practise placing vacuum or forceps.

One of the students will be given a delivery complicated by shoulder dystocia, and through this demonstration, management is reviewed: calling for help, McRoberts maneuver, suprapubic pressure, and an explanation and demonstration of the maneuvers to resolve the shoulder dystocia.

Indications for cesarean section and basic neonatal resuscitation are reviewed.

Evaluation

The effectiveness of the session has been evaluated using the comparison of the pretest and posttest. The students' attitudes toward the session are evaluated using the standard evaluation form used by the Faculty of Medicine.

APPENDIX 21.B

Pap Smear with Hybrid Simulation

STATION 1—SP INSTRUCTIONS

NAME: Mrs. Danielle A.

Age: 25–35 years

Scenario: Gynecology

Type: Physical examination—hybrid patient

CANDIDATE'S INSTRUCTIONS: Danielle A. is a married flight attendant who presents to your office for a routine pelvic examination and Pap test. It has been two years since her last visit, which included a Pap smear that was normal. *Please perform a focused physical examination and communicate with the patient appropriately.*

SP INSTRUCTIONS

SP opening statement: "I'm here for my Pap smear."

SP attire: casual, with a sheet over legs, wearing shorts.

SP starting position: Sitting with legs crossed on an examination table, with a model pelvis below her legs under the sheet. When examination starts, put legs up in stirrups on either side of model.

Chief concern/complaint in patient's words: None.

Patient's behavior, affect, and mannerisms: The patient appears a bit nervous about the pelvic examination but is cooperative and well-spoken.

History of present situation: Danielle is a married, sexually active woman on oral contraceptives. She has no history of illness or surgery; she is on no other medications and has no allergies. Her period is regular, but she has occasional midcycle and postcoital spotting. She has not had a physical examination or Pap smear for two years. Her prior Pap tests were normal, although she had one year ago, which was "mildly abnormal"—this was simply repeated six months later and had resolved.

Danielle became sexually active at age 16 years and has had three sexual partners. She has had no known STDs, genital warts, or infection. She has used the condom and contraceptive pill in the past and is currently on the pill. Menarche (first menses) was at age 13 years, and last menstrual period was three weeks ago and regular.

SOCIAL HISTORY: Danielle's husband of six months is a lawyer who is healthy. They've been together for a year and a half. Danielle lost her mother to cancer of "unknown origin" when the mother was 45 years old.

STATION 1—EXAMINER'S CHECKLIST

Examiner's Instructions: Score a point only for those items performed satisfactorily, not for items unsatisfactorily attempted. Only provide feedback after the intermittent buzzer.

> **Candidate's Instructions:** Danielle A, is a married flight attendant who presents to your office for a routine pelvic examination and Pap test. It has been two years since her last visit, which included a Pap smear that was normal. *Please perform a focused physical examination (speculum examination, including Pap and cultures, and bimanual examination) and communicate with the patient appropriately.*

Done Satisfactorily √

1. Introduces self to patient	
2. Explains what examinations will be performed	
3. Prepares/organizes/checks equipment (speculum, Pap container, brush, gloves, cultures)	
4. Positions model appropriately at foot of table, positions patient's legs appropriately	
5. Puts on gloves	
6. Warms speculum (either warm water or hands), +/– lubricant	
7. Inspection of external genitalia—vulva, vagina	
8. Communicates to patient that she will feel the speculum	
9. Speculum inserted appropriately (examiner may offer to hold flashlight)	
10. Cultures x 2 done correctly (gonorrhea and chlamydia)	
11. Pap test done correctly	
12. Describes the normal findings they are looking for—cervix appears normal	
13. Talks to patient throughout speculum examination, explaining what is being done, normal findings	
14. Removes speculum appropriately	
15. Uses lubricant (silicon) to perform bimanual examination	
16. Checks for cervical motion tenderness	
17. Palpates size of uterus, mobility, position	
18. Palpates adnexa, comments on size, asks if it is tender	
19. Communicates with patient during bimanual examination, reassures patient with normal findings	
20. Redrapes patient when examination complete	

Global rating of candidate performance relative to a graduating fourth year student

Unsatisfactory			Satisfactory		
Inferior	Poor	Borderline	Borderline	Good	Excellent
4	4	4	4	4	4

Examiner: _____

Station 1

CANDIDATE'S INSTRUCTIONS

Danielle A. is a married flight attendant who presents to your office for a routine pelvic examination and Pap test. It has been two years since her last visit, which included a Pap smear that was normal.

Please perform a *focused* physical examination (speculum examination, including Pap and cultures, and bimanual examination) and communicate with the patient appropriately.

Please treat the pelvic model as you would a real patient.

CHAPTER 22

Hybrid Simulation

Jean Forsha Byrd, Fabien Pampaloni, and Linda Wilson

INTRODUCTION

Communication is an essential skill for all health professionals. Simulation provides an opportunity for nursing students to experience communication in complex situations guided by the mentorship of their faculty. Hybrid simulation helps fill this gap in the educational process by allowing students to practice complex skills and therapeutic communication simultaneously. Hybrid simulation is the combination of a human patient using a mannequin and simulation using a standardized patient.

In hybrid simulation, you combine mannequins of any fidelity and tabletop simulators with a standardized patient to create a complex, high-level learning activity. This type of simulation can be used in a variety of settings. The addition of a real person to augment the simulator creates a life-like element that increases the complexity of performing a particular skill. No longer can the student think only about the procedure, but they also have to think about what they are saying and addressing the needs of not only the patient, but in certain cases, the entire family. The addition of a standardized patient with a mannequin decreases the awkwardness of talking to a mannequin. An example of hybrid simulation for advanced practice was shared in an article by Higham, Nestel, Lupton, and Kneebone (2007), in which bench-top pelvic simulators and standardized patients afforded students opportunities to practice complex skills and integrate them with the social skills needed when dealing with patients. In this simulation activity, artificial legs were positioned around the bench-top simulator, and the standardized patient was positioned behind the simulator in such a way to give a realistic body contour. The student now faced the challenge of simultaneously performing a pelvic examination and communicating in a therapeutic manner. A proctor in the room gave cues to the standardized patient regarding what was physically going on, allowing for realistic communication between the standardized patient and the student.

Another area in which this type of simulation works well is when working with an infant and family. A low-fidelity infant doll can be used with a standardized patient acting as the caregiver. This type of scenario allows the student to practice physical assessment on the infant while demonstrating the social and communication skills needed to work with the parents. Depending on the specific objectives needed for the simulation, this particular type of simulation can be very portable, being used in a laboratory or classroom setting.

Hybrid simulation can also be performed using the adult mannequins in a bedside setting. In these simulations, the standardized patient acts as a family member at the bedside. A real example of this type of simulation scenario is the student who is caring for a client after a right hemicolectomy. The client, who is a mid-fidelity mannequin with a microphone, and the wife, who is the standardized patient, is in the room at the bedside. During the scenario, the nurse comes in and performs an assessment on the patient. During the assessment, the patient and wife ask the nurse various questions. The student's assessments reveal pain and swelling in the patient's right lower leg. During the implementation of this scenario, the student saw this as an issue but was thrown off by some of the wife's questions. For example, the student wanted to go call the doctor to share the clinical findings, but when the student asked, "Is there anything I can get or answer for you before I leave?" The standardized patient said, "Yes, the doctor hasn't told us when we will be able to have sex again." This particular question perplexed the student, who knew that this was an important question—I can't ignore it, but I am struggling with how to answer her question, prioritize findings, and not panic the patient in regards to why that is not the priority at this time.

Another area that presented difficulty was when the student was preparing to hang a heparin drip. During the preparation, the student expressed difficulty in being able to say, "I am not going to talk right now, I just want to focus to make sure I have the correct drug calculation and drug dosage." In the debriefing from this simulation, the students did an excellent job in performing the task but verbalized that the struggle was in dealing with the families' questions and reactions. In the clinical setting, there was always someone else in the room to help with that element while they were performing various procedures.

There are some hybrid simulations that have already been created by various vendors. You may have some of these, but they are generally not listed as hybrid simulations. On the supply list of the simulation, under participants, it will list *family member*. This may be listed as a student role. For an effective hybrid simulation, training and orientation is key for whoever is involved in the simulation. The faculty and standardized patient need to be aware of what the expectations and goals are for the simulation. This training should include any cues they need to be aware of or if there are any leading questions that should be asked at different times during the scenario. This preparation before the implementation of the scenario creates a better learning experience. This type of scenario can be difficult for the student depending on how much "distraction" is presented by the standardized patient, and, depending on the student's skill level, will judge how much the standardized patient will need to be refocused. A brief practice run in the training for this type of scenario is a key element to a successful simulation: it helps ensure that all participants are looking for the same markers and cues, and it helps prevent overexaggeration and distraction.

Oftentimes, a vendor-created simulation may not fit your educational needs or budget, thus leading to the creation of a hybrid simulation. The first piece in developing a hybrid simulation is to look at your goals and needs. Ask yourself, what would you like to see from the students? What area or areas do the students need more experience in? Is there an experience we would like every student to have? By writing down the answers to these questions, specifically in regards to the psychomotor skills desired for the students, you will have a starting point to create a hybrid simulation. At the end of the chapter, you will find a sample hybrid simulation that was developed to meet the needs of the Community College of Philadelphia as defined by these questions.

The next step is to look at your resources. When looking at your resources, look at everything from low-fidelity mannequins, tabletop simulators, training devices, high-fidelity mannequins, and things as simple as a baby doll. For example, a tabletop simulator used to teach central line dressing changes, drug administration, and blood draws can be used for a hybrid simulation. Any of the previously mentioned skills can be applied in a hybrid simulation by placing a standardized patient behind the simulator and adding a patient gown. If the simulator is on the heavy side, place it on a bedside table with the standardized patient behind it in a chair. As a history, the client can have chronic obstructive pulmonary disease and be sitting in a tripod position to facilitate oxygen. This relatively simple setup makes a much more complex learning experience for our students and requires them to apply more information.

Once you have created specific psychomotor skills and reviewed your available resources, the next step is to create your specific objectives. Your specific scenario may only have four or five specific objectives; this does not include things that are part of standard practice, such as hand washing and introductions, unless these are the focus of the simulation.

From here, narrow your selection to a basic case and history. This would include the name, age, and race of the client, allergies, admitting diagnosis, physician, medical history, history of the present illness, primary medical diagnosis, and a history of any surgical procedures.

After having collected a basic history, it is time to start writing the scenario. In this specific case, and to assist in writing the scenario, we used a detailed simulation design template created with the help of our fellow simulation experts from Drexel University College of Nursing and Health Professions in Philadelphia, PA. The benefit of this template is that it lists multiple items that could possibly be needed to complete the scenario; these lists work as a trigger to add the necessary items into the scenario. Using the template as your guideline while developing the scenario will keep you from getting lost during the experience. Even with complex scenarios, the template will allow you to go back and review the objectives to keep yourself focused.

It is easy to make a scenario too complex. As an expert, you see many more details than the novice so, if while writing the scenario, it looks too elaborate, it probably is. Remember, the goal of a hybrid simulation is for the student to perform a task, whether it is an assessment or procedure, and communicate therapeutically at the same time. Other things to keep in mind are your resources, if you have three scenarios going on simultaneously but only have one EKG machine, that skill might not be the best psychomotor skill to have in the scenario, and other options for equipment and treatment. At the very end of this chapter, you will find a completed, detailed simulation design template for a hybrid simulation experience testing the students on pyloric stenosis.

After completing the detailed simulation design template, the next step is to pilot the simulation. By running through the simulation, essentially a dress rehearsal, using all of the needed equipment allows an opportunity to adjust the props and identify any missing elements. This dress rehearsal also allows the standardized patient and facilitator to work on cues and timing. Once the dress rehearsal is completed and any necessary modifications have been made to the simulation scenario, you are ready to introduce the students to this type of simulation.

Each facility has its own theory on what information the students should have before entering a simulation. For a hybrid simulation, students should know the objectives and that there will be a simulator and a standardized patient. If the standardized patient has a tabletop simulator or training device attached to them, the student should be made aware of this. This awareness will help take some of the shock factor away, calming the student and allowing them to "buy into" the scenario. Creating this awareness gives the students a sense of comfort and allows them to receive the most out of this educational experience.

The experience during a simulation can be changed significantly by changing the conversation. For example, in the sample simulation, *pyloric stenosis*, the scenario can be significantly changed by having the mother demonstrate signs of postpartum depression, or by using moulage techniques and applying bruises on the standardized patient or the low-fidelity mannequin that could be indicative of domestic abuse. These changes would add additional goals to the scenario, but it easily adds diversity and increases the complexity of the scenario.

CONCLUSIONS

In conclusion, hybrid simulation fits a specific need in the realm of simulation. The outcomes following hybrid simulation experiences are of an incredible benefit to health professions students and faculty and include higher skill performance, increased knowledge, elaborated critical thinking, and strong self-confidence (Jeffries, 2005). Hybrid simulation allows students to practice skills and communication techniques simultaneously and gives them the multitasking experience that they would get on the clinical floor. Hybrid simulations can increase the diversity and complexity of simulation activities that can be offered to students to cover complex scenarios and ensure patient safety, respect, and dignity during real-life encounters.

PYLORIC STENOSIS STUDY CASE

One of the areas defined by the Community College of Philadelphia, Department of Nursing was to expose the students to various pediatric scenarios. In our program, the students have many interactions with children but few with mothers and their new babies, thus narrowing the scope of the scenario to be built. In our program, we have low-fidelity infant mannequins; the scenario we chose to develop was on the topic of pyloric stenosis. The physical key assessments we wanted the students to find were a movable olive-shaped mass, sunken fontanels, and a decreased weight gain when charted on a growth chart. The movable olive-shaped mass was created by a ball of tape attached to the doll and then covered with a pair of panty hose (this simulated the skin and allowed us to hide the tape ball). To simulate the sunken fontanels, a note was taped to the infant's fontanels stating that they were sunken; the students would only discover this if they removed the infant's hat and looked. As for the infant's length and weight, if the student placed the infant on the scale, they were given a card listing the infant's weight. If they attempted to measure the infant, they were given a card from the proctor listing the infant's length. The objectives of this scenario were focused on the assessment pieces regarding the abdomen and fontanels, and applying the information regarding the length and weight. At this time, the objective was not to see if the student knew how to use a scale or measure an infant's length, but more so how to apply the information.

NAME: Mr. Thomas R.

CASE: Pyloric stenosis

SCENARIO: The patient is an 8-week-old baby boy brought to the clinic by his concerned mother, with a general complaint of spitting up and vomiting after every feeding. The mother is also worried about him not gaining any weight. The student has 15 minutes to complete the encounter.

TRAINING QUESTIONS

▩ DOB: 8 weeks ago
▩ Gender: Male
▩ Weight: 10 lbs.
▩ Height: 48 cm
▩ Attending physician pediatrician: Dr. Harris
▩ Medical history: Noncomplicated vaginal birth
▩ Immunizations up to date: Yes
▩ Any allergies: NKDA
▩ Social history: Thomas lives with me and my husband.
▩ Previous pregnancies: No, Thomas is our first baby.
▩ Primary medical diagnosis: Pyloric stenosis

STUDENT GRADING

Communication

▩ Introduced self
▩ Good eye contact
▩ Spoke clearly in terms the patient can understand
▩ Active listener
▩ Asked about patient's work history
▩ Obtained a past health history in an organized systematic format
▩ Asked about a family history
▩ Asked about previous hospitalizations
▩ Asked about allergies
▩ Asked about current medications that the mother/parent is taking
▩ Provided reassurance and tried to alleviate my concerns and fears
▩ Reported assessment findings to the pediatrician

PHYSICAL EXAMINATION

▩ Washed hands before examination
▩ Used appropriate terms for the mother
▩ Performed a focused assessment on the infant
▩ Identified signs of dehydration in the infant
▩ Used a growth chart

REFERENCE

Higham, J., Nestel, D., Lupton, M., & Kneebone, R. (2007). Teaching and Learning Gynaecology examination with hybrid simulation. *The Clinical Teacher.* 4:238–243.

Jeffries, P. R. (2005). A framework for designing, implementing, and evaluating simulations used as teaching strategies in nursing. *Nursing Education Perspectives, 26*(2), 97–103.

CHAPTER 23

Human Simulation for Rehabilitation Sciences

*Sarah Wenger, Margery A. Lockard,
and Maria Benedetto*

INTRODUCTION

The use of standardized patients (SPs) in physical therapy (PT) education programs began during the 1990s and was developed primarily from applications in medical education, where they have been used in the teaching and evaluation of students since the 1960s (Barrows, 1993) (Harden & Gleeson, 1979). SPs, described by Barrows (1993) as persons who have been carefully trained to portray a particular patient with a specific medical history and condition, are now used in the education of many types of health professionals, including physical and occupational therapists. Using them offers many advantages over using students' classmates to depict patients. SP responses are realistic and reproducible so that all students can experience the same clinical encounter. The complexity of a patient encounter can be designed to match the students' level of education. Inexperienced students can learn to manage high-risk or complex situations without risk to patient safety (Ladyshewsky, Baker, Jones, & Nelson, 2000). A study that surveyed entry-level PT programs in the United States and Canada reported on the prevalence and usage of SPs in their curricula (Paparella-Pitzel, Edmond, & DeCaro, 2009). The survey data were collected in 2005, and analyses showed that 33% of respondents were using SPs in their programs and over half of these programs had implemented SP usage since 2000. Only 11% of the responding programs reported that they were not interested in using SPs. These data provide evidence of a growing trend to include SPs in entry-level PT education. This is consistent with the American Physical Therapy Association's Educational Strategic Plan (2006–2020) that encourages academic and clinical faculties to investigate the effectiveness of SPs as a pedagogical strategy (American Physical Therapy Association, 2006). For those programs that reported including SPs in their curricula, the two most common educational objectives associated with SP usage were the teaching or evaluation of students' interview and musculoskeletal skills. Other clinical skills taught or assessed by using SPs included psychosocial, communication, and functional skills. Programs that are not using SPs offered the following reasons (in order of prevalence): lack of funding, inadequate time for training SPs, constraints on faculty time, and not having access to SPs.

Medical educators developed the "objective structured clinical examination" (OSCE) to evaluate clinical performance by using SPs to assess students' mastery of a set of important clinical skills required for clinical competence (Barrows, 1993; Harden & Gleeson, 1979). An OSCE typically includes multiple stations of approximately 5 to 10 minutes each that require students to demonstrate a particular clinical skill at each station. However, OSCEs do not demonstrate if the student is able to select the skill appropriately when presented with a clinical problem (Barrows, 1993). For this purpose, Barrows (1993) suggests a clinical practice examination. This type of clinical simulation has a longer (20–30 minutes), less directed format that requires students to select and perform all the components of examination that are necessary for a particular patient problem presented in the simulation scenario. This format requires students to demonstrate integration of basic science with clinical knowledge and skills. They are required to process the data collected during examination, to formulate clinical decisions, and to communicate effectively with the SP. Today's PT education programs must prepare practitioners for autonomous practice. Although a high level of technical competence is required, it is not sufficient for competent clinical performance. To achieve clinical competence, students must simultaneously (Panzarella & Manyon, 2008):

1. Consider pathophysiologic mechanism
2. Take a history
3. Formulate an initial hypothesis
4. Perform a physical examination
5. Select clinical tests
6. Reprioritize hypotheses
7. Make a diagnosis
8. Prescribe treatment
9. Educate the patient

SPs are proving to be a successful and cost-effective method to help students transition from the classroom to the clinic by building their competence and confidence (Black & Marcoux, 2002). In this chapter, we will discuss important issues to consider when deciding to integrate simulated clinical experiences with SPs into your PT curriculum and how to develop and plan for a clinical simulation event.

DECIDING TO ADD CLINICAL SIMULATION WITH SPS TO YOUR CURRICULUM

Using a standardized simulated clinical environment with SPs for teaching or assessment of clinical performance has many advantages that have been described earlier in this text. However, making the decision to include clinical simulation with SPs in a particular PT curriculum requires careful thought, planning, and coordination. There are a wide variety of goals and formats for using SPs; it is important to define the overarching purposes, to develop specific goals, and to select formats that integrate well into your program's curriculum. Thus, we strongly encourage faculty who wish to use SPs in teaching or performance assessment to start with the program's curriculum committee. The curriculum committee should identify the overall purposes and develop specific learning objectives and desired outcomes, similar to how learning objectives would be coordinated across the curriculum. Clinical simulation is often used for the general purpose of teaching or assessing clinical performance or competence. The skills required for clinical competence have been described and include knowledge and technical skills, patient management skills, humanistic dimensions (e.g., empathy, respect, confidentiality, communication), and professionalism (Lockyer & Violato, 2004; Violato, Marini, Toews, Lockyer, & Fidler, 1997). Clinical simulation encounters with SPs can be designed to address any or all of these domains. Table 23.1 provides a few examples of learning objectives that have been used by some PT curricula to guide the development of clinical simulation events.

Another decision that should be discussed and made by the curriculum committee concerns how the encounters will be used in the curriculum. Specifically, will the experience be used as an assessment or as a teaching opportunity? If it will be an assessment, the committee must determine if it will be a summative or formative evaluation. Formative assessments provide feedback on performance to the students from experts (usually faculty), SPs (patient receiving care), and sometimes peers. The feedback process can also include self-assessment and self-reflection to facilitate identification of strengths and areas in need of attention and to develop a plan for improvement. Formative assessments usually do not have grades or consequences for advancement in the program.

Summative evaluations require students to meet a predetermined standard of "minimum competence" and have consequences. Consequences for failing to achieve

Table 23.1 *Examples of Learning Objectives for Standardized Patient Experiences in PT Curriculum*

Citation	Learning Objectives or Outcomes
Panzarella and Manyon (2008)	o Performs an appropriate history and physical examination for a particular patient with a musculoskeletal (herniated disc) and neuromuscular (CVA) complaint o Demonstrates integration by answering patient questions that requires explanation of symptoms, explaining rationale for interventions, and discussing prognosis
Ladyshewsky, Baker, Jones, and Nelson (2000)	o Performs a complete history and physical examination for a patient with a common musculoskeletal problem (rotator cuff) o Demonstrates clinical reasoning by describing the differential diagnosis and diagnosis, delineating and explaining management plans, and demonstrating application of knowledge of pathophysiology
Hale et al. (2006)	The student demonstrates: o Confidence and skill in interviewing, screening, and appropriate physical examination o Ability to recognize relationships between diabetes and visual changes o Ability to appropriately refer patients o Knowledge of diabetes standards of care o Familiarity with commonly used adaptive equipment for visually impaired persons o Attitudes toward working on multidisciplinary health care teams
Hayward et al. (2006)	o To teach and reward student development of core professional values: accountability, communication and respect, professional duty, social responsibility, and integrity o To assess student acquisition of clinical evaluation skills including interview, screening, examination and evaluation, special tests, clinical decision making, home exercise, and education

a minimum pass score may be high stakes (failing a course or not being permitted to progress in the program) or low stakes (requiring remediation and retesting or performance of additional activities with no impact on progression in the program). When consequences for failing to meet a minimum standard are high stakes, it is important to verify the validity and reliability of the cases and assessment instruments. Specific policies and procedures should be carefully thought-out and developed by the curriculum committee. Some curricula have clinical simulations with SPs that have both formative and low-stake summative features. Specific issues that must be considered regarding the consequences of clinical simulation encounters are discussed in the Planning the SP clinical simulation event section.

Clinical simulation events with SPs may be course based, focusing on skills related only to one course, such as musculoskeletal examination, or they may be more integrative, requiring students to integrate and use skills and knowledge learned in multiple courses. In the latter case, the curriculum committee should determine the timing of the event in the curriculum and the level or degree of synthesis that is reasonable for the students to demonstrate on the basis of where they are in the overall curriculum. One of the primary outcomes of clinical simulation with SPs that has been reported is improved student confidence (Black & Marcoux, 2002; Boissonnault, Morgan, & Buelow, 2006; Hale, Lewis, Eckert, Wilson, & Smith, 2006; Hayward, Blackmer, & Markowski, 2006). However, presenting students with simulated clinical encounters that require knowledge, performance, or decision-making skills at a level that is beyond their current abilities may have a negative impact on developing clinical confidence and performance.

Time allotment within the curriculum for SP encounters is another factor that should be considered by the curriculum committee. When SPs are used for teaching purposes, the events can be incorporated into the appropriate course's allotted laboratory time. However, integrative SP encounters with formative assessments require a significant amount of time for the encounters themselves as well as for debriefing, feedback sessions, self-assessment, and reflection. Commitment by the curriculum committee to provide adequate time for the SP encounters as part of the curriculum—not just something added in or inserted between classes as usual—is necessary to ensure the desired positive impact on student learning, development of confidence and competence, and accurate assessment of their clinical performance.

In addition to assessing individual student's clinical abilities, the SP encounters can help faculty assess the effectiveness of the curriculum in teaching clinical skills and decision making. For example, if most students do poorly on a particular case or fail to perform certain tests that the faculty feels are essential, the problem is probably not a student deficit but is more likely a problem with the curriculum or methods of teaching. Overall student performance on simulated clinical encounters can be used to identify unrecognized curricular issues and trigger curricular review or revision as needed.

Involvement of the curriculum committee is necessary when making global decisions about introducing the use of SPs into the curriculum. However, it is more practical for the development of the cases, materials, and other tasks related to the simulation event to be performed by a designated faculty member or, preferably, a faculty SP committee. Once educational goals and objectives are set by the curriculum committee, the faculty SP committee can determine how to practically and effectively develop SP experiences. The faculty SP committee has several things to do, including the development of valid, realistic, and reliable cases and checklists; the training of SPs to be authentic; and all the administrative work of scheduling and coordinating the events. This is very time consuming and must be distributed and recognized in faculty work load.

Selecting the Type of SP Encounter to Meet the Learning Objectives

There are various formats in which students can interact with SPs in clinical simulation. The format used must be selected on the basis of the overall curricular purpose for the encounters: summative or formative performance assessment or learning and practice experiences without evaluation. If the goal is to assess students' ability to perform and interpret basic clinical skills, the OSCE format may be selected. In this format, faculty develop a series (5–20) of short, directed scenarios that require students to select and perform a specific skill at each station.

Each station usually requires only approximately 5 to 10 minutes, and the student receives information about the client that directs the student to the appropriate clinical task before meeting the SP. For example, one station in an OSCE examination may provide a chief complaint and brief history and ask the student to perform the special tests to diagnose the problem. There is usually a station following the encounter in which the student is asked to apply or interpret their SP examination findings or identify an appropriate action on the basis of the findings. These are used extensively in medical education and licensure testing (Whelan et al., 2005; Williams, 2004). They have also been used in PT education (Wessel, Williams, Finch, & Gemus, 2003). OSCEs are most often used in summative evaluations of clinical performance and use checklists to identify behaviors that are required to achieve or exceed a preestablished numerical "passing" score.

A group debriefing session usually follows the encounters so students can learn what was expected. Students may or may not be permitted to review their scored checklists. If the encounters were videotaped, students can be permitted to review the videos of their performances. In this format, students usually do not receive individual feedback. However, there is some evidence that verbal feedback and the opportunity to discuss what a student was thinking during the encounter enhances both student learning and satisfaction with the experience (Rose & Wilkerson, 2001).

Clinical competence requires more than just the ability to perform and interpret clinical skills. Some educators have designed extended clinical encounters that require students to demonstrate integrative skills. They do this by having students perform an examination during the encounter that requires them to sort through their knowledge "in real time" and to select appropriate information to make clinical decisions that they will then communicate to their patients (Panzarella & Manyon, 2007). The descriptive study of the use of SPs in physical therapist education programs by Paparella-Pitzel et al. (2009) reports that about half of the programs that are using SPs use encounters that last between 10 and 30 minutes, and another 44% report that their encounters last longer than 30 minutes. Thus, it appears that most physical therapist education programs are using the extended format.

Although checklists are the most frequently used tool to assess performance (about 60%), most programs also provide students with feedback in addition to their performance checklists. Feedback may include direct oral or written feedback from faculty, as well as direct oral feedback from their SP (Paparella-Pitzel et al., 2009). This extended SP format with multiple sources of feedback provides a formative assessment method that may help students transition from the classroom to clinic (Black & Marcoux, 2002; Ladyshewsky et al., 2000; Panzarella & Manyon, 2007).

SPs encounters are also used within courses as a learning tool. With this application, the SP activity is designed not to assess performance but to teach a skill or inform development of professional values, attitudes, or beliefs. The use of SP encounters in the classroom or laboratory provides students with "opportunities to grapple with uncertainty in the context of performance" and requires students to "think on their feet" to respond to unexpected circumstances (Jensen, 2009). Educators in rehabilitation professions have used SP learning experiences as a tool to teach clinical decision making in complicated situations, ethics, medical screening, diabetes counseling, interviewing, and affective domain stills, such as interpersonal communication, sensitivity to cultural differences, and responses to ethical and moral dilemmas (Boissonnault et al., 2006; Hale et al., 2006; Hayward et al., 2006; Jensen, 2009; Velde, Lane, & Clay, 2009). In these learning experiences, students typically engage the SPs as dyads or triads of students or in small groups, where one student plays the therapist role while the others observe and provide feedback.

Group reflection and discussion typically follow the encounter, and decision making is performed collectively. Students have expressed a higher level of satisfaction with this teaching method as compared with traditional, less active formats (Boissonnault et al., 2006; Hale et al., 2006; Velde et al., 2009). One study that used SP encounters to teach medical screening and physician communication found that students who participated in the SP activity performed better on follow-up examination questions that required application than peers who learned the same material with traditional methods (Boissonnault et al., 2006).

Resourcing the SP Encounters

There are a variety of ways in which educators manage the physical and technical aspects of setting up and implementing SP experiences for their students. Some programs may have access to centralized offices that assist in the administration and coordination of SP experiences. When available, these offices may offer a central facility (private examination rooms with videotaping capability) and staff who secure the SPs and assist with their training, as well as equipping and setting up the rooms and running the encounters on the day of the SP event. Some human simulation centers offer digital videotaping so that the videos can be viewed by students and faculty online, as well as in specially equipped rooms for small or large group debriefing sessions (www. ems-works.com). This software may also provide the ability to include computer-based pre- and post-encounter activities, as well as online completion of checklists.

In the survey conducted by Paparella-Pitzel et al. (2009), only 31% of the respondents who reported using SP encounters in their curricula had access to a central simulation office, but more than 50% reported using videotaping. Thus, although access to a central office is helpful and may reduce the demands on faculty time, it is not a requirement for introducing assessments or learning experiences with SPs into your curriculum. There are many "low-tech" ways to implement SP experiences. For example, if you do not have access to a separate space, a departmental clinical teaching laboratory space may be used and in some cases may be more desirable. Central clinical simulation facilities often have examination rooms that are designed to mimic a physician's examination room; thus, space for walking and observing functional activities is often quite limited. These rooms also are usually equipped with the typical doctor's office examination table that makes moving the patient, as is necessary in many therapists' examination procedures, awkward. It may also be difficult to realistically simulate other types of practice settings frequently used by therapists, such as a home or rehabilitation facility.

An advantage of a central simulation center is that the staff can help in finding, screening, training, and paying for the individuals who will be the SPs. Large programs and medical schools hire professional actors and have staff for SP training. Smaller schools or programs not associated with medical schools that may not be able to hire professional actors have other options.

For example, some programs use program faculty as the SPs. Upper-level students in the program have been used as SPs as well as students from other professional programs within the college or university, such as physician assistant students (Boissonnault et al., 2006; Hale et al., 2006). One program that used upper-level PT students as SPs for a first year experience reported that "the students who volunteered to role-play patients expressed getting significant value and satisfaction from their experience" (Boissonnault et al., pp. 28–34). Programs that reside in colleges or universities with theater or performance arts departments may recruit students within these majors for their SPs (Black & Marcoux, 2002). Another possible source for SPs is retired persons. Many colleges have centers for learning in retirement or lifelong learning institutes. These programs bring healthy, active retirees to campuses to attend classes or courses. These retired individuals are often motivated to assist in the education of future health care providers and typically are excellent SPs.

There are many ways to find individuals who are willing to be SPs, but all will require careful training and assessment of their ability to authentically portray the case "patient." The time required for SP training for a particular case varies considerably as reported in the literature—from as little as 2 hours to as many as 30 hours (Black & Marcoux, 2002; Ladyshewsky et al., 2000). Training time will vary depending on what is expected of the SP. For example, if the SP is required to present gait abnormalities and movement disorders, more training time may be required than if the simulation scenario only requires verbal responses as in an interview. More time may also be needed for training if SPs are required to identify clinical behaviors and complete a checklist. Because SP training is critical to the realism of the SP experience, this topic is discussed in more detail later in this chapter (Planning for the Clinical Simulation Event).

Despite variations in sources for SPs and their training, most studies report that SPs are able to reliably and authentically portray patients as rated by both experienced clinicians and students (Black & Marcoux, 2002; Boissonnault et al., 2006; Hayward et al., 2006; Ladyshewsky et al., 2000; Panzarella & Manyon, 2008). In addition, most students who have worked with SPs in learning or assessment situations are highly satisfied with their experiences with their SPs and feel that the simulated encounters enhanced their learning (Black & Marcoux, 2002; Boissonnault et al., 2006; Velde et al., 2009). Some students who participated in an integrated SP encounter described the experience "as an extremely valuable experience that provoked anxiety and challenged them to think on their feet like no other experience ever had" (Panzarella & Manyon, 2008, pp. 24–32).

The cost of adding simulated clinical experiences with SPs to a curriculum must also be considered and evaluated. Cost can be evaluated in terms of money spent as well as in faculty time. Monetary costs are usually associated with paying for SP training and encounter time, sending faculty to training seminars or conferences, or renting time and space in a central simulation center (e.g., in a nearby medical school). The cost of paying SPs may vary by geographical location (variation in typical local wages), as well as by whether professional actors or students or individuals from the community are hired (Black & Marcoux, 2002; Panzarella & Manyon, 2008).

The time spent by faculty in developing simulation experiences with SPs is also variable. If the SP encounters are designed as learning experiences to enhance laboratory activities, additional faculty time beyond that required to develop usual course activities may be minimal (Black & Marcoux, 2002). However, the faculty time required to develop simulation experiences that involve summative or formative assessment, debriefing, checklists, and multiple sources of feedback is considerable (Hayward et al.,

2006; Ladyshewsky et al., 2000; Panzarella & Manyon, 2008). Faculty time is required for case development, validation of the case for authenticity, developing SP scripts and training protocols, either training the SPs or training the trainers, developing the checklists and determining their reliability, developing or administering the debriefing sessions, standardizing and coordinating the various feedback sessions, and scheduling for and coordinating the day of the event. Careful attention to each of these activities is essential for a satisfactory and successful SP simulation event. These areas are discussed in more detail in the Planning the SP clinical simulation event section.

If more than one SP event occurs during an academic year, the cost in faculty time is substantial and must be taken into account when considering the cost of implementing a program. Multiple summative or formative SP events may occur in an academic year, when students participate in an SP clinical simulation in each of their academic years of study. Programs with a large number of students and those that have multiple yearly simulation events may need to provide dedicated administrative support or teaching release time to the faculty who supervise the SP programs. The next section presents the details of planning for, developing, and carrying out a clinical simulation event.

PLANNING THE SP CLINICAL SIMULATION EVENT

The faculty SP laboratory (SPL) committee needs to take the following steps to create a blueprint that outlines the organization of the SPL experience and then to develop specific cases that follow that blueprint. Curricular goals should guide your decisions.

Determine the Specific Goals for the Encounter—Cognitive, Psychomotor, and Affective Domains

For cognitive goals, students are evaluated on constructs such as clinical decision making and differential diagnosis. For psychomotor goals, the encounter can be structured as an OSCE that requires students to perform specific tests, measures, or treatments. For affective goals, students are presented with interpersonal challenges so that they can experience and be evaluated on verbal and nonverbal communication, patient instruction, recognition and negotiation of cultural differences, and challenging patient interactions.

Determine the Number of Cases for Each Experience

There are several formats that may be considered: (a) one case that all students complete; (b) several different cases, but each student completes only one of the cases; or (c) several different cases and each student completes all of the cases. An advantage of all students experiencing the same case is the efficient use of faculty time. This format also allows for post-encounter comparisons and discussion among students. A drawback of this choice is the narrow focus and the potential for information sharing by students before completion of the case by all students. To broaden the scope and make information sharing less likely, several cases can be offered, with each student assigned to one of the cases. This will allow students to compare their performance across different cases and have more content exposure. The main drawback of this method is additional preparation time by the faculty SPL committee and the need for faculty to be familiar with more than one case. The third option, to have each student complete more than one case during the experience, is recommended when the experience is high stakes. This structure presents the same drawback of increased preparation time and the need for faculty to learn more than one case. However, when there are high stakes, it is imperative that students have several opportunities to demonstrate their competence (Norcini & Boulet, 2003; Whelan et al., 2005).

Identify the Tasks Students Will Perform During the Encounter

It is important to determine what you want the students to do. Consider what psychomotor tasks to evaluate and what constructs students should be exposed to. Common tasks include taking a history, performing an examination, establishing a plan of care, providing interventions, summarizing findings, fielding patient questions, and providing patient education.

Determine the Length of the Encounter

The length of the encounter will depend on the level of academic preparation and amount and type of clinical exposure of the students. Questions to consider include the following: (1) Are they in their first, second, or third year of study in the curriculum? (2) Have they had a clinical education experience? (3) What content has been covered in the curriculum at the time of the experience? (4) What tasks are students required to complete? For example, if the encounter is for first year students who are required to take a history only, the case may be completed in 15–20 minutes. Second year students who are required to complete an entire initial evaluation may require 45–60 minutes. Students who have completed clinical rotations may be able to complete the same case in 30 minutes. In addition, encounters that require synthesis and decision making during the experience may require more time.

Develop Learning Activities to Accompany the Encounter

Learning activities are an important part of the SPL experience and can be positioned before and after the encounter. Pre-encounter activities can range from student surveys on perceived competence (strengths and weaknesses) or confidence levels to written assignments.

Post-encounter activities can range from evaluative assignments for grades to reflection papers for meta-cognitive learning processes. Students can complete a reflective assignment, create case documentation, participate in peer assessment activities, or perform any number of other learning assignments. Debriefing and feedback activities are important formative post-encounter activities that are typically included following SP experiences.

Determine the Methods for Feedback and Debriefing

Debriefing and feedback require faculty–student interaction to enhance student learning. During group debriefing, a faculty member meets with students to review important aspects of the case. This allows students to identify and understand the "clinical bottom line" and important "take-home points." The one-on-one feedback process allows a faculty member to evaluate an individual student's meta-cognitive processes and provides the opportunity to engage in rich formative interaction (Rose & Wilkerson, 2001). Feedback is essential for the development of clinical decision-making skills and clinical competence (Lockyer, 2003; Lockyer et al., 2006). It can foster reflective practice that encourages students to create a plan for improvement across all domains, including cognitive, psychomotor and affective (Babyar et al., 2003; Hayward et al., 2006; Musolino, 2006).

Feedback can be provided in many ways, including checklists, face-to-face meetings, written summaries and group debriefings. Providing multiple sources of feedback is an effective way to enhance acceptance of feedback and facilitate willingness to change. Useful types of feedback include self, peer, SP, and faculty/expert feedback (Fereday & Muir-Cochrane, 2006; Hayward et al., 2006; Lockyer, 2003; Lockyer et al., 2006).

When students review their own performance, they build self-assessment skills that are valuable for improving their clinical practice (Violato & Lockyer, 2006). Assessment from a peer provides students with feedback from someone who was "in the trenches" with them and may have alternative approaches to the same clinical problem. It also allows students to practice providing feedback to others. Feedback from SPs provides input from the patient's perspective and is highly valued by students (Panzarella & Manyon, 2008; Rose & Wilkerson, 2001; Velde et al., 2009). It is especially helpful for the development of communication and other affective skills (Guiton, Hodgson, Delandshere, & Wilkerson, 2004). Feedback from a faculty expert helps students identify errors in their problem-solving processes as well as understand academic expectations (Rose & Wilkerson, 2001).

Develop Methods for Student Assessment

Once the encounter content and goals have been established, assessment procedures should be designed. Evaluations are typically formative, summative, or a hybrid of both. Whether the encounter is formative or evaluative, it is important to have a well-developed plan for feedback so that student learning is maximized. If a summative component is included in the experience, grading standards and retake policies should be developed (Norcini & Boulet, 2003; Williams, 2004). Common grading options include a numerical score or a rating of satisfactory or unsatisfactory based on performance of required behaviors listed on a checklist. The faculty SP committee should consider the range of consequences for a nonpassing grade for each encounter, such as a lower grade in a specific course, special remediation, extended clinical time with a learning contract, or dismissal from the program. For high-stakes consequences, the evaluation tool and passing standards must be valid and reliable (Norcini & Boulet, 2003; Whelan et al., 2005; Williams, 2004). The Angoff method, which uses a panel of experts to establish a "cut score" for passing, is one way of standardizing checklist scoring (Talente, Haist, & Wilson, 2003). Regardless of the method of determining the minimum passing score, evaluation standards must be transparent and clear to both faculty and students.

Most SP experiences, whether formative or evaluative, include a checklist. Checklists are used for assessment when encounters are graded because they establish clear performance expectations. They are also used to provide immediate and standardized feedback to students.

Developing good case-specific checklists can be difficult. The key is to keep them short, simple, clear, and behaviorally based. Items may be scored dichotomously with a yes/no (did or did not do) response or by using a three-option scale: "did effectively," "did poorly or incompletely," or "didn't do" (Ladyshewsky et al., 2000). SP encounters designed to measure students' ability to integrate what they have learned in the curriculum have used scales with four options: detrimental, below expectations, meets expectations, or exceeds expectations (Panzarella & Manyon, 2007). Regardless of the specific grading scale used, content and curricular experts should develop or select the items that are included in the checklist to ensure that the items are consistent with the curriculum and reflect current evidence-based practice.

For summative encounters, remediation and retake policies must be developed and made clear to students and faculty before the experience. Remediation can be accomplished in a variety of ways to guide students in their preparation for the retake experience.

Develop the Case(s)

In consultation with content experts, develop a specific case that meets the educational goals, desired complexity and conforms to the selected case parameters. Decide if and when to give students additional case information such as a referral or an intake form. If additional materials are provided, students may receive this material immediately before the encounter or days in advance. A sample intake form is provided in Box 23.8.

Props, special equipment, and cosmetics for the SPs (to simulate wounds, bruising, and so forth) must be considered to ensure authenticity. The availability and practicality of using these items can be a limiting factor in case development. There are many wonderful case ideas that are unusable because of the impracticality of realistic simulation.

Develop SP Training and Materials

Effective SP training is essential for case reliability and accurate portrayal of the patient. Before training, each SP should receive a detailed description of the case in lay language, a basic script, and information about required dress and affect. A sample of the SP training materials we use in Drexel University's Physical Therapy and Rehabilitation Sciences Department is provided in Boxes 23.5 and 23.6. Specific information and training about how to act the physical presentation of the case is critical. Training should include live demonstration and videos that show how to portray painful responses, altered gait patterns, or other patient conditions. It is important to set aside time for SP rehearsal and role-playing with feedback from faculty. Trainers should allow time for questions and clarification of SP concerns during practice sessions. The reliability and standardization of SP acting may be improved by providing multiple training sessions and by testing SP performance for accuracy and consistency (Kavanagh & Morrison, 2005). Accurate portrayal of the patient scenario is important for standardization among student experiences and has been demonstrated in numerous studies (Black & Marcoux, 2002; Ladyshewsky et al., 2000; Williams, 2004).

Develop Student Materials and Instructions

Students generally demonstrate anxiety about SP encounters. However, this anxiety can be minimized by providing detailed and explicit instruction as to what to expect and how performance evaluation will be conducted. It is also helpful for students to understand why the experience is important for their education. Start by presenting an overview of how the SP experience enhances the curriculum and a description of the learning objectives. Provide a schedule and step-by-step instructions about how the encounter will be conducted, including any pre- and post-encounter activities that are required. A schedule of events that lists specific activities with due dates is also helpful. Students need to know faculty expectations for their performance and the evaluation methods that will be used. At Drexel University, in the Physical Therapy and Rehabilitation Sciences Department, we have developed a course or site within the university's online course management system to house information for both faculty and students. An outline of the information provided to students via the course management site is provided in Box 23.1. Students can "click" into each folder to retrieve detailed information in a question-answer format.

Develop the Checklist(s)

Content experts should create checklists that are short, clear, action oriented, and focused on the encounter's specific goals (Whelan et al., 2005). It is helpful to split the checklist into categories and organize items so that they follow a typical examination sequence. Several checklists can be developed, depending on who will complete them (e.g., self, peer, SP, or faculty). If several checklists are completed by different evaluators, it is helpful to choose parallel organization and wording for each checklist so students can easily compare observations from different sources. Specific performance items may be labeled as "need to do" or "nice to do" to help students identify specific areas for improvement. Checklist items may also be weighted differently to distinguish performance behaviors that are essential from those that are less important. Another option is to identify key checklist items that must be completed to pass the experience. Depending on the case and its goals, checklists may include items regarding the sequencing of actions and the time to perform an action. Samples of SP, faculty, self, and peer checklists can be found in Boxes 23.4 and 23.7. Another assessment method that may be used with or as an alternative to checklists is a global rating scale (Regehr, MacRae, Reznick, & Szalay, 1998; Solomon, Szauter, Rosebraugh, & Callaway, 2000). A global rating scale asks the evaluator to rate overall student performance in selected categories, such as interpersonal skills, communication, or examination. Raters may simply choose a "pass/fail" designation or a descriptive scale that indicates the quality of student performance (e.g., exceeds expectations, meets expectations, below expectations) may be used (Panzarella & Manyon, 2008). There is some evidence that global rating scales, when used by content experts, are equivalent to checklists (Regehr et al., 1998; Solomon et al., 2000).

Provide Information to Faculty

Faculty evaluators need the case description, evaluation materials, and detailed expectations for student performance. Faculty should have enough time to ask questions, gain clarification, and build consensus for standardized feedback and evaluation. It is advisable to have a faculty training session before each SP experience. Feedback and assessment styles will vary among faculty members. Although some differences in style are acceptable, all feedback should be nonjudgmental and evaluations must be standardized among all faculty evaluators (Rudolph, Simon, Dufresne, & Raemer, 2006). Finally, the faculty need a detailed schedule. Schedule tables are helpful as they provide, at a quick glance, all important due dates. An outline of the Drexel University Physical Therapy and Rehabilitation Sciences Department's online course management system course or site for faculty is provided in Box 23.2. A sample of faculty case information is provided in Box 23.3. Faculty are able to "click" into each folder in the online faculty course or site to retrieve detailed information.

Develop the Schedule

This seemingly simple task almost always becomes complicated. It is important to consider all parties involved. SP, student, and faculty schedules must be considered, along with the availability of the space and equipment you plan to use. Consider all of the pre-encounter and post-encounter activities when creating a schedule, as these activities can be time consuming for students and faculty. Allow sufficient time for individual meetings between students and faculty. If the experience is graded, allow enough time to complete remediation and retesting before the end of the term. It is important that students who are struggling are not distracted from their examinations. When the schedule has been established, publish it to all who are involved so that the expectations are clear and deadlines can be met.

EVALUATING THE SPL EXPERIENCE

After an event is completed, evaluation of the experience is necessary to determine if the goals and learning objectives have been met and if case revisions are required. The SPL event and results should be assessed to answer the following questions:

- Were the patient portrayals by different SPs standard and consistent with the requirements of the case?
- Was the simulated clinical experience authentic?
- If checklists were used, are they valid, reliable, and meaningful?
- What impact did the experience have on the students?
- Did the performance of the students as a whole reveal any areas for curricular review?

Assessment of the consistency and accuracy of the acting among the SPs who present a case is easier to do if the students have been videotaped. An evaluator can view randomly selected videos from each SP across the event and rate their performance of key aspects of the case. If videos are not available, the evaluator can directly observe randomly selected encounters for each SP. If the prevalence of inaccuracy or inconsistency is high, solutions may include revising the SP training methods, selecting other SPs for future cases, or revising the case so that it is less difficult to portray.

Box 23.1 *FAQs, Case Documents, and Case-Specific Information Provided to Students in an Online Course Format*

General Information
1. What is the standardized patient laboratory (SPL)?
2. What is a standardized patient (SP)?
3. What is arcadia?
4. Why do we have SPL encounters?
5. Overview of SPL curriculum.
6. What do I need to prepare for the SPL encounter?
7. How do I get to the SPL?
8. What should I bring with me to the SPL?
9. What should I wear to the SPL?
10. What examination equipment will be available in the SPL room?
11. How should I expect the SPL experience to run?
12. Can I discuss my SPL experience with my classmates?
13. What happens after the SPL encounter?
14. How will I be evaluated?
15. How do I evaluate myself?
16. Why do I have to do self-assessments before and after the SPL?
17. What is reflective practice and why is reflection part of the SPL experience?
18. How do I give and receive feedback?
19. What is a personal plan for improvement?
20. Categories of evaluation.

SPL Documents
1. Instructions for accessing online student materials, including videos of the encounter, checklists and other student documents
2. Pre-SPL self-reflection survey
3. Post-SPL self-reflection survey
4. Peer feedback form

SPL Experience 2 (example)
1. Schedule of events
2. Day-of schedule
3. Experience 2 SPL expectations

Box 23.2 *General Information, Case Documents, and Case-Specific Information for Faculty Provided in an Online Course Format. Detailed Information Is Available Inside Each Folder.*

General Information
1. SPL curriculum overview
2. SPL curriculum goals
3. SPL research agenda
4. The student process
5. Pre-SPL encounter activities
6. SPL encounter activities
7. Post-SPL encounter activities
8. SPL evaluation
9. Faculty feedback
10. Personal plan for improvement
11. Categories of SPL evaluations (based on CPI)

Instructions for Accessing Online Student Videos, Checklists and Other Student Documents

SPL Experience 2 (Example)
1. Schedule of events
2. Day-of schedule
3. Faculty assignments
4. Case Folders

Special Tests: This folder contains information on the special tests we expect students to perform in case you are not familiar with all of them.

Box 23.3 *Sample Faculty Case Information*

Case Structure
Students will have 10 minutes when they arrive in the SPL to review an intake form for this patient. The students will have 35 minutes to conduct their examination and to provide a brief explanation of their findings and Plan of Care. They will then have 10 minutes at the wallaroo (computer outside the examination room) to answer the question below. Afterward, they will receive 10 minutes of verbal feedback from the SP.

Case Description
This is a patient who fell on their shoulder while playing tennis. The students will do an initial evaluation and should diagnose AC joint sprain. The SP will ask when they can return to playing tennis, and the students should respond in the range of 3–6 weeks, including an appropriate description of tissue healing. For more details about the case, look over the SP training materials. Expectations for performance are outlined in the checklist.

Post Encounter Question
On the basis of the examination you just completed, write an assessment paragraph for your patient. Include your diagnosis, prognosis, and general POC (you do not need to list specific exercises).

Box 23.4 *Sample SP Checklist*

- Student introduced self, including full name and professional designation.
- Student balanced professionalism and friendliness well.
- Student made me feel comfortable.
- Student's manual handling was not too rough or too timid.
- Student used good communication skills and was easy to understand.
- Student used nonmedical terminology and explanations.
- Student gave you a chance to speak and did not interrupt.
- Student exhibited natural varied eye contact.
- Student demonstrated appropriate nonverbal communication for the situation.
- Student appeared confident, did not display nervous or distracting behaviors.
- Student was dressed professionally, including Drexel ID badge.
- Student asked you about your goals.
- Student asked if you had any questions.
- Student summarized findings and provided explanation of plan of care.
- Explanation to patient of findings and POC is simple, clear, and complete.
- Student started each interview area with an open-ended question.

Box 23.5 *Sample Case: SP Script*

Presenting complaint: "I have pain right here" (point to top of shoulder).
  Planned question: "When will I be able to go back to playing tennis?"

Box 23.6 *Sample Case: SP Case Details*

BACKGROUND INFORMATION

Age: 30–50

Occupation: Make it up. There should be something that is more difficult to do after your injury. It would be some kind of reaching, lifting, pushing, or pulling activity. Verify the occupation that you select with the case trainer to insure that it is appropriate and that it fits with the case presentation.

Setting: Outpatient PT clinic.

Affect: Nothing special, cooperative, make up the details.

Appearance: Street clothes; you will be expected to remove your shirt. Women need to have a sports bra or tank top on so that the shoulder can be exposed.

Presenting Complaint: Your shoulder hurts when you lift your arm and hand above your head or across your body.

Medical History: None.

Medications: Advil on occasion when the pain is bad.

Social Information: Make up the details. Verify the social information you select with the case trainer to confirm that it fits with the case presentation.

Recreational Activities: You play tennis three times per week. You work out two times per week. You lift some weights and do some cardio training. You have not been playing tennis or lifting weights since you hurt yourself. You have been doing your cardio. You have not tried to play tennis because it hurts, especially with serves or backhands. You did try to lift some weights but had pain every time you elevated your arm higher than your nose and so have not done any more weight lifting. You have been trying to do lifting, reaching, pushing, and pulling activities at home and work with your good arm.

History of Present Illness: One week ago, you fell when you slipped on the tennis court and landed on your shoulder. You have noticed pain when you lift your arm above your nose and when you bring your arm across your body. Because it has not improved over the last week, you decided to see a physical therapist. You are going directly to the physical therapist and have not consulted a physician.

(continued)

(continued)

EXAMINATION INFORMATION

Pain: Now 4/10, best 3/10, worst 6/10. You have not taken Advil today. The pain is on top of your shoulder. It hurts when you elevate your arm above your nose and when you bring your arm across your body. You have no pain when you use your arm at waist or shoulder level. You would describe the pain as a deep ache that throbs when it gets bad. It feels better when you rest and take Advil. It feels worse when you try to lift, reach, pull, or push and when you tried lifting some weights at the gym and when you play tennis.

Palpation: You have pain when the therapist pushes on the bony spot on the top of your shoulder.

Vital Signs: Whatever you normally have, but it you have high blood pressure please let me know.

Range of Motion: Everything is normal except your left shoulder. You cannot elevate above your nose or move your arm across your body without pain. Tell the physical therapist that it hurts. You can push into the pain a little but have to stop because of increasing pain.

Strength: You have normal strength in your good arm and in the elbow, wrist, and hand of your bad arm. Your bad arm is strong when it is not elevated. When it is elevated higher than your nose, you are only able to take minimal resistance before your arm gradually lowers with discomfort.

Posture: You have rounded shoulders.

Special Tests: Every time the physical therapist lifts your arm above your nose or brings the left arm across your body, you should wince and report pain. You will also have pain when the physical therapist squeezes your shoulder. Anything else you should report feeling fine.

SPECIAL INSTRUCTIONS:

Please be prepared to expose your shoulder. You will not be able to wear a gown so please come dressed appropriately so that your shoulder can be exposed. Women will need to wear a tank top or sports bra.

The students are expected to complete a history, do an examination, and provide you with an explanation of their findings. They have been instructed to excuse themselves when they are finished by saying something like "it was a pleasure to meet you." They have also been instructed that they may wear watches and reference them to pace themselves as there are no clocks in the rooms. Please overlook these somewhat awkward social behaviors when grading and giving feedback.

Box 23.7 *Sample Case: Faculty/Self/Peer Checklist*

Need to do (required) = Standard text
Nice to do = italics

Safety:
Used good body mechanics

Professional Behavior and Communication:
Introduced self, including full name and professional designation
Balanced professionalism and friendliness well
Used good communication skills and was easy to understand
Used nonmedical terminology and clear explanations
Gave patient opportunity to speak and did not interrupt
Exhibited natural varied eye contact
Demonstrated appropriate nonverbal communication for the situation
Appeared confident and did not display nervous or distracting behaviors
Was dressed professionally, including Drexel ID badge
Asked patient about their goals/reason for visit
Asked if patient had any questions
Summarized findings and provided explanation of plan of care
Explanation to patient of findings and POC is simple, clear, and complete

(continued)

(continued)

History Taking:
Started each area of interview with an open ended question
Used directed follow up questions
Reviewed reason for visit and mechanism of injury
Discovered that patient fell and landed on shoulder
Asked patient to rate pain on a scale of 0–10
Observed patient locating their symptoms on themselves
Discovered if patient's symptoms radiate or change location
Asked patient to describe quality of pain
Discovered patient's recreational activities and ADLs
Discovered that patient has pain with weight lifting and when playing tennis
Discovered patient's occupation
Discovered patient has pain with specific work activities
Confirmed PMH and medication(s) listed on intake form

Screening:
Took BP and HR
Visually inspected shoulder without clothing
Observed active range of motion at both upper extremity joints (at least one motion at each joint)
Applied over pressure to all nonpainful motions
Performed sensory screen for BUE (sampling at least five dermatomes on each side)
Tested at least one upper and one lower extremity deep tendon reflex

Examination:
Progressed examination from gross measures to specific/special tests
Palpated involved shoulder without clothing
Measured involved shoulder ROM with goniometer for elevation, external rotation, and internal rotation
Performed MMT of involved shoulder elevation, external rotation, and internal rotation
Performed MMT of noninvolved shoulder elevation, external rotation, and internal rotation
Performed one test for AC joint involvement (sheer, horizontal adduction)
Performed one test for rotator cuff involvement (Hawkins, Neers)

Evaluation and Diagnosis:
Identified that pt presents with signs of AC joint sprain
Identified limited ROM, decreased strength, and pain as impairments
Identified functional limitations in weight lifting and tennis

Plan of Care:
Includes a period of rest with activity modification (i.e., limitation of elevation and horizontal adduction)

Box 23.8 *Sample Physical Therapy Intake Form*

1. Describe the symptom(s) or problem(s) that brought you to physical therapy today.
2. When did these symptoms start?
3. Who referred you to physical therapy for this problem?
4. Who is your family doctor or primary care provider (address)?
5. Have you seen another other health care provider for this problem? If yes, who have you seen and list any tests or treatments you have received.
6. Do you take any prescription or nonprescription medications? If yes, please list them. If you don't recall the name of the medicine, list the condition for which you are taking it.
7. Medical and surgical history: Please check if you have ever had

(continued)

(continued)

___Arthritis
___Broken bones/fractures
___Osteoporosis
___Blood disorders
___Circulation/vascular problems
___Heart problems
___Asthma
___High blood pressure
___Lung problems
___Stroke
___Diabetes/high blood sugar
___Low blood sugar/hypoglycemia
___Head injury
___Depression, metal health problem

___Multiple sclerosis
___Muscular dystrophy
___Parkinson disease
___Seizure/epilepsy
___Allergies
___Developmental/growth problems

___Thyroid problems
___Cancer of_____
___Liver problem
___Kidney problems
___Ulcers/stomach problems
___Skin diseases
___Other_____

8. Family history (indicate whether mother, father, brother/sister, aunt/uncle, or grandmother/grandfather, and age of onset if known)
  a. Heart disease:
  b. Hypertension:
  c. Stroke:
  d. Diabetes:
  e. Cancer:
  f. Psychological:
  g. Arthritis:
  h. Osteoporosis:
  i. Other:

9. Check any of the following symptoms that you have experienced during the last year. Check all that apply.

___Chest pain
___Heart palpitations
___Persistent cough
___Hoarseness
___Shortness of breath
___Dizziness or black-outs
___Coordination problems
___Weakness in arms or legs
___Loss of balance
___Difficulty walking
___Joint pain or swelling
___Pain at night

___Difficulty sleeping
___Loss of appetite
___Nausea/vomiting
___Difficulty swallowing
___Bowel problems
___Weight-loss or gain
___Urinary problems
___Fever/chills/sweats
___Headaches
___Hearing problems
___Vision problems
___Other_____

10. Have you ever had surgery? Please circle one: Yes   No
  If yes, please list the operation(s) and when you had them.

Assessing the authenticity of a case includes determining if the case presentation is consistent with an actual or typical patient, as well as assessing the realism of the physical space, equipment and environment. To determine the realism of the case presentation, recruit clinicians who practice in the specialty area presented to view videos. Have them rate how well the case emulates real patient behavior and how well the setting and environment emulate an actual patient visit. It may also be helpful to ask clinicians to rank the difficulty of the case for novice clinicians. These rankings may help with case selections for future SP events.

When checklists are developed by collaborations between content and curricular experts, it is important to evaluate the checklist's performance as a measurement tool before using it again. Content validity is established by careful construction, including input from therapists involved in current practice in the case content area. However, if the checklist is used to determine competence or level of skill, its ability to discriminate between the test students and those with more experience or entry-level novice therapists must be determined. This can be done by comparing the checklist scores of a cohort of more experienced students or novice therapists to those of the test students. Internal consistency measures how well each item in the checklist correlates with the others and with the whole test. It can be measured using a statistical tool, Cronbach's alpha. If there is poor internal consistency, checklist items should be reviewed and appropriate revisions made.

Typically, checklists are completed by various evaluators for different students. For example, to complete checklists for a class of 50 students, 10 different faculty members may complete checklists for 5 students each. When this occurs, evaluator reliability must be confirmed. This can be tested by determining the correlations among item responses and overall scores from different evaluators observing the same case performance. Poor inter-rater reliability may require rewriting items—to make them clearer or simpler—or improving rater training. If the checklist scores are used to determine student classification, such as satisfactory, borderline pass, borderline fail, or unsatisfactory, a global rating scale can be completed at the end of the checklist, and correlations between the scores and classifications can be investigated.

To evaluate the impact of the SP encounter on the students, pre-encounter and post-encounter surveys can be used to assess the effect of the experience on their confidence and self-assessment of their competence. Focus groups are also useful in learning about the perceptions of the students.

Another important assessment is to perform an item analysis on the checklist. When an expected action on the checklist is not performed by most students, it probably does not reflect individual student failure. Possible reasons that should be investigated include the following: the standard was too high; there was a failure of the encounter design, such as the case was too difficult for the time provided; and the curriculum did not sufficiently present the topic or issue. The curriculum committee will need to study the issue and modify the case or how the topic is presented in the curriculum.

Some researchers have tried to determine if student performance in SP experiences can be used to predict student performance in other areas. Correlations between SP encounter scores and outcome measures such GPA, performance measures in clinical internship, or licensure scores have been reported (Panzarella & Manyon, 2008; Wessel et al., 2003; Williams, 2004). However, all of these correlations have been low, which suggests that each measures a different phenomenon, all of which are necessary for clinical competence but not the same.

CONCLUSION

Although the initial development and implementation of clinical simulation with SPs is time consuming and labor intensive, there are many rewards. Although initially anxious, students typically rate SP experiences very positively. Most report that the practice with feedback is invaluable and state that they would like more simulation opportunities during their education. Development and evaluation of simulation experiences requires the participation and cooperation of all faculty, which may prompt discussion and recognition of curricular weaknesses and lead to greater integration of content across the curriculum.

REFERENCES

American Physical Therapy Association. (2006). *Education strategic plan (2006–2020).* Retrieved 08/24, 2010, from http://www.apta.org/AM/Template.cfm?Section=Home&TEMPLATE=/CM/ContentDisplay.cfm&CONTENTID=43038

Babyar, S. R., Rosen, E., Sliwinski, M. M., Krasilovsky, G., Holland, T., & Lipovac, M. (2003). Physical therapy students' self-reports of development of clinical reasoning: A preliminary study. *Journal of Allied Health, 32*(4), 227–239.

Barrows, H. S. (1993). An overview of the uses of standardized patients for teaching and evaluating clinical skills. AAMC. *Academic Medicine, 68*(6), 443–451; discussion 451–453.

Black, B., & Marcoux, B. C. (2002). Feasibility of using standardized patients in a physical therapist education program: A pilot study. *Journal of Physical Therapy Education, 16*(2), 49–56.

Boissonnault, W., Morgan, B., & Beulow, J. (2006). A comparison of two strategies for teaching medical screening and patient referral in a physical therapist professional degree program. *Journal of Physical Therapy Education, 20*(1), 28–34.

Fereday, J., & Muir-Cochrane, E. (2006). The role of performance feedback in the self-assessment of competence: A research study with nursing clinicians. *Collegian, 13*(1), 10–15.

Guiton, G., Hodgson, C. S., Delandshere, G., & Wilkerson, L. (2004). Communication skills in standardized-patient assessment of final-year medical students: A psychometric study. *Advances in Health Sciences Education: Theory and Practice, 9*(3), 179–187. doi:10.1023/B:AHSE.0000038174.87790.7b

Hale, L. S., Lewis, D. K., Eckert, R. M., Wilson, C. M., & Smith, B. S. (2006). Standardized patients and multidiscplinary classroom instruction for physical therapist students to improve interviewing skills and attitudes about diabetes. *Journal of Physical Therapy Education, 20*(1), 22.

Harden, R., & Gleeson, F. (1979). Assessment of clinical competence using an objective structured clinical examination (OSCE). *Medical Education, 13*(1), 41–54.

Hayward, L. M., Blackmer, B., & Markowski, A. (2006). Standardized patients and communities of practice: A realistic strategy for integrating the core values in a physical therapist education program. *Journal of Physical Therapy Education, 20*(2), 29–37.

Jensen, G. (2009). Exploration of critical self-reflection in the teaching of ethics: The case of physical therapy. Retrieved August 26, 2011, from http://www.eric.ed.gov/PDFS/ED478992.pdf

Kavanagh, M., & Morrison, L. (2005). *Quality control: Establishing and maintaining SP reliability.* Retrieved from http://www.aspeducators.org/webinar/webinar_051105_archive.htm

Ladyshewsky, R., Baker, R., Jones, M., & Nelson, L. (2000). Evaluating clinical performance in physical therapy with simulated patients. *Journal of Physical Therapy Education, 14*(1), 31–37.

Lockyer, J. (2003). Multisource feedback in the assessment of physician competencies. *Journal of Continuing Education in the Health Professions, 23*(1), 4–12. doi:10.1002/chp.1340230103

Lockyer, J., Blackmore, D., Fidler, H., Crutcher, R., Salte, B., Shaw, K., et al. (2006). A study of a multi-source feedback system for international medical graduates holding defined licences. *Medical Education, 40*(4), 340–347. doi:10.1111/j.1365-2929.2006.02410.x

Lockyer, J. M., & Violato, C. (2004). An examination of the appropriateness of using a common peer assessment instrument to assess physician skills across specialties. *Academic Medicine, 79*(10 Suppl), S5–S8.

Musolino, G. M. (2006). Fostering reflective practice: Self-assessment abilities of physical therapy students and entry-level graduates. *Journal of Allied Health, 35*(1), 30–42.

Norcini, J., & Boulet, J. (2003). Methodological issues in the use of standardized patients for assessment. *Teaching and Learning in Medicine, 15*(4), 293–297.

Panzarella, K. J., & Manyon, A. T. (2007). A model for integrated assessment of clinical competence. *Journal of Allied Health, 36*(3), 157–164.

Panzarella, K. J., & Manyon, A. T. (2008). Using the integrated standardized patient examination to assess clinical competence in physical therapist students. *Journal of Physical Therapy Education, 22*(3), 24–32.

Paparella-Pitzel, S., Edmond, S., & DeCaro, C. (2009). The use of standardized patients in physical therapist education programs. *Journal of Physical Therapy Education, 23*(2), 15–23.

Regehr, G., MacRae, H., Reznick, R. K., & Szalay, D. (1998). Comparing the psychometric properties of checklists and global rating scales for assessing performance on an OSCE-format examination. *Academic Medicine, 73*(9), 993–997.

Rose, M., & Wilkerson, L. (2001). Widening the lens on standardized patient assessment: What the encounter can reveal about the development of clinical competence. *Academic Medicine, 76*(8), 856–859.

Rudolph, J. W., Simon, R., Dufresne, R. L., & Raemer, D. B. (2006). There's no such thing as "non-judgmental" debriefing: A theory and method for debriefing with good judgment. *Simulation in Healthcare, 1*(1), 49–55.

Solomon, D. J., Szauter, K., Rosebraugh, C. J., & Callaway, M. R. (2000). Global ratings of student performance in a standardized patient examination: Is the whole more than the sum of the parts? *Advances in Health Sciences Education: Theory and Practice, 5*(2), 131–140.

Talente, G., Haist, S. A., & Wilson, J. F. (2003). A model for setting performance standards for standardized patient examinations. *Evaluation and the Health Professions, 26*(4), 427–446.

Velde, B. P., Lane, H., & Clay, M. (2009). Hands on learning: The use of simulated clients in intervention cases. *Journal of Allied Health, 38*(1), E17–E21.

Violato, C., & Lockyer, J. (2006). Self and peer assessment of pediatricians, psychiatrists and medicine specialists: Implications for self-directed learning. *Advances in Health Sciences Education: Theory and Practice, 11*(3), 235–244.

Violato, C., Marini, A., Toews, J., Lockyer, J., & Fidler, H. (1997). Feasibility and psychometric properties of using peers, consulting physicians, co-workers, and patients to assess physicians. *Academic Medicine, 72*(10 Suppl. 1), S82–S84.

Wessel, J., Williams, R., Finch, E., & Gemus, M. (2003). Reliability and validity of an objective structured clinical examination for physical therapy students. *Journal of Allied Health, 32*(4), 266–269.

Whelan, G. P., Boulet, J. R., McKinley, D. W., Norcini, J. J., van Zanten, M., Hambleton, R. K., et al. (2005). Scoring standardized patient examinations: Lessons learned from the development and administration of the ECFMG clinical skills assessment (CSA). *Medical Teacher, 27*(3), 200–206.

Williams, R. G. (2004). Have standardized patient examinations stood the test of time and experience? *Teaching and Learning in Medicine, 16*(2), 215–222.

CHAPTER 24

Human Simulation for Physician Assistants

James R. Carlson

INTRODUCTION

*P*hysician assistants (PAs) have been providing patient care as part of the medical team for more than four decades (Stead, 1966). Although still a relatively new profession, the number of PAs in practice has grown considerably. The American Academy of Physician Assistants (AAPA, 2009) estimates that there are more than 70,000 PAs practicing in the United States. PAs are currently licensed to practice in all 50 states and work in a variety of specialties including primary care fields, medical subspecialties, general surgery and surgical subspecialties, and emergency medicine. PAs are employed in hospital-based practices, group and solo physician practices, urban health centers, rural locations, and within military settings (Dehn, 2010).

PAs are entrusted to carry out a broad range of clinical duties similar to those of physicians, including gathering and reviewing clinical data, establishing a diagnosis, and enacting treatment plans (AAPA, 2010). The scope of practice varies from state to state and practice to practice, but PAs may perform comprehensive as well as focused history and physical examinations, order and interpret diagnostic studies, and may be given prescriptive authority. PAs provide patient education, perform a variety of clinical procedures ranging from simple suturing to more complex procedures, such as chest tube placement, or may first assist during surgical procedures.

PAs are qualified and well trained to perform the above skills, but only under the guidance, delegation, and licensure of a supervising physician (AAPA, 2010). PAs are similar to Advanced Practice Nurses (Bryant-Lukosius, DiCenso, Browne, & Pinelli, 2004) but offer a slightly different perspective, adhering to a core philosophy in which care is provided through a physician-dependent relationship (Jones, 2007). PAs see patients individually or as a key part of the medical team, but their scope of practice is limited to physician-delegated authority and is, by definition, collaborative practice. This differs from many Advanced Practice Nurses, who may be licensed to practice individually with or without collaborative practice agreement (McCabe & Burman, 2006). PA education follows a medical model similar to that of physician education, and the collaborative nature of the PA/physician team is emphasized (AAPA, 2010).

PA Training

The first PA training program was established by Dr. Eugene Stead at Duke University School of Medicine, graduating its first class in 1967 (Carter & Strand, 2000). There are currently 142 PA training programs in the United States and additional programs are being developed internationally (Physician Assistant Education Association, 2010). Entry-level education typically ranges from 24 to 36 months and may result in a certificate, associate, baccalaureate, or master's degree. Although a master's degree is not required for practice, 87% of current PA training programs award a master's degree at the completion of training.

The focus on providing a strong foundation in primary care is likely appropriate given that PAs are able to move between specialties during their career (Hooker, Cawley, & Leinweber, 2010), but interesting in light of the fact that in 2008 more than 50% of new PA graduates took a job in a non-primary care specialty (Physician Assistant Education Association, 2010). This trend poses a significant training and licensing challenge as entry-level trainees must acquire a broad set of clinical skills useful in many clinical settings during a relatively short training time. This includes learning how to take an appropriately focused history and physical exam, providing patient education, and performing an array of clinical procedures with accurate technique. Given the broad range of settings and diverse tasks PA graduates could be responsible for, PA programs must carefully structure their curricula so that time and resources allow new graduates to be proficient in an array of clinical skills and procedures. As this chapter will show, PA programs seem to increasingly rely on a wide range of simulated modalities to meet this challenge.

Licensure and Certification

The National Commission on the Certification of Physician Assistants (NCCPA) is the public agency charged with credentialing PAs entering the health care workforce and verifying clinical competency (Hooker, Carter, & Cawley, 2004). The NCCPA accomplishes this primarily through administering the Physician Assistant National Certifying Examination to all new PA graduates entering practice and then verifying competency at regular intervals through the Physician Assistant National Recertifying Examination or the Pathway II Examination. Although performance on these examinations is considered the gold standard for verifying PA competency, and is universally recognized by all 50 states as a part of granting licensure, it is important to note that these measures are computer-based examinations focused on testing knowledge domains (NCCPA, 2010). Currently, there is no national standardized performance-based examination used by the NCCPA to verify the ability of a PA to actually carry out the clinical tasks essential for patient care.

Without an NCCPA-instituted performance-based exam, PA training programs currently carry the *sole responsibility* of documenting that PAs entering the workforce are competent to perform the clinical skills necessary to appropriately practice. This practice was not always the case. Starting in 1978, PAs were required to pass a practical element of their board examinations known as the Clinical Skills Portion, in which candidates were presented with a patient scenario and then asked to perform an appropriate examination for the case. The Clinical Skills Portion was discontinued in 1997 because of the logistical and psychometric concerns associated with administering this form of evaluation (Hooker et al., 2004). This is in contrast to current practices in both allopathic and osteopathic physician training, in which candidates are required to pass a national board-level simulation-based performance examination before licensure (National

Board of Osteopathic Medical Examiners, 2010; U.S. Medical Licensing Examination, 2010).

PAs are trained in a medical model; the absence of a current performance-based board examination as part of credentialing is of interest. PA programs charged with verifying skill competency increasingly rely on simulation not only to provide formative learning experiences, but also for simulation-based, institution-specific performance examinations as components of summative assessment (Coplan, Essary, Lohenry, & Stoehr, 2008). The remainder of this chapter will provide an overview of current practices and trends regarding the use of simulation in PA education, discuss recommendations for simulated case and exam development in PA education, and provide examples of case scenarios beneficial to PA training.

Overview of Simulation in PA Education

The types of simulation provided during PA training are similar to those offered to physicians during their initial education (Cooper & Taqueti, 2008; Williams, 2004). Both models emphasize the acquisition of basic clinical skill sets early in training, with progression to more advanced skills and mastery in later training (Ericsson, 2008). A majority of medical schools now use simulation to meet these goals. This trend may have increased access to simulation within PA education, as PA programs affiliated with medical schools tend to run more simulated exercises (Coplan et al., 2008). Literature describing the specific use of simulation in PA education is sparse but it seems that PA programs use a range of simulated modalities, including training standardized patient (SP) cases, part task trainers, and full-body, mannequin-based simulation.

The Use of SPs in PA Training

The most comprehensive literature documenting the integration of simulation in PA education highlights the use of SPs (Calhoun, Virbin, Gryzybicki, 2008; Coplan et al., 2008). The Association of Standardized Patient Educators (2010) defines an SP as:

> (A) person trained to portray a patient scenario, or an actual patient using their own history and physical exam findings, for the instruction, assessment, or practice of communication and/or examining skills of a health care provider. In the health and medical sciences, SPs are used to provide a safe and supportive environment conducive for learning or for standardized assessment.

It is important to stress the *standardized* component when defining an SP as one of the intended goals of SP cases is to provide reproducible learning activities and reliable measurement processes. This is usually best done through calibration and training under the guidance of an experienced SP educator. Some settings may use students or faculty to portray a case, but best practices include using a patient with experience and training to standardize case portrayal and assessment (Mavis, Ogle, Lovell, & Madden, 2002; Wallace, 2007). An overview of the training and use of SPs can be found in an earlier chapter of this book.

Calhoun et al. (2008) and Coplan et al. (2008) found that approximately 80% of PA programs use SPs within their curricula. Of the PA programs using SPs, nearly all (98%) report using SPs as a component of didactic training, and 67% use SPs within the clinical curriculum. PA training emphasizes the mastery of skills essential to general clinical practice, so it is not surprising that SPs appear to be frequently involved in teaching history and physical examination skills as an adjunct to problem-based learning, and introducing more challenging concepts such as cultural competency (Calhoun & Chambers, 2004; Fleek, 2003; Luce, 2001; Parkhurst & Ramsey, 2006). In some programs, SPs provide direct feedback to students on the basis of their performance and are used to provide small group and individualized instruction. In addition, a majority of PA programs use specialty-trained SPs to teach sensitive examinations such as breast, pelvic, and rectal examinations (Calhoun & Chambers, 2004; Calhoun et al., 2008).

It is estimated that 80% of PA programs using SP methodologies include SP-based examinations as a component of summative evaluation (Calhoun et al., 2008; Coplan et al., 2008). Summative evaluations tend to focus on the achievement of core clinical skills such as performing a history and physical, providing patient education and counseling, and demonstrating effective interpersonal communication. Literature documenting the reliability and validity of SP examinations in PA education is sparse but encouraging. Asprey, Hegmann, and Bergus (2007) documented that clinical level medical and PA students performed comparably on an SP examination designed to measure history, physical examination, and communication competencies. Additional studies have provided evidence of SP examination reliability and described the credibility of various standard-setting processes used to document and track student performance during SP examinations (Carlson, Tomkowiak, & Knott, 2010; Carlson, Tomkowiak, & Stilp, 2009). However, it remains unclear if PA programs are routinely following best practices when developing, designing, and implementing SP examinations.

SPs provide realistic scenarios that allow students to perform a patient interview and examination, but are limited in that they often do not have or cannot mimic certain findings, such as abnormal heart and lung sounds or vitals. This is a significant training issue, as PAs are expected to be able to interpret the clinical information that they collect (NCCPA, 2010). Also, it is clearly not appropriate to perform more invasive procedures such as suturing, airway management, or central line placement on SPs. SPs are well-suited to engage a variety of clinical skills in PA education, but part-task trainers and mannequin-based encounters provide PA educators with additional options to engage and assess competencies that SP methodology cannot fully address.

Use of Simulation to Teach Clinical Procedures

It is largely up to each individual PA program under the review of the Accreditation Review Commission on Education for the Physician Assistant (2010) to determine which clinical procedures to include in their curricula. As noted earlier, this can be challenging because PAs routinely perform a wide variety of procedures in actual practice. To compound this challenge, the frequency with which PAs are delegated to perform specific procedures is not clear and varies greatly between practice settings. Procedures such as suturing and basic life support are commonly understood to be essential skills that most, if not all PAs, should master because of their importance in a wide range of practice settings, but the need for proficiency in other skills is less clear. For example, endotracheal intubation or chest tube insertion may be important for a critical care or emergency medicine PA to learn but far less important for PAs practicing in family medicine or orthopedics. Similarly, PAs may receive training in highly common procedures such as venipuncture, bladder catheterization, or intramuscular injections, but rarely, if ever, perform the skill if it is routinely delegated to another member of the team.

The results from one recent peer-reviewed study are far from definitive but do identify which procedural skills are emphasized in a majority of PA curricula (Carlson, Laack, & Stilp, 2006). For educators interested in simulation-based training, this study was also able to identify which procedures were taught primarily through hands-on laboratory exercise or simulation, which were primarily practiced on actual patients during clinical rotations, and which procedures were emphasized through both simulation and practice on actual patients. Table 24.1 highlights the clinical procedures most frequently prioritized in PA education. A priority procedure was defined as a procedure that more than 50% of responding programs reported as being addressed through a formal laboratory exercise or simulation or could verify that all students had the opportunity to perform on actual patients during clinical training.

It is interesting to note that, other than the four procedures listed in Table 24.1 (suturing, Papanicolaou test and endocervical culture, local anesthesia, and venipuncture), less than half of the responding programs could verify that all graduates actually performed this list of skills during clinical training. This is despite the fact that all students are required to rotate through core rotations representative of a range of practice settings, including internal medicine, family medicine, emergency medicine, surgery, pediatrics, and obstetrics and gynecology. Thus, PA programs relied primarily on laboratory and simulated exercises to ensure that all graduates had experience in performing a great majority of the procedures surveyed. This finding is certainly not optimal, as simulations are meant to introduce and reinforce appropriate clinical behavior, not to replace experiential learning with actual patients. This finding is also not surprising, as many advocates of simulation have long noted that one of the advantages of simulated exercises is to provide clinical experiences to trainees in cases or skills that they might not ordinarily see or may not have the opportunity to practice on their clinical rotations (Issenberg, MaGaghie, Petrusa, Gordon, & Salese, 2005).

Table 24.1 *Clinical Procedures Most Frequently Prioritized in PA Education*

Priority Procedures	Hands-on Laboratory Exercise or Simulation (%)	All Students Perform during Clinical Training (%)
Simple suturing/laceration repair	96	86
Casting	91	45
Venipuncture	90	59
IV catheter insertion	88	45
Fracture/dislocation immobilization (splinting)	86	45
Bladder catheterization	81	44
Endotracheal intubation	81	17
ACLS	79	45
Complex suturing/laceration repair	73	32
Papanicolaou test and endocervical culture	71	71
Local anesthesia	62	67
Nasogastric intubation	64	19
Spirometry/pulmonary function testing	53	14

Source: From Carlson et al. (2006).

Although far from complete, the items noted in Table 24.1 represent a set of core skills that PA educators seem to be primarily addressing through some form of medical simulation. Precise details and common simulated modalities used to address each task are not clear, but faculty and simulation centers involved in PA training may find these data helpful when choosing to purchase simulation equipment and plan simulation curriculum. In addition, these data might be helpful to faculty and staff responsible for designing and carrying out simulated activities proposed to verify PA competency in a core set of clinical procedures before graduation. PA programs focused on a specific training area, such as a postgraduate residency in a surgical subspecialty or orthopedics, may wish to emphasize additional procedures specific to the respective discipline.

The most cost-effective way to simulate most of the procedures listed in Table 24.1 is through the use of part-task trainers. Part-task trainers are artificial body parts designed to simulate performing a specific procedure or technique (Maran & Glavin, 2003). This contrasts with full-body mannequin simulation (also known as high-fidelity simulation), in which the simulator may allow for multiple procedures to be performed in the context of a full case scenario. Task trainers are often designed to look and feel like the regional anatomy and provide learners with the opportunity to gain comfort with the equipment and dexterity necessary to perform the clinical procedure (Maran & Glavin, 2003; Scalese, Obeso, & Issenberg, 2007). For example, airway trainers generally consist of an upper torso and head with an anatomically correct mouth and oropharynx to allow the learner to realistically place an oropharyngeal airway or perform endotracheal intubation. A vast number of similar part-task trainers exist, including simulated arms for intravenous insertion or venipuncture, breast models that are capable of simulating a mass, or pelvic trainers used to teach the bimanual examination and endocervical biopsy.

Part-task trainers are also frequently described as low-fidelity because they are inanimate, provide a minimally realistic experience, or are not sophisticated enough to provide performance feedback (Maran & Glavin, 2003). Low-fidelity task trainers are inexpensive but capable if the training goal is to orient the learner to equipment and steps for completing the procedure. If the procedure requires that the mannequin is animated (e.g., simulated breathing or heart tones, pulse, bleeding) or is capable of capturing student data (e.g., hand location and breadth of coverage during the bimanual exam) then a higher fidelity task trainer or full-body mannequin might be used. For example, Issenberg, Gordon, Stewart, and Felner (2000) describe the use of Harvey, a high-fidelity task-specific simulator focused specifically on teaching and assessing cardiovascular examination, including accuracy when interpreting cardiac auscultation findings. Higher fidelity trainers, such as Harvey, may be most necessary when training for mastery in which a procedure or finding needs to be highly realistic (Scalese et al., 2007). When designing and allocating resources for simulation, PA faculty should consider the cost–benefit of higher fidelity simulators, as higher fidelity often equates with higher initial cost, maintenance, and greater technical expertise to operate.

Full-Body Mannequin-Based Simulation in PA Education

Full-body mannequin-based simulators, often referred to as *high-fidelity simulators* or *human patient simulation*, are used with increasing frequency in medical and health professions education (Cooper & Taqueti, 2008; Multak, Euliano, Gabrielli, & Layon, 2002). As with SPs, most full-body mannequins provide the opportunity to engage history and physical examination competencies, but also are capable of allowing for abnormal cardiopulmonary findings, performance of procedures, and administration of medication in real-time during a case scenario. They can be used to run simple bedside teaching scenarios for individuals or groups of learners as a strategy to augment traditional content delivery, or to engage a health care team in the complexities of a dynamically evolving crisis situation (Issenberg et al., 2005).

High-fidelity mannequin-based simulation could be used to deliver cases and content in a format similar to traditional SP scenarios, but with the ability to embed abnormal cardiopulmonary findings. However, its true benefit to PA education might be recognized through the potential for interprofessional team training (Devita, Shaefer, Lutz, Wang, & Dongilli, 2005). PAs regularly interact with physicians, nurses, respiratory therapists, emergency medical technicians, and a host of other health care professionals, and PAs entering the workforce need to be proficient when communicating and interacting with their fellow team members.

Errors within the medical team have been cited in the analysis of root cause events, and team-training programs have focused on improving team communication and structure as a mechanism to improve patient safety. There is substantial literature documenting the use of team training as an effective method to improve patient safety (Chakraborti, Boonyasai, Wright, & Kern, 2008; Salas, DiasGrandados, Weaver, & King, 2008; Shapiro et al., 2004). Teams may work together to coordinate care during a mannequin-based case and then be debriefed on the quality of their teamwork. Standardized participants can be used in conjunction with mannequin-based simulation to take on the role of another health care provider (confederate) scripted to challenge team cohesion through deliberate action. For example, a scripted but standardized supervising physician may commit an error, order the team to take an action inappropriate to the patient case, or display unprofessional behavior during the simulation. In this way, a PA may learn when and how to appropriately challenge the decisions of a senior staff member.

In summary, the literature clearly demonstrates the use of SP-based simulation in PA education. It is also evident that PA programs rely on task trainers and mannequin-based simulation for teaching and possibly assessing clinical competencies, but the extent to which these methods are fully utilized is not completely understood. Educational researchers interested in the use of simulation in PA education should focus efforts on gaining a better understanding for how and when these learning experiences are used within PA training and if PA programs are following best practices when integrating them into the curriculum.

DEVELOPMENT OF SIMULATED CASE STUDIES IN PA EDUCATION

Simulation-based learning and assessment activities can be costly in terms of faculty time and departmental budgets (Carlson et al., 2010). To make the most of these valuable resources, PA educators should follow recommended practices for case development and when using case scenarios with high-stakes assessment. The methods PA programs use to design and implement simulation in their respective curricula are unclear, and the remainder of this chapter will focus on best practices when developing simulated case scenarios and exams.

The development of simulation-based activities in PA education should take steps to construct valid and credible simulations (Downing & Haladyna, 2008; Yudkowsky,

Downing, & Wirth, 2008). The greater the stakes of the simulated encounter (e.g., performance measures influence grading decisions, need for authentic experiences to train for mastery), the greater the need to provide and document validity evidence (Downing & Haladyna, 2008). This process includes the design-appropriate content blueprint, development of case stations with reliable case portrayal and assessment protocols, and providing sufficient sources of validity evidence to evaluate the trustworthiness of examination data (Yudkowski, 2009).

Figure 24.1 highlights a hypothetical blueprint for simulation within a traditional PA curriculum. A blueprint is a tool faculty might use to broadly design a curriculum or outline the specific domains of emphasis for a learning and assessment activity (Downing & Haladyna, 2008; Yudkowsky et al., 2008). The blueprint in Figure 24.1 highlights sample learning activities and assessments at different points in training. Each activity or assessment should be blueprinted in greater detail to outline the specific content and methods that will be employed.

Let us consider the common example of a PA program desiring to design and carry out a summative clinical year simulation-based examination with the intended purpose of verifying student clinical competency before graduation (Coplan et al., 2008). Involved faculty will need to design an examination blueprint by selecting content domains, case scenarios to address those domains, and the number of stations necessary to reliably measure competency in this level of learner. The blueprint should be designed in such a way

Figure 24.1 *Hypothetical Blueprint for Simulation Use Within a Traditional PA Curriculum.*

Early Training (didactic phase) Introducing basic clinical principles and acquisition of core skill sets.	Later Training (clinical phase) Introduce advanced clinical principles and verify continued development of care clinical skill sets.
Sample learning activities – SP case studies engaging basic history, physical examination, interpersonal communication for common clinical presentations. – Task training laboratories designed to teach and allow for practice of core procedures that will be performed while on clinical rotations (suturing, IV insertion, venipuncture, bimanual exam, etc.) – Human patient simulator or computer-based simulation to train cardiopulmonary auscultation and interpret abnormal vs. normal findings.	**Sample learning activities** – SP case studies reinforcing sound history, physical examination, and interpersonal communication. Patient education, behavioral medication, and challenging topics (substance abuse recognition and counseling, health care literacy, medical errors, etc.) – Procedures reinforced in clinical context (e.g., hybrid SP/suture task trainer to emphasize patient communication during procedure, dynamic mannequin-based simulation requiring advanced airway management). – Team-based human patient simulation focused on interactions with other providers and collaborative decision-making across professional boundaries.

Sample performance assessment activities
– Long case at completion of Physical Examination course (complete a full examination with appropriate technique).
– End of didactic training/preclinical multistation Objective Structured Clinical Exam. Short stations with distinct clinical tasks. Examples might include:
  – "Elicit a sexual history from this patient."
  – "Demonstrate a full neurologic examination."
  – "Appropriately throw three simple interrupted sutures on the task trainer."
	Sample performance assessment activities
	– End of clerkship multistation examinations focused on key content and principles relevant to core rotations (e.g., family medicine, pediatrics, surgery, emergency medicine). Grade on examination is factored into overall clerkship grade.
	– Comprehensive summative clinical skills examination before graduation. Broad emphasis on integration of multiple skills within a case scenario and clinical judgment, as opposed to short stations with distinct highly directed clinical tasks. See blueprint in Figure 24.2 for eight case-summative clinical skills examinations and case examples for further information.

that the combination of and number of stations has adequate validity evidence (e.g., does the examination credibly measure the knowledge and skills necessary to determine if a PA student can successfully engage in clinical practice? Downing & Haladyna, 2008).

Examination Domain(s) to be Measured

As noted previously, the Physician Assistant National Certifying Examination and the Physician Assistant National Recertifying Examination credibly capture clinical knowledge but not clinical behavior because they are computer-based multiple-choice examinations (NCCPA, 2010). The eight content domains currently emphasized by the NCCPA on these examinations provide a good starting point for the development of a local institution-specific, simulation-based examination blueprint so that PA programs can verify behavioral skill in these areas. The eight domains include history and physical examination, using laboratory and diagnostic studies, formulating the most likely diagnosis, clinical interventions, pharmaceutical therapeutics, health maintenance, applying basic science concepts, and professional practice (Arbet, Lathrop, & Hooker, 2009; NCCPA, 2010). Many of these domains, such as history and physical examination or clinical interventions (suturing, airway management, etc.), lend themselves to simulation-based examination through SP, task trainers, or mannequin-based simulation.

Case Selection

The purpose of the case or scenario station is to provide an authentic opportunity to practice a skill or to engage the content domains to be assessed. Case selection should be intimately related to the domains emphasized and, where possible, evidence should be used to help faculty select case scenarios most appropriate and likely to engage students in the desired domains. A recent practice analysis conducted by Arbet et al. (2009) highlighted that content domains are of varied importance depending on the type of patient and presenting problem. For example, managing patients with chronic progressive problems such as Type 2 diabetes mellitus or rheumatoid arthritis often require greater proficiency in the use of pharmacologic therapeutics, whereas managing patients with life-threatening emergencies requires greater use of history and physical examination skill and determining a most likely diagnosis.

Practice analysis data can be used to inform the content of performance examinations. For example, if a simulated exercise or examination is meant to evaluate and engage the ability to develop a differential diagnosis or determine a most likely diagnosis, a patient scenario presenting with a potential life-threatening emergency (e.g., chest pain, myocardial infarction vs. angina vs. gastroesophageal reflux disease) or an acute but limited problem (e.g., cough, upper respiratory infection vs. seasonal allergic rhinitis) would likely be best used. If the intended goal of the examination is to address the pharmaceutical therapeutics domain, it might be best to use a case dealing with a chronic progressive problem, such as a follow-up visit for a hypertensive patient whose blood pressure is poorly controlled using current medications. Table 24.2 highlights the prioritized content domains for three hypothetical SP case scenarios by type of patient and patient acuity based on practice analysis findings reported by Arbet et al. (2009).

For example, each of the above cases could also include elements of professional practice by engaging and assessing interpersonal communication. What is most important to remember is that the examination blueprint and case selection should be deliberately designed with specific competencies and content domains in mind so that students

Table 24.2 *Prioritized Content Domains for Three Hypothetical Case Scenarios and Level of Patient Acuity*

Acuity: Acute Limited Case scenario: 3-year-old girl and mother present to an outpatient clinic with fever, cough, and shortness of breath.	Acuity: Chronic Progressive Case scenario: 45-year-old woman presents for annual evaluation of her rheumatoid arthritis. Patient is experiencing a worsening of symptoms.	Acuity: Life Threatening Case scenario: 60-year-old man presents to the emergency room with chest pain for 3 hours, tachycardia, and a history of cardiovascular disease.
1. Most likely diagnosis 2. Pharmaceutical therapeutics 3. Applying basic science 4. History and physical 5. Clinical interventions 6. Professional practice 7. Using laboratory and diagnostic studies 8. Health maintenance	1. Pharmaceutical therapeutics 2. Applying basic science 3. Clinical interventions 4. Most likely diagnosis 5. History and physical 6. Health maintenance 7. Using laboratory and diagnostic studies 8. Professional practice	1. Most likely diagnosis 2. History and physical 3. Pharmaceutical therapeutics 4. Applying basic science 5. Using laboratory and diagnostic studies 6. Clinical interventions 7. Professional practice 8. Health maintenance

Source: Adapted from Arbet S., Lathrop J., & Hooker R.S. (2009). ©2009 American Academy of Physician Assistants and Haymarket Media Inc.

actually perform (or are given every reason to perform) the skills that align with the objectives of the simulated exercise. Figure 24.2 outlines the content domains and selected case studies in a blueprint for a sample clinical year performance examination in PA training.

Number of Case Stations

It is essential that multiple case stations are used for high-stakes examinations or when performance data are needed for research purposes (Yudkowsky et al., 2008). Single station experiences may be appropriate for formative learning activities, but if grading decisions are to be made, multiple stations should be used to promote examination reliability. It is generally recommended that a minimum of 10 case stations are necessary to achieve the reliability necessary to meaningfully interpret student performance (Epstein, 2007). Although reliability can be attained with fewer stations, a performance examination needs to include enough stations in the blueprint to reliably measure the desired content domains. This means that content domains should be evaluated across many stations, not just one station for each domain. If an examination is proving unreliable, adding additional stations that measure similar domains may be able to increase examination reliability (Yudkowsky et al., 2008). Figure 24.2 demonstrates a blueprint designed to promote reliable assessment data by using multiple cases to measure each domain multiple times.

Case Development, Selection of Appropriate Simulated Modality, and Training

Once examination domains and case topics have been established, detailed case scenarios and assessment tools should be scripted and defined. The processes for case and assessment tool development is beyond the scope of this chapter, but it is generally recommended that a systematic process is used in which a faculty panel defines and develops the scenario and assessment tools based, when possible, on literary evidence (Downing & Haladyna, 2008). Appropriate modalities should be selected for each case station. Now, SP cases appear to be most frequently used in PA education because the training emphasis is on history, physical exam, and patient education, but task trainers and high-fidelity mannequin-based simulators may be appropriate if the assessment of clinical skills, such as suturing or Advanced Cardiac Life Support (ACLS), is desired.

Figure 24.2 *Hypothetical Blueprint for an Eight Case Summative Clinical Performance Examinations Near Completion of PA Education.*

	History-Taking and Performing Physical Examination	Using Laboratory and Diagnostic Studies	Formulating Most Likely Diagnosis	Health Maintenance	Clinical Intervention	Pharmaceutical Therapeutics	Applying Basic Science Concepts	Professional Practice
Acute Abdominal Pain—SP Case* Initial work-up (history, physical, labs, differential diagnosis, and plan) in emergency department for female of child-bearing age.	X	X	X				X	X
Diabetes—SP Case* Follow-up visit after initial treatment with oral hypoglycemic agent. Patient experiencing signs of hypoglycemia. Current labs provided. Provide patient education.	X	X	X	X		X	X	X
Suture Station—Hybrid SP/Part Task (Suture) Trainer* Candidate to suture simple laceration while explaining procedure to patient.	X			X	X	X		X
Hypertension—SP Case Outpatient evaluation for patient presenting with history of high blood pressure readings on multiple visits. Consider primary vs. secondary hypertension and recommend lifestyle modifications.	X	X		X			X	X
Shortness of Breath—SP Case Outpatient work-up. Care requires interpretation of pulmonary function testing, development of a differential diagnosis, and recommendations for pharmacologic management.	X	X	X			X	X	X
IV Insertion Station—Part Task Trainer (IV Arm) Start an IV on task trainer. Station will also include dosing calculation of several IV medications.					X	X	X	
Postoperative Encounter—Hybrid Mannequin-based/SP Case* Evaluate postoperative patient experiencing mild chest pain 1 day after laparoscopic cholecystectomy. 12-lead EKG, noninvasive monitoring, and basic labs provided. Present findings to resident who enters the room toward the end of the encounter.	X	X	X				X	X
Headache—SP Case Evaluate patient presenting with recent headaches. During interview, patient displays drug-seeking behavior.	X		X	X		X	X	X

*See Appendix 24.A, sample case studies for use in PA education, for a more detailed description of these cases.

Care should be taken to ensure that SP training is done in a way to standardize case portrayal and maximize examination reliability (Wallace, 2007).

Assessment Processes and Instruments

Feedback is an essential component of any simulated exercise (Issenberg et al., 2005; Hills & Pollard, 2003). Although feedback in formative learning activities may be verbal, high-stakes examinations also rely on specific measurement instruments and processes to document PA student performance, justify grading decisions, and provide feedback to PA faculty to drive curricular change (Calhoun & Chambers, 2004; Carlson et al., 2010; Coplan et al., 2008; Whitman & Pedersen, 1998). It is therefore necessary that assessment tools are systematically developed to allow student performance to be appropriately interpreted. A number of guidelines exist in the medical literature regarding the appropriate use of assessment methods during simulated experiences (Gorter et al., 2000; Hodges, 2002; Yudkowsky et al., 2008). In-depth discussion of these methods is beyond the scope of this chapter, but the degree to which PA programs are using these processes is not well-reported. It is worth discussing a few key points when designing assessment instruments used with SP encounters.

First, the mechanism of assessment must be decided. With regard to SP cases frequently used during general PA education, performance on an SP case is generally documented using a case-specific checklist (Gorter et al., 2000; Huber et al., 2005). A case-specific checklist is a set of key elements that are implied to define a standard of medical care for a specific case and task as defined by the PA faculty. As an example, a case designed to engage history and physical examination competency would allow PA students to experience an SP case and then rate them on whether or not they performed the maneuvers documented using the checklist. See Appendix 24.A for examples of case-specific checklists for a variety of case scenarios.

Although the rating scale for case items can vary depending on the case or institution, history items are typically rated as done/not done (student performed the item or not), physical examination items might be rated as done/not done, but with incorrect technique, or omitted, and interpersonal communication items might be rated on a Likert scale (strongly disagree → strongly agree). Dichotomous items (done/not done) generally demonstrate higher interrater reliability. In addition, the number of items on a case-specific checklist is important to consider, as too few items may fail to adequately capture student performance, whereas too many items can decrease examination reliability because of poor rater recall (Huber et al., 2005; Vu et al., 1992). There is no firm number detailing the optimal amount of case checklist items, but 15 to 20 items may provide enough items to sufficiently document skill without significantly impairing rater recall (Goiter et al., 2000; Huber et al., 2005).

Second, it must be determined who is completing student performance ratings for the domains measured. Within PA education, grading on SP cases is likely best completed by a combination of the SP portraying the case and PA faculty (Carlson et al., 2010; McLaughlin, Gregor, Jones, & Coderre, 2006). There is strong evidence to suggest that well-calibrated SPs can document student performance on case-specific checklists as reliably as PA faculty; however, each individual PA program must decide which content is most effectively and efficiently assessed by faculty, SPs, or simulation operators based on the examination blueprint and stakes of the examination. For example, it may be reasonable for an SP to complete a faculty-developed case-specific checklist used to document student performance of key history, physical examination, and interpersonal communication items, where the SP is simply recording if a student asked a series of specific history questions or performed a few specific maneuvers (Huber et al., 2005).

In some instances, an SP or highly trained nonfaculty observer has also been shown to be able to appropriately document student performance of specific clinical skills such as suturing. In many cases, it may be more appropriate for faculty to evaluate the quality and accuracy of a case differential diagnosis and management plan (Han, Kreiter, Park, & Ferguson, 2006). Simply put, the performance of specific concrete behavioral case items may be reliably assessed by SPs or nonfaculty raters, whereas higher level skills, such as diagnostic reasoning, are best assessed by experienced faculty. Regardless, faculty and nonfaculty SP raters should be properly trained and calibrated to maximize scoring reliability and the meaningful interpretation of student performance during high-stakes examination (Downing & Haladyna, 2008; Hodges, 2002).

Standard Setting and Denoting Minimal Competency

When simulation is used for high-stakes assessment, PA educators also need to consider what standard is considered passing on the examination. This is an important, although often somewhat overlooked, element of the case and examination development process. PA faculty need to consider if items on the case checklist are to represent a minimal standard of care where completion of *all* items denotes competency. If not, faculty must determine what percentage of checklist items is considered passing or minimal competence. Although an arbitrary percentage of 70% or greater could be assigned as passing, it is more acceptable to use a systematic standard-setting process (Downing, Tekian, & Yudkowsky, 2005).

A number of standard-setting methods appropriate for use with simulation-based examinations are reported in the medical literature, including the Angoff, Borderline Group, Ebel, and Hoffstee methods (Downing et al., 2005; Yudkowksy, Downing, & Wirth, 2008). There is growing evidence documenting the credibility of these standard-setting methods within PA-focused simulated exercises, but the extent to which PA faculty regularly engage in these practices is unclear (Carlson et al., 2009, 2010). This is of particular importance within PA education because PA programs are charged with verifying skill competency through local institution-specific measures including simulation-based assessment, as opposed to a national board level examination similar to the U.S. Medical Licensing Examination Step 2 clinical skills. No single method may be appropriate to all simulated exercises because successful integration can depend on a number of factors, including available faculty time, access to technology to facilitate video review, and the intended purpose of the exam. Whatever the method used, the PA faculty responsible for integrating simulation into their curricula for examination purposes should select and implement a defensible standard-setting process so that examination performance can be meaningfully interpreted (Downing & Haladyna, 2008).

There are a number of other factors important to the design of simulated encounters in PA education. Using case blueprints, careful selection of case scenarios, the development of reliable assessment instruments, and credible standard setting processes are but a few of the factors faculty should consider. PA faculty involved in the design of simulated activities should become familiar with these processes and sources of validity evidence so that simulation resources are appropriately employed.

SAMPLE CASE SCENARIOS

Appendix 24.A provides five sample case scenarios for use in PA education. Each case provides a brief summary, list of student tasks, suggested modality (SP, task trainer, mannequin-based, hybrid simulation, etc.), suggested modifications to tasks based on level of learner, content domains engaged, and sample assessment checklists. Case examples are scripted with minimal detail and are only to serve as a brief template and example. Full cases should include sufficient detail to promote case reliability by minimizing the SP's or simulation operator's need to improvise. This frequently results in case scenarios consisting of 10 pages or more and is obviously impractical to include in this chapter. Faculty wishing to use the provided scenario templates may do so, but a detailed script designed to specifically engage the learning objectives within their respective setting will need to be compiled.

REFERENCES

Accreditation Review Commission on Education for the Physician Assistant. (2010). *Accreditation standards.* Retrieved from http://www.arc-pa.org/acc_standards/

American Academy of Physician Assistants. (2009). *AAPA Physician Assistant National Report.* Retrieved from http://www.aapa.org/images/stories/Data_2009/2009aapacensusnationalreport.pdf

American Academy of Physician Assistants. (2010). *Our practice areas.* Retrieved from http://www.aapa.org/about-pas/our-practice-areas

Arbet, S., Lathrop, J., & Hooker, R. (2009). Using practice analysis to improve the certifying examinations for PAs. *Journal of the American Academy of Physician Assistants, 22*(1), 31–36.

Asprey D, Hegmann T, & Bergus G. (2007). Comparison of medical student and physician assistant student performance on standardized-patient assessments. *Journal of Physician Assistant Education, 18*(4), 16–19.

Association of Standardized Patient Educators. (2010). *Definition of an SP.* Retrieved from http://www.aspeducators.org/sp_info.htm

Bryant-Lukosius, D., DiCenso, A., Browne, G., & Pinelli, J. (2004). Advanced practice nursing roles: Development, implementation, and evaluation. *Journal of Advanced Nursing, 48*(5), 519–529.

Calhoun, B., & Chambers, D. (2004). Standardized patients and simulated patient encounters in the evaluation of students. *Perspective on Physician Assistant Education, 15*(2), 99–101.

Calhoun, B., Vribin, C., & Grzybicki, D. (2008). The use of standardized patient in the training and evaluation of physician assistant students. *Journal of Physician Assistant Education, 19*(1), 18–23.

Carlson, J., Laack, S., & Stilp, C. (2006). *What primary care procedural skills are PA schools teaching and how are they teaching them.* Poster session presented at the 2006 American Association of Physician Assistants Annual Conference, Toronto, Canada.

Carlson, J., Tomkowiak, J., & Knott, P. (2010). Simulation-based examination in physician assistant education: A comparison of two standard-setting methods. *Journal of Physician Assistant Education, 21*(2), 7–14.

Carlson, J., Tomkowiak, J., & Stilp, C. (2009). Using the Angoff method to set defensible passing levels for standardized patient performance evaluations in PA education. *Journal of Physician Assistant Education, 20*(1), 15–23.

Carter, R., & Strand, J. (2000). Physician assistants: A young profession celebrated the 35th anniversary of its birth in North Carolina. *North Carolina Medical Journal, 61*(5), 249–256.

Chakraborti, C., Boonyasai, R., Wright, S., & Kern, D. (2008). A systematic review of teamwork training interventions in medical student and resident education. *Journal of General Internal Medicine, 23*(6), 846–853.

Cooper, J., & Taqueti, V. (2008). A brief history of the development of mannequin simulators for clinical education and training. *Postgraduate Medical Journal, 84*, 563–570.

Coplan, B., Essary, A., Lohenry, K., & Stoehr, J. (2008). An update on the utilization of standardized patients in physician assistant education. *Journal of Physician Assistant Education, 19*(4), 14–19.

Devita, M., Shaefer, J., Lutz, J., Wang, H., & Dongilli, T. (2005). Improving medical emergency team (MET) performance using a novel curriculum and a computerized human patient simulator. *Quality and Safety in Health Care, 14*, 326–331.

Dehn, R. (2010). The development of varying physician assistant roles in the United States. *Journal of the American Academy of Physician Assistants, 23*(1), 53–54.

Downing, S., & Haladyna, T. (2009). Validity and it's threats. In S. Downing & R. Yudkowsky (Eds.), *Assessment in health professions education* (pp. 217–243). New York: Routledge.

Downing, S., Tekian, A., & Yudkowski, R. (2005). Procedures for establishing defensible absolute passing scores on performance examinations in health professions education. *Teaching and Learning in Medicine, 18*(1), 50–57.

Epstein, M. (2007). Assessment in medical education. *New England Journal of Medicine, 356*, 387–396.

Ericsson, K. A. (2008). Deliberate practice and acquisition of expert performance: A general overview. *Academic Emergency Medicine, 15*(11), 988–994.

Fleek, K. (2003). The benefits of using standardized patients with didactic-year physician assistant students. *Perspective on Physician Assistant Education, 14*(2), 74–77.

Gorter, S., Rethans, J., Scherpbier A., van der Heijde, D., Houben, H., van der Vleuten, C., et al. (2000). Developing case-specific checklists for standardized patient-based assessments in internal medicine: A review of the literature. *Academic Medicine, 75*, 1130–1137.

Han, J., Kreiter, C., Park, H., & Ferguson, K. (2006). An experimental comparison of rater performance on an SP-based clinical skills exam. *Teaching and Learning in Medicine, 18*(4), 304–209.

Hills, K., & Pollard, S. (2003). Focused teaching for focused learning: An approach to teaching clinical medicine using standardized patients. *Perspective on Physician Assistant Education, 14*(3), 145–148.

Hodges, B. (2002). Creating, monitoring, and improving a psychiatric OSCE. *Academic Psychiatry, 26*(3), 134–161.

Hooker, R. S., Carter, R., & Cawley, J. R. (2004). The National Commission on Certification of Physician Assistants: History and role. *Perspective on Physician Assistant Education, 15*(1), 8–15.

Hooker, R. S., Cawley, J. F., & Leinweber, W. (2010). Career flexibility of physician assistants and the potential for more primary care. *Health Affairs, 29*(5), 880–886.

Huber, P., Baroffio, A., Chamot, E., Herrmann, F., Nendaz, M., & Vu, N. (2005). Effects of item and rater characteristics on checklist recording: What should we look for? *Medical Education, 39*(8), 852–858.

Issenberg, B., Gordon, D., Stewart, G., & Felner, J. (2000). Bedside cardiology skills training for the physician assistant using simulation technology. *Perspective on Physician Assistant Education, 11*(2), 99–103.

Issenberg, B., MaGaghie W., Petrusa, E., Gordon, D., & Scalese, R. (2005). Features and uses of high fidelity medical simulation that lead to effective learning: A BEME systematic review. *Medical Teacher, 27*(1) 10–28.

Jones, E. (2007). Physician assistant education in the United States. *Academic Medicine, 82*(9), 882–887.

Luce, D. (2001). Teaching students to take the history: An overview. *Perspective on Physician Assistant Education, 12*(2), 100–106.

Maran, N., & Glavin, R. (2003). Low-to high-fidelity simulation—A continuum of medical education. *Medical Education, 37*(Suppl. 1), 22–28.

Mavis, B., Ogle, K., Lovell, K., & Madden, L. (2002). Reproducibility of clinical performance assessment in practice using in cognito standardized patients. *Medical Education, 36*, 827–832.

McCabe, S., & Burman, M. (2006). A tale of two APNs: Addressing blurred practice boundaries in APN practice. *Perspectives in Psychiatric Care, 42*(1), 3–12.

McLaughlin, K., Gregor, L., Jones, A., & Coderre, S. (2006). Can standardized patients replace physicians as OSCE examiners? *BMC Medical Education, 6*(1), 12.

Multak, N., Euliano T., Gabrielli A., & Layon J. (2002). Human patient simulation: A preliminary report of an innovative training tool for physician assistant education. *Perspective on Physician Assistant Education, 13*(2), 103–106.

National Board of Oseteopathic Medical Examiners. (2010). COMLEX-USA Level 2-PE (Performance Evaluation) Fact Sheet. Retrieved from http://www.nbome.org/docs/PEFactSheet.pdf

National Commission on the Certification of Physician Assistants. (2010). *Certification exams.* Retrieved from http://www.nccpa.net/exams.aspx

Parkhurst, D., & Ramsey, C. (2006). The marriage of problem-based learning with standardized patients: An evaluation of physician assistant students' cultural competency in communication. *Journal of Physician Assistant Education, 17*(1), 58–62.

Physician Assistant Education Association. (2010). *Twenty-Fifth Annual Report on Physician Assistant Educational Programs in the United States.* Retrieved from http://www.paeaonline.org/index.php?ht=d/sp/i/243/pid/243

Salas, E., DiasGranados, D., Weaver, M., & King, H. (2008). Does team training work? Principles for healthcare. *Academic Emergency Medicine, 15*(11), 1002–1009.

Scalese, R., Obeso, V., & Issenberg, B. (2007). Simulation technology for skills training and competency assessment in medical education. *Journal of General Internal Medicine, 23*(1), 45–49.

Shapiro, M., Morey, J., Small, S., Langford, V., Kaylor, C., Jagminas, L., et al. (2004). Simulation based teamwork training for emergence department staff: Does it improve clinical team performance when added to an existing didactic teamwork curriculum? *Quality and Safety in Health Care, 13,* 417–412.

Stead, E. (1966). Conserving costly talents: Providing physicians' new assistants. *Journal of the American Medical Association, 198,* 1108–1109.

U.S. Medical Licensing Examination®. (2010). *Step 2 Clinical Skills (CS).* Retrieved from http://www.usmle.org/Examinations/step2/step2cs.html

Vu, N., Marcy, M., Colliver, J., Verhulst, S., Travis, T., & Barrows, H. (1992). Standardized (simulated) patients' accuracy in recording clinical performance checklist items. *Medical Education, 26*(2), 99–104.

Wallace, P. (2007). Training the standardized patients: An overview. In P. Wallace (Ed.), *Coaching standardized patients for use in the assessment of clinical competence* (pp. 156–162). New York: Springer Publishing.

Whitman, N., & Pedersen, D. (1998). The use of standardized patients to evaluate a physician assistant program curriculum. *Perspective on Physician Assistant Education, 9*(2), 93–96.

Williams, R. (2004). Have standardized patient examinations stood the test of time and experience. *Teaching and Learning in Medicine, 16*(2), 215–222.

Yudkowsky, R. (2009). Performance assessment. In S. Downing & R. Yudkowsky (Eds.), *Assessment in health professions education* (pp. 217–243). New York: Routledge.

Yudkowsky, R., Downing, S., & Wirth, S. (2008). Simpler standards for local performance examinations: The yes/no Angoff and whole-test Ebel. *Teaching and Learning in Medicine, 20*(3), 212–217.

APPENDIX 24.A: SAMPLE CASE STUDIES FOR USE IN PA EDUCATION

Station topic/case chief complaint: Acute abdominal pain—emergency department setting.

Presenting situation and case summary: Woman of child-bearing age presents to the emergency room with acute abdominal pain. Pain is in the right lower quadrant, associated nausea, no history of similar symptoms. Past medical history of sexually transmitted disease, patient is sexually active. Patient is hemodynamically stable but in obvious pain during encounter.

Student tasks: Perform a focused history and physical examination on SP (15 minutes).

Write a SOAP note to document the patient encounter (10 minutes).

Station modality/requirements: Intended for use as SP case—SP should have no abdominal scars related to prior abdominal surgery or significant abdominal pathology.

Task modification(s): If used with early level students, task may direct student to perform a focused abdominal examination. For more advanced students engaged in team simulation, this case may also be modified for use with a full-body mannequin simulation to integrate monitoring and hemodynamic instability requiring initial patient stabilization (because of ruptured ectopic pregnancy or ruptured appendix).

Content Domains and Suggested Case Objectives

Content Domain	Sample Learning/Assessment Objectives
History and physical examination	– Elicit history of present illness for acute pain, medical history for STD, and social history suggestive of potential pregnancy. – Perform a focused and technically precise cardiovascular, focused abdominal examination, genitourinary examination considered.
Using laboratory and diagnostic studies	– Order appropriate laboratory work-up for acute abdomen including pregnancy testing during postencounter exercise. – Order appropriate imaging studies (ultrasound or CT [after negative pregnancy test]).
Formulating the most likely diagnosis	– List appropriate DDx for acute abdomen on postencounter note including possible GI (appendicitis) OB/Gyn (ectopic pregnancy, ovarian torsion), and GU (nephrolithiasis) pathology.
Pharmaceutical therapeutics	– Recognize the need for and list an appropriate pain medication for situation.
Applying basic science concepts	– Apply understanding of gastrointestinal (GI), obstetric (OB), gynecologic (Gyn), and genitourinary (GU) pathology.
Professional practice	– Use effective interpersonal communication skills with SP, appropriately interact with a patient in acute pain through effective questioning and offering reassurance, accurately document the patient encounter on SOAP note.

Sample case-specific items if used for assessment: The following checklist items are intended to be completed by a trained SP immediately after the encounter or trained rater or monitor while observing. Postencounter to be graded by faculty.

Done	Not Done	Sample history items for acute abdominal pain case Did the examiner ask about the following? (mark item as either done or not done)
		1. Where is the pain located?
		2. Has the pain been in the right lower quadrant the whole time or did it move there?
		3. Describe the pain.
		4. Nausea, vomiting, or diarrhea.
		5. History of associated fever.
		6. Pain or discomfort with urination.
		7. History of sexually transmitted disease.
		8. Recent sexual activity.
		9. Last menstrual period.
		10. Medical history of similar.

Correct	Incorrect	Omitted	Sample physical exam items for acute abdominal pain case Did the examiner perform the following with correct technique? (mark item as correct, incorrect, or omitted)
			Washed hands with soap and water before performing exam.
			Auscultated the abdomen in all four quadrants.
			Palpated the abdomen in all four quadrants.
			Performed psoas or obturator signs.
			Performed rebound testing.
			Stated that a pelvic and rectal examination would be performed.

SD	D	N	A	SA	**Sample interpersonal communication items** (mark responses on a five-point scale)
					Initiating the encounter
					Organization
					Questioning and listening
					Patient-centered atmosphere (in this case, was the fact that the patient was in pain addressed)
					Ending the Encounter

SD = strongly disagree, D = disagree, N = neutral, A = agree, SA = strongly agree.

Station topic/case chief complaint: Diabetes—outpatient primary care setting.

Presenting situation and case summary: Follow-up visit after initial treatment with oral hypoglycemic. Patient experiencing symptoms and signs of hypoglycemia due to inappropriately taking prescribed medication. Patient has not been using home glucose monitoring. Labs provided showing that blood glucose is still elevated.

Student tasks: Perform a focused history/provide appropriate patient education (15 minutes).

Write a SOAP note to document the patient encounter (10 minutes).

Station modality/requirements: Intended for use as SP case.

Task modification(s): If used with early level students, task may include providing a more detailed background history on the patient chart and asking the student to spend the encounter specifically screening for medication compliance and lifestyle factors. For more advanced students, case may include a challenging element of patient illiteracy related to improperly taking oral hypoglycemic and noncompliance with home glucose monitoring.

Content Domains and Suggested Case Objectives

Content Domain	Sample Learning/Assessment Objectives
History and physical examination	– Elicit history of present illness for recently diagnosed diabetic on new medication experiencing signs and symptoms of hypoglycemia.
Using laboratory and diagnostic studies	– Recognize that glucose readings at today's visit are elevated. – Elicit information pertaining to frequency and readings associated with home glucose monitoring.
Formulating the most likely diagnosis	– Identify hypoglycemia as cause of signs and symptoms. – Recognize diabetes is not treated to target goals. – If applied to case, recognize health care literacy issues pertaining to case.
Health maintenance	– Address the importance of home glucose monitoring and glycemic control. – Negotiate behavioral modification with patient to improve glycemic control.
Pharmaceutical therapeutics	– Identify hypoglycemia secondary to oral hypoglycemic. – Consider the need for modification of or replacement of oral hypoglycemic.
Applying basic science concepts	– Apply understanding of Type 2 diabetes mellitus, risk factors associated with underlying cardiovascular disease, and hypoglycemia.
Professional practice	– Use effective interpersonal communication skills with SP. – Provide effective patient education within the context of this case. – If applied to case, appropriately address patient noncompliance in the context of literacy issues.

Sample case-specific items if used for assessment: The following checklist items are intended to be completed by a trained SP immediately after the encounter or trained rater or monitor while observing. Postencounter to be graded by faculty.

Done	Not Done	Sample history/patient education items for diabetes follow-up case Did the examiner ask about the following? (mark item as either done or not done)
		1. Recent symptoms of hypoglycemia (dizziness, shaking, sweating)?
		2. When (what time during the day) hypoglycemia symptoms occur?
		3. Onset: when did you first notice these symptoms?
		4. Tell me exactly how you are taking your medications.
		5. Have you been taking your blood sugar at home?
		6. Informed you that your symptoms are likely because of improperly taking medication.
		7. Have you been monitoring your blood sugar at home?
		8. Why you have not been taking your blood sugar at home?
		9. Informed you how to monitor your blood sugar at home/suggested meeting with diabetes educator to discuss this.
		10. Elicited that the patient has poor reading ability/illiteracy.

SD = strongly disagree, D = disagree, N = neutral, A = agree, SA = strongly agree.

SD	D	N	A	SA	Sample Interpersonal Communication items (mark responses on a five-point scale)
					Initiating the encounter
					Organization
					Questioning and listening
					Patient-centered atmosphere (in this case, was the fact that the patient could not read addressed in a respectful manner)
					Ending the encounter

Station topic/case chief complaint: Suture station.

Student tasks: Throw three simple interrupted sutures with appropriate technique.

Demonstrate appropriate sterile technique.

Provide appropriate patient education/communication while performing procedure.

Station modality/requirements: Hybrid simulation: suture task trainer (low-fidelity suture arm) in proximity to SP. Standardized nurse or medical assistant could also be involved to assist with procedure and serve as rater to observe and score procedure performance.

Task modification(s): If used with more advanced students or faculty would like to put the task within a clinical context, consider hybrid simulation with SP. Student to perform suturing on task trainer but interact with and provide education to the SP.

Content Domains and Suggested Case Objectives

Content Domain	Sample Learning/Assessment Objectives
History and physical examination	– Elicit history related to injury, recent tetanus, general medical problems, allergies, etc.
Clinical intervention	– Select appropriate suture materials for anatomic region. – Demonstrate appropriate wound irrigation. – Provide adequate wound closure with three simple interrupted sutures. – Use sterile technique while performing procedure.
Health maintenance	– Inquire about last tetanus and identify factors that may impair wound healing. – Provide appropriate instructions for wound care including when to return to clinic for suture removal.
Pharmaceutical therapeutics	– Identify appropriate anesthetic for anatomic region. – Consider the need for antibiotic prophylaxis based on injury history.
Applying basic science concepts	– Dermatology, wound healing, infectious disease.
Professional practice	– Use effective interpersonal communication skills with SP. – Use effective interpersonal communication skills with simulated RN/Medical Assistant. – Provide effective patient education regarding wound care.

Sample case-specific items if used for assessment: The following checklist items are intended to be completed by a trained SP immediately after the encounter or trained rater or monitor while observing. Postencounter to be graded by faculty.

Done	Not Done	Sample assessment items for suture station Did the student demonstrate the following? (mark item as either done or not done)
		1. Selection of appropriate suture material for case/anatomical location.
		2. Irrigated wound with appropriate technique.
		3. Administered regional anesthesia appropriately.
		4. Properly put on sterile gloves.
		5. Maintained sterile field at all times during procedure.
		6. Suture needle was loaded into needle driver as 2/3 ratio.
		7. Needle consistently entered perpendicular to patient skin.
		8. Needle consistently entered skin 2 to 5 mm from wound margin.
		9. Needle consistently exited skin at 2 to 5 mm from wound margin.
		10. Suture material wrapped twice around needle driver to begin knot.
		11. Final knots were square.
		12. Wound margins were approximated with appropriate tension.

SD	D	N	A	SA	Sample Interpersonal Communication items (mark responses on a five-point scale)
					Initiating the encounter
					Organization
					Questioning and listening
					Patient education: clear instructions and information was consistently offered during the encounter
					Interaction with colleague (standardized RN or medical assistant) was clear, appropriate, and respectful
					Ending the encounter

SD = strongly disagree, D = disagree, N = neutral, A = agree, SA = strongly agree.

Station topic/case chief complaint: Trauma—emergency department setting.

Presenting situation and case summary: Twenty-something man or woman presents to the emergency department after motor vehicle accident. Multiple problems including head laceration, c-spine immobilization, chest and abdominal contusions, right lower extremity fracture. PA student is part of the interprofessional team accepting care from emergency medical services (paramedics). Additional team members might include attending physician, chief resident, other PAs, nursing staff, ED tech, and radiology tech. Case requires rapid primary and secondary survey, prioritization of most severe injuries first with highest priority on potential cardiovascular compromise (pericardial tamponade, tension pneumothorax), and acute management to promote patient stability. This case is intended for simulation targeted at team-based training.

Team tasks: Initiate primary (ABC) and secondary survey.

Identify problems prioritize must urgent problems first.

Recognize and institute appropriate treatment (BLS, ACLS, ATLS, and definite treatment as case evolves.

PA student: Appropriately fulfill roles and responsibilities as assigned by team leader.

Tasks: Effectively communicate and collaborate with other team members.

Monitor fellow team member performance and assist teammates as necessary.

Station modality/requirements: Mannequin-based simulation with potential for integration of multiple trainees or standardized participants (standardized RN, physician, etc.). Patient will be portrayed by mannequin to allow for dynamic monitoring, recognition of abnormal findings (e.g., muffled heart tones, hemorrhage), and performance of procedures in context (e.g., airway management, pericardiocentesis).

Task modification(s): Depending on available trainees, the encounter may integrate other types of students as a form of interprofessional education or use standardized participants to portray other team members. If standardized participants (confederates) are used, they can be scripted to engage the student(s) in very specific team behaviors pending the objectives of the simulation (e.g., trigger conflict, provide misinformation, fail to perform assigned duties). It is recommended that if team training is instituted, highly specific team objectives are identified and standardized participants institute a behavioral trigger to make sure the team objective is addressed. For example, a confederate RN might hand the PA student the wrong medication to administer if the team goal of the simulation is to engage the student in cross-monitoring behaviors.

Content Domains and Suggested Case Objectives (for PA Student)

Content Domain	Sample Learning/Assessment Objectives
History and physical examination	– As directed by team leader, perform heart and lung auscultation and report findings to team. – Listen to discussion of historical and physical examination information provided by other team members to gain an understanding of the patient presentation.
Formulating the most likely diagnosis	– *Upon prompting by chief resident,* list the differential diagnosis for a patient with presenting injuries and prioritize which injuries should be addressed first.
Pharmaceutical therapeutics	– Listen to pharmacologic interventions discussed by the team. – Recognize the appropriate pharmacologic interventions for the problem.
Clinical interventions	– Assist the chief resident with endotracheal intubation. – At the direction of the team leader, properly fulfill a task associated with ACLS (chest compressions, use of a defibrillator, etc.)
Applying basic science concepts	– Apply understanding of cardiopulmonary, neurologic, orthopedic, and abdominal pathology as it relates to acute injury.
Professional practice	– Use effective interpersonal communication skills with other team members. – Verbally intervene to prevent a medication error (if scripted into case). – Monitor other team members and recognize the need to provide task assistance (e.g., helps prep intubation equipment and assist before the need for prompting from the chief resident).

If used for assessment, sample case-specific checklist items: Team-based simulation can be very difficult to formally assess and is likely not appropriate for high-stakes summative assessment. Data collected to inform debriefing and formative assessment may be very valuable. The following checklist items might be used to evaluate general team performance or individual PA student performance during this type of case.

Done (note time)	Not Done	Sample key case items (evaluated at the team level) Did the team perform the following? (mark item as either done or not done and note time to action)
		1. Recognized the primary problem (e.g., cardiac tamponade).
		2. Initiated appropriate treatment (e.g., pericardiocentesis).
		3. Recognized pulseless arrest (ventricular tachycardia).
		4. Rescue breathing and chest compressions were performed at intervals consistent with BLS guidelines (30:2 ratio).
		5. Defibrillated patient.

SD	D	N	A	SA	Sample Generic Teamwork Evaluation (mark responses on a five-point scale)
					Clear leadership was established
					Communication was clear, brief, and meaningful
					Team members monitored and assisted one another
					Roles and responsibilities were clear and evenly distributed across team

SD = strongly disagree, D = disagree, N = neutral, A = agree, SA = strongly agree.

Done	Not Done	**Sample PA student-specific items** Did the PA student perform the following? (mark item as either done or not done
		1. Recognized that the medication to be administered was inappropriate based on team leader instructions (atropine handed to PA student instead of epinephrine).
		2. Did not administer atropine.
		3. Asked RN confederate for epinephrine instead.
		4. Assisted chief resident with intubation without the need to be asked.
		5. When directed to perform chest compressions, compressions were at appropriate rate and depth.

Station topic/case chief complaint: Postoperative evaluation—inpatient surgery floor.

Presenting situation and case summary: Fifty-year-old man, 1 day after uncomplicated laparoscopic cholecystectomy. Student to enter the room and perform a standard postoperative evaluation. Patient recovering as expected except for mild fever and new onset of mild shortness of breath/cough the morning of the visit. Morning labs provided. During the last 5 minutes of the encounter, the surgery resident (standardized participant—confederate) will enter the room. Student will be responsible to provide a brief bedside presentation and is prompted to make recommendations regarding patient status and further work-up.

Student tasks: Perform a focused postoperative evaluation (10 minutes).

Present case to resident (5 minutes).

Write a note to document the encounter (10 minutes).

Station modality/requirements: Mannequin-based case (patient) set to have signs of right lung consolidation (atelectasis vs. pneumonia). Standardized participant (resident) trained to portray case and evaluate student performance.

Task modification(s): If used with early level students, emphasis might solely be on the patient encounter and forego the resident presentation. Students with increasing levels of expertise might be questioned in detail by the resident to justify their rationale for clinical decisions. Scenario might also be reversed for use with a physician resident and standardized PA student to engage physician candidates with mentoring techniques to improve bedside teaching.

Content Domains and Suggested Case Objectives

Content Domain	Sample Learning/Assessment Objectives
History and physical examination	– Perform the essential historical and physical examination elements of a standard postoperative work up. – Recognize and interpret normal and abnormal findings on the cardiopulmonary examination.
Using laboratory and diagnostic dtudies	– Recognize normal laboratory findings and consider further labs of use within the patient scenario. – Order appropriate imaging studies (plain film of chest)
Formulating the most likely diagnosis	– List appropriate DDx for postoperative shortness of breath, including infectious pathology. – Other than shortness of breath, recognize normal postoperative recovery.
Applying basic science concepts	– Apply understanding of gastrointestinal (GI) and cardiopulmonary pathology.
Professional practice	– Use effective interpersonal communication skills and presentation with surgical resident.

Sample case-specific items if used for assessment: The following checklist items are intended to be completed by a trained SP immediately after the encounter or trained rater or monitor while observing. Postencounter to be graded by faculty.

Done	Not Done	Sample history items for postoperative case Did the examiner ask about the following? (mark item as either done or not done)
		1. How is your pain level (surgical site)?
		2. Have you been using incentive spirometer?
		3. Have you been having shortness of breath/chest pain?
		4. Have you been able to eat/hold down food or liquid?
		5. Nausea/vomiting?
		6. Have you had a bowel movement?
		7. Have you been urinating?
		8. Have you been walking?
		9. Describe (in greater detail) the shortness of breath/chest pain.

Correct	Incorrect	Omitted	Sample physical examination items for postoperative case Did the examiner perform the following with correct technique? (mark item as correct, incorrect, or omitted)
			Washed hands with soap and water before performing exam
			Auscultated the heart.
			Auscultated the lungs
			Fully exposed and inspected all wound sites on abdomen
			Auscultated the abdomen in all four quadrants
			Palpated the abdomen in all four quadrants

SD	D	N	A	SA	Case Presentation to Resident (mark responses on a five-point scale)
					Current situation as clearly presented and new symptoms (shortness of breath/cough emphasized)
					Student provided background appropriate for situation and to justify recommendations made
					Recommendations were clearly presented (with or without prompting from resident) and demonstrated sound clinical reasoning
					Interpersonal communication was clear, concise, and well-organized

SD = strongly disagree, D = disagree, N = neutral, A = agree, SA = strongly agree.

CHAPTER 25

Human Simulation in Couple and Family Therapy Education

Stephanie Brooks and Racine Henry

For almost two decades, the issue of provider competency has been linked to significant problems in the delivery of health care services (Pew Health Profession Commission, 1993). According to the Institute of Medicine, health care education has a profound impact on quality of care and concomitant health care disparities (Committee on Crossing Quality Chasm: Adaption to Mental and Health Addictive Disorders, 2006; Committee on Quality Health Care in America, 2001; President's New Freedom Commission on Mental Health, 2003). Previously, the health care professions such as nursing and medicine made significant attempts to critique and change their curricula (Cassel, 2004; Diekelmann, 2002; Freeman, Voignier, & Scott, 2020; Whitcomb, 2004). The literature clearly describes the multitude of drivers and challenges in designing and executing a curriculum that is responsive to educational and health care accreditation institutions, shifts in health care systems, and more importantly, patient demographics and care (Hamner & Wilder, 2001; Hayden, Dufel, & Shih, 2002; LaMantia & Panacek, 2002).

Until recently, behavioral health care professions have been negligent and slow to make the necessary changes to modernize outdated and uncorroborated training methods as well as address the increasing problem of workforce retention (Hoge, 2002; Hoge & Morris, 2002; Roberts, Borden, Christiansen, & Lopez, 2005). In 2004, the Substance Abuse and Mental Administration, the Annapolis Coalition (a partnership between the American College of Mental Health Administration and the Academic Behavioral Health Consortium), the consumers, and the health care providers convened a meeting to address the problems behavioral health care professions must confront to ameliorate workforce competency issues.

In 2004, the American Association for Marriage and Family Therapy (AAMFT) introduced its first draft of core competencies for the Couple and Family Therapy (CFT) profession (AAMFT, Clinical Competencies Task Force, 2003). Subsequently, in 2005, the Commission on Accreditation for Marriage and Family Therapy Education (COAMFTE) developed new outcome-based accreditation standards to be implemented by all accredited programs by 2007 (COAMFTE, 2006). (MFT) at minimum will require programs to become more proficient at measuring CFT students' clinical competency and development over time (Brooks, 2010). The shift to outcome-based accreditation standards in Master of Family Therapy (MFT) programs further requires CFT educators to reevaluate their program requirements and design.

This chapter thus describes how the CFT Department at Drexel University integrated human simulation into the COAMFTE-accredited CFT program. Included is an overview of the educational program, with goals and objectives, and how human simulation is used in a clinical seminar course as a formative evaluative tool and as an instructional method in a therapist training course. Case examples illustrate both the planning and the technical aspects of human simulation and the robust experience it provides students.

IMPLICATIONS OF NEW OUTCOME-BASED EDUCATIONAL STANDARDS

History and Role of Accreditation

The profession of CFT is a relatively young discipline in relation to its health care counterparts. The CFT educational standards were first published in 1949 (COAMFTE Site Visitor Handbook; Nichols, 1979). Since that time, the standards have been revised at least 12 times. Before 2005, the standards had an "input orientation." In other words, in the previous COAMFTE Version 10.3, programs had to demonstrate the curriculum-met baseline standards, and students were exposed to certain types of clients, completed 500 clinical contact hours, and had at least 100 supervision hours. Outside conventional and traditional methods of evaluation, the COAMFTE standards did not require programs to provide "evidence" of student learning and subsequent competency. Although educational programs worked diligently to adhere to the standards, student competency was assumed and rarely challenged. Nonetheless, Kniskern and Gurman (1979) expressed concern regarding the lack of empirical data to support educational standards and learning practices. Despite the concern about education and training outcome research, data emerged supporting that COAMFTE CFT programs more than COAMFTE nonaccredited programs were perceived by faculty and students to adhere to the mission of socializing students to the CFT profession, as well as committed to maintaining standards of practice (Henry, Sprenkle, & Sheehan, 1986).

The Relationship Between the Competency-Based Movement and the CFT Education

The AAMFT competency-based movement has implications for the economical survival of the profession (Miller, Todahl, & Platt, 2010). In an effort to ensure the profession remains viable, it needs to compete for its market share and to continue to demonstrate its value to gatekeepers of services such as insurance companies and legislative bodies (Bowers, 2004).

Although AAMFT did not require educational programs to integrate the MFT into the curriculum, the COAMFTE Version 11 outcome-based standards were developed in response to new movement. Undoubtedly, the development of the COAMFTE outcome-based standards is influencing how educators and supervisors are conceptualizing and evaluating student competency (Miller et al., 2010; Perosa & Perosa, 2010). Over the past 2 years, a number of articles have described the use of experiential teaching strategies and observational evaluative methods to teach as well as evaluate clinical competencies

(Miller, 2009; Miller, Linville, Todahl, & Metcalfe, 2009). Standardized patients or simulated clients were initially used to evaluate and train physicians (Barrows, 1993). Human simulation has also been successfully adopted by other health care professions such as physicians assistants, rehabilitation science, and nursing programs as a method to develop skills and to evaluate clinical skills and formal testing (Hale, Lewis, Eckert, Wilson, & Smith, 2006; Hills & Pollard, 2003; Yoo & Yoo, 2003). Although other health care professionals have embraced human simulation, it has not been readily adopted by CFT educators.

In a recent survey study of COAMFTE-accredited master's degree programs, CFT faculty identified lectures, small group work, and independent study as the top three educational strategies. Almost 15% of the sample reported using standardized patients (Brooks, 2010). CFT faculty in the same study reported over the past year the most common evaluation methods were videotapes, written reports, and role-plays. Simulated laboratory experiences were reported by 58% of the sample; however, the study did not differentiate between simulated laboratory experiences with standardized patients, simulation laboratory experiences using faculty, and students in role-plays.

Hodgson, Lamson, and Feldhousen (2007) formerly introduced the profession to use of simulated laboratory and standardized patients as a teaching tool for managing high-risk clients. They used the simulated experience as a formative evaluation to assess students' skills in cases with suicidal, homicidal, child maltreatment, and domestic violence situations.

THE CFT DEPARTMENT

The CFT Department consists of four programs: MFT, Post-Master's Certificate, PhD in CFT, and Online Medical Family Therapy Certificate Programs. The CFT program was first established at Hahnemann University in 1976 and received its COAMFTE initial accreditation in 1985. The Post-Master's Certificate program was established in 1999 and received its COAMFTE initial accreditation in 2000.

From the inception of the program, students simultaneously engaged in their clinical practicum and coursework. The overall mission of the CFT program is to develop highly trained CFT clinicians by exposing and teaching them the CFT classic approaches and postmodern and evidenced-based models. The department is committed and uses cultural awareness and sensitivity, social justice, and Person of the Therapist as metaframeworks for conceptualizing problems and therapeutic strategies. In the MFT program, students are engaged in practicum for 2 years in conjunction with intensive individual and group supervision. Over the course of the program, students complete one continuous 12-month practicum and one 9-month practicum.

Clinical Practice

During the first quarter, the MFT students attend a weekly 2-hour clinical seminar. The clinical seminar is a component of the practicum course, which includes 16–20 hours at a clinical site along with a minimum of 4 hours of individual and group weekly supervision. Students must accrue a minimum of 350 total clinical contact hours to graduate from the program. At least 250 of the 350 hours must be with couples, families, or multifamily or multicouple groups. Unlike many CFT programs, the Drexel

University CFT program does not operate a training clinic where faculty can provide students with live supervision. Instead actual clinical experience is gained in external practicum sites.

The purpose of the first year practicum is for the student to develop foundational skills necessary for the practice of CFT. The program expects students to be able to do the following:

First Year Goals and Objectives for MFT Students
- Demonstrate caring respect for the client
- Demonstrate a basic knowledge of system theory and attentive to the relational context of the presenting problem
- Demonstrate the ability to develop a rapport and effectively join with clients.
- Demonstrate a working knowledge of the *Diagnostic and Statistical Manual of Mental Disorders, Fourth Edition, Text Revision*
- Demonstrate sensitivity and understanding of sociocultural issues
- Develop a theoretical framework for the treatment case
- Recognize one's emotions and how those emotions influence their behavior while conducting therapy
- Use supervision as a mechanism to expand the students thinking and work with a particular case
- Demonstrate knowledge about the function and practice of AAMFT Code of Ethics and Agency Policies

Creating a Learning Environment: Lessons Learned From Supervision

A major strength of the program is the structure and process for clinical supervision. The CFT core faculty members function as both group and individual supervisors for students, along with practicum site and off-site individual supervisors. This program component enables faculty to have access to the students' clinical work through direct observation supervisory modalities such as audio and videotape.

Historically, in practice and in teaching CFT, both videotape and live supervision have been held out to be the gold standard of supervisory practice (Nichols, Nichols, & Hardy, 1990; Lee, Nichols, Nichols, & Odom, 2004). Generally speaking, there seems to be divergent opinions and research about to what degree either modality is useful in CFT training (Lee & Everett, 2004; Locke & McCollum, 2001; McCollum & Wetchler, 1995). For example, live and videotape supervision are purported to increase supervisees, performance anxiety and has the potential for creating a toxic learning environment (Lee & Everett, 2004). In a recent study, supervisees found live supervision more beneficial and perceived therapy as progressing more than their clients (Silverthorn, Bartle-Haring, Meyer, & Toviessi, 2009). Faculty must exercise care and use caution when developing and implementing a simulation curriculum.

Obvious differences exist between live supervision and simulation. For example, actual clients are involved in live supervision; therefore, client care is always the primary purpose for each live supervision encounter. Second, every live supervision is unique and unpredictable, thereby creating a rich learning environment but uneven clinical experience for evaluating students' clinical competencies. The benefit of the simulation with standardized patient families enables the program to emphasize and prioritize the students' educational and training needs without risking client care. Contrary to in-class role-plays where students generally have a preexisting relationship with their colleague or faculty members, using standardized patients reduces bias in the encounter. The standardized patient actors at the College of Health Profession in Drexel University all have previous work experience as standardized patients for medical professions and have additional professional acting experience. In addition, unlike most role-plays, all standardized patients are provided with a script and engage in at least two hours of case training. This helps to create continuity in the case as well as create foci for the encounter. These core elements facilitate the learning outcomes that organize our evaluative process.

GENERAL CONSIDERATIONS FOR IMPLEMENTING HUMAN SIMULATION

The following sections will describe what we consider to be the essential elements to successfully introduce simulation in a CFT program. Both the education and the planning human simulation requires a time commitment from faculty. Identifying at least one faculty member to serve as the coordinator will help in educating the program faculty as well as implementing the simulations. Planning to implement simulation should begin one year before the first encounter, and the faculty coordinator should expect to spend an equivalent of three hours a week devoted to simulation.

Faculty Development

Developing a human simulation curriculum is labor intensive and requires faculty endorsement and commitment of resources. Before a program begins planning simulation, it is recommended they spend time learning about the range of education and training experiences this modality affords educators. The literature in nursing and medicine has an abundance of publications describing the use of human simulation in clinical programs.

The second task for faculty is to become familiar with the technical aspects of the simulation laboratory. This includes familiarity with the variety and the capacity of the hardware and software systems. This would include forms of recordings, available database for storing data, and report writing. All of these factors shape how you develop specific simulations and your overall simulation curriculum.

The third task for faculty who are unfamiliar with human simulation and standardized patients is to seek mentorship from an experienced faculty member in simulation. The Interdisciplinary Simulation Committee at the College of Health Profession became a learning laboratory and a resource for the primary author.

Finally, consider developing some tips for faculty feedback. Generally, as professionals, we regard ourselves as experts in communicating with others. However, simulation feedback should be handled with the same level of care that has been recommended in the CFT supervision literature. In medicine, it has been found that the quality of feedback and the opportunities to establish educational targets are associated with positive and negative learning environments (Berbano, Browning, Pangaro, & Jackson, 2006; Menancery, Knight, Kolodner, & Wright, 2006). Lee and Everett (2004) offer a comprehensive list of concerns for supervisors who engaged in group and live supervision. These lists of guidelines are full with useful guidelines for organizing and delivering feedback to students engaged in simulation. It is the faculty members' responsibility to remember that simulation is a very public encounter involving student's peers, standardized patient families, simulated laboratory technical staff, and program faculty. It is important not to create a toxic environment that impedes a student's ability to risk learning. If simulation is executed with care, it can be a very safe learning environment for students to test not only their knowledge but to engage and find their therapeutic voice.

Case Writing and Training Standardized Patient Families

We have only used couple and family case studies in our simulation program. The writing of the case study is a fairly simple exercise. It is important to continuously evaluate whether the case content will achieve the desired educational outcomes. Checking with the design of your evaluation methods for the simulated encounter will help you with the first task. The standardized patient actors can assist you in making sure the construction of the case has enough depth, and will enable you to develop each character and plot.

The success of your simulation in part is contingent on how well you prepare your standardized patient families for their roles. Second to witnessing a student successfully navigating an encounter, the development of cases with standardized patient actors can be both an enjoyable and rewarding process. It is essential for case development to be a collaborative venture between the program and the standardized patient actors. One way to assess if a case study is well put together is by evaluating how your standardized patient actors respond to the story line and characters. Experienced standardized patient actors know if a propose story or role is credible or is too theatrical. It is advisable to really partner with the standardized patient actors and work with them to build each character. This is a time-consuming process but one which will make the case study more authentic. In addition, the degree to which you are able to concentrate on building a story line and characters assists the standardized patient actors own their roles and consistently reproduce the performance for each encounter. Finally, whenever possible, create some rest time between encounters and train two sets of standardized patient actors for each scenario. The latter will help to safeguard against problems during simulation related to an actors' illness or role fatigue. Playing a depressed mother in a family for 4- to 50-minute sessions per day requires a different use of self than acting a role of a patient with lower back pain for 4- to 20-minute encounters. Two unanticipated consequences for standardized patient actors may be emotional fatigue as well as an increased awareness about painful family of origin issues. Careful debriefing with the standardized patient family helps them identify and articulate impasses.

Finally, standardized patient actors should be trained on how to give feedback to CFT students. Standardized patient actors should not offer feedback to students about technique, such as "it would have been better if you asked like this" or attempt to correct student's behavior. Instead, we find it more useful if they provide students with feedback about what it was like to be a client. Limiting the standardized patient actor's feedback within this framework minimizes the tendencies to get into right or wrong polarizing conversations with students, which can become a negative learning experience.

DREXEL UNIVERSITY HUMAN SIMULATION CURRICULUM

Our first year CFT students take MFT Ethics and Legal Practices, Historical and Sociocultural Influences in CFT, Introduction to Systems Thinking, Person-of-the-Therapist Training (POTT), and Practicum. The clinical seminar course is one of three components of practicum. The other two components are engagement in a 16- to 20-hour/

week clinical practicum site and individual and group supervision. For the past 2 years, the program implemented a curricula including human simulation in both our clinical seminar and person of the therapist courses. Currently, we are finalizing the planning for including simulation in the curriculum for our second-year MFT students.

Clinical Seminar Course

This clinical seminar course replaced the previous prepracticum 40-hour weeklong clinical readiness course. That course was developed to introduce and to prepare students for clinical practicum as well as to ensure program compliance with our old COAMFTE Version 10.3 standards. The clinical seminar is taught by our Director of Clinical Training. The course is an extension of our clinical orientation and is highly experiential. Specifically, this course affords students additional opportunities to become adept at documentation, practice assessment, diagnostic skills, recognizing and applying systemic theory, interviewing skills, and genogram construction.

Second, the clinical seminar provided another feedback loop for the Director of Clinical Training to assess how students were adjusting to the clinical practicum and monitor their progression. Third, the CFT program has specific outcomes students must achieve by the end of the first year. Using the competency-based evaluation form, all clinical feedback regarding a student's progression was provided every quarter by their individual and group supervisors. Majority of the time, this structure worked very well; however, occasionally a student who was really struggling and required program intervention would fall through the cracks. Faculty therefore agreed it would be prudent to develop a program evaluation for all incoming students with a multidimensional feedback component.

Phase 1

During week 8 of the clinical seminar, students are scheduled to see a standardized patient family in the simulated laboratory. The clinical cases are developed by the Director of Clinical Training and Program Director on the basis of the course and program outcomes. Students conduct a 50-minute session with the family that is recorded. Directly after the session, they receive feedback from the standardized patient family about what it is like for them to be their client. The feedback is not technical in nature—it is designed to provide the student about how they manage the therapeutic environment, engage the family, and manage anxiety. The student is encouraged to ask the standardized patient family-specific questions about their session. After the debriefing session, the student completes a progress note of the session. The progress note is later evaluated for content and ability to adhere to a prescribed format. The student receives some verbal feedback from the director of training or program director about their session, including whether we would like them to repeat the exercise at a later date.

The simulated laboratory experience is not a test. It is designed to give students feedback about their development. Thus, any student who uncharacteristically performs poorly is asked to repeat the exercise to address specific concerns. Furthermore, a portion of the recorded section will be shown to a faculty pod, and repeating the exercise allows the student to choose what they consider is their best work. The student is then given an assignment to review the recording and from their vantage point write and conduct a self-evaluation on the basis of the objectives of the exercise and set learning goals for themselves. This is one of many ways the program promotes self-evaluation in an effort to prepare students for lifelong learning.

Phase 2

Students are scheduled for a feedback session with a faculty pod. The faculty pod generally consists of a least three core faculty members who meet with the student about their progression in the program. Efforts are made to schedule students with faculty with whom they have had little to no contact with during the quarter. On the day of the evaluation, the student briefly presents their learning goals for the next quarter. Faculty and student dialogue about their learning goals and then review a brief portion of their simulated laboratory recording. Students are then evaluated on five core competencies: (1) ability to engage in systemic and relational thinking; (2) ability to recognize, understand, and be sensitive to cultural differences; (3) ability to identify and understand how person-of-the-therapist issues interface with the case; (4) evolving professionalism and developing a professional identity as an MFT; and (5) ability to demonstrate ethical and professional integrity. Each competency is evaluated using a rubric of satisfactory, fair, and unsatisfactory. The feedback form also provides faculty to make narrative comments about strengths, concerns, and recommendations (Appendix 25.A). These recommendations are included in the student's learning objectives. All students receive a formal letter from the program, summarizing the impression of their overall program progression, future learning goals, and if appropriate remediation, plan (Appendix 25.B).

The following is a case example used in our clinical seminar. It is designed for evaluating the degree to which students have learned the necessary assessment and treatment planning skills.

CASE STUDY EXAMPLE: R.-C. FAMILY

Maria is a 39-year-old Puerto Rican woman who recently became a grandmother. Her daughter Alexandria, now 18 years old, had a baby 6 months ago that was fathered by her 24-year-old boyfriend. Alexandria's father is African American, works in construction, and lives in the Philadelphia area. He would see Alexandria on holidays and has always been financially supportive. Alexandria and her 6-month-old daughter Jamie live in Maria's home. The grandmother initiated therapy because she is still trying to seek legal action against her daughter's boyfriend. She believes it is statutory rape but has not been able to get the police involved. The boyfriend has not been emotionally or financially supportive, and recently they found out he has fathered another daughter who is 4 months old. She does not understand why her daughter refuses to proceed with child support petition and is still willing to see him. The daughter also has a problem with her mother because she wants her mother to watch the child while she goes out with friends. Her mother refuses because she believes Alexandria should take care of her own child. Mother and daughter frequently argue about parenting Jamie. Maria feels that her mother tells her what to do and does not allow her to make any mistakes.

Person-of-the-Therapist Training

All Drexel CFT students take three courses in POTT. The approach is based on Harry Aponte's Person-of-Therapist Training Model, which until 2002 was only available in private training institutions (Aponte & Winter, 2000). The philosophy of POTT calls for students to develop mastery of self to have more access and control of self in the therapeutic process. Students are taught how to be more self-aware, including their own unresolved life struggles in the service of being able to both identify and differentiate from their clients. Students identify their own signature themes and learn how they can use them as a therapeutic tool. The model advances that growth, and healing is a lifelong process and therefore requires the therapist to take active steps toward managing their struggles while simultaneously becoming more accepting of self. A full description of the POTT model is beyond the scope of this chapter (see Aponte et al., 2009; Lutz & Irizarry, 2006).

Human Simulation and POTT Model

In the first quarter, students are introduced to the POTT model and learn about the concept of signature themes. Signature themes emerge from our personal histories, family of origin, and sociocultural attributes (spirituality, gender, sexual orientation, race, culture, etc.) that influence our development. Our signature themes organize us to behave in particular ways and subsequently influence our attitudes, behaviors, and emotions in both our personal and professional lives (Aponte, Powell, Brooks, Watson, Litzke, Lawless et al., 2009). Each student presents at least once on their signature theme and how it influences their clinical work. The POTT clinical outline is as follows:

- Your signature theme:
  (Briefly describe how you conceptualize your signature theme(s) today)
- Case identification and Information
- Your genograms: therapist and clients
- Focal issues in therapy
- Clinical hypotheses
- Treatment process—clinical strategy and use of self
- Person of the therapist
  (How are you meeting the personal challenges you face in this case about both the focal issue of the case and the relationship with the client?)
- Questions you have about the case and self
  The goal of the second quarter POTT course is to increase the student's awareness of their signature theme while they are conducting therapy. The 2-hour class is held in the simulated laboratory, and each student conducts a full clinical session with a standardized patient family. The format is as follows:
- Five to 10 minutes reorienting the therapist to the exercise. They are instructed not to get overly focused on "solving problems" but to try to connect and join with each family member
- Students conduct a 50-minute clinical session. All sessions are recorded, and the coinstructors provide direction to the student via a bug in the ear. The class is also viewing the encounter in a separate room. Note that the simulated laboratory technical support also views the encounter in real time.
- The student receives feedback from the standardized patient family for 10 to 15 minutes. The tone of the feedback is conversational and more of a dialogue between the family and the student. However, the standardized patients are required to complete an evaluation form answering a series of yes or no questions.
- After the standardized patient family gives the student feedback, a debriefing meeting is held with the coinstructors, students, and class observers.
- Class members are allowed to offer the presenting student therapist supportive comments about the session but are not allowed to critique their session. Instead, each class member is asked to reflect and share how the session affected them using their signature theme as a guide.

The third and final POTT class takes place in the simulated laboratory with the focus on how to use your signature themes as a therapeutic tool. The goal is to help the students recognize their signature theme and learn how to use them in therapy. This is probably the most challenging but rewarding part of the learning process for students. The second quarter format for the simulated sessions is repeated for the POTT III course.

The following are two case examples used in the POTT course. The J. family case study is designed to simulate weekly therapy (Brooks & Allen, 2008a, 2008b).

THE J. FAMILY

Carolyn J. is a 45-year-old African American woman who was recently diagnosed with major depression. Carolyn's depression took over after her 19-year-old son was murdered. Carolyn has been married to Garvin for 16 years. Garvin is Jeffrey's (her son's) stepfather. However, Garvin, age 45 years, thought of Jeffrey as his own son and has been devastated since his death. He now feels he is losing Carolyn to depression and has reached out to her sister Michele for support.

Two years ago, Carolyn's son was sitting on the front porch and was shot during a random drive-by shooting. For approximately 6 months, before her son's death, the neighbor had been taken hostage by a group of dealers and killers. Carolyn's son was a good kid who worked part-time and was in his first year at Villanova.

Since Jeffrey's death, Carolyn has stopped working, cut herself off from friends, and stays at home—mostly in her bedroom. Garvin or the younger children (a boy and a girl, 13 and 15 years old, respectively) are unable to get her involved or interested in the family. Garvin has been able to get Carolyn to a psychiatrist; however, she flat out refuses to take medication and refuses to go into the hospital. Garvin has confided in Michele (age 50 years), Carolyn's sister, and Kevin (age 39 years), her brother, about the problem. He told them how helpless he has been feeling and that he is afraid she may hurt herself. He wonders if she has a will to live.

Michele was able to talk Carolyn into seeing a family therapist. She had tried to have her make an appointment after Jeffrey's murder, but Carolyn refused. This time, Michele would not take no for an answer. Both Michele and Kevin are involved in the therapy.

Progression of Therapy Sessions
>   Sessions 1–5: husband, wife, and brother
>   Session 6: husband, wife, and sister
>   Sessions 7 and 8: husband, wife, sister, and brother

The S. family case study is designed to simulate a course of therapy over two quarters. The case example provides a description of the case for POTT III. The S. family background information for the POTT II and POTT III training can be found in Appendix 25.C (Allen & Brooks, 2008).

The S. Family—POTT II

- Anne S. is a 71-year-old widowed woman of Irish decent recently discharged from the hospital. For the past 5 years, she has lived alone. Five years ago, Anne's husband, who was very physically active, died of a massive heart attack. Anne has a medical history of insulin-dependent diabetes and hypertension and frequently violates her dietary limits and forgets to take her medication. More recently, she fell down the stairs in her home and fortunately did not suffer any fractures, although she did hit her head.

- Anne's daughter Maddie (age 49 years) wants her to move to an apartment or into an assisted living arrangement. Her other daughter Clare (age 45 years), who lives in an apartment in Chicago, thinks her mother should move in with Maddie and her husband. She is worried about her mother and is opposed to her living alone or in an assisted living situation. She believes her sister is selfish and has always been loyal to her father. She cannot believe her sister is this cold. George (age 51 years) is Maddie's husband (Allen & Brooks, 2008b).

CONCLUSIONS

Human simulation is an untapped resource for CFT education. Faculty could use simulation as a teaching method to help students improve interviewing, assessment, and intervention skills. It can also be easily incorporated as a teaching method for clinical courses such as narrative family therapy or structural therapy. In addition, human simulation offers COAMFTE programs new and observable ways to improve program and student evaluations. Lastly, the simulated laboratory technology creates opportunities for conducting research about education and training of students and educators. Faculty development is an unexplored but critical area as the profession moves into an outcome-based era.

REFERENCES

Allen, A., & Brooks, S. (2008). *C[...]-R[...] Family.* Philadelphia, PA: Couple and Family Therapy Department, Drexel University.

American Association for Marriage and Family Therapy, Clinical Competencies Task Force. (2003). *Proposed clinical competencies.* Washington, DC: Author.

American Association for Marriage and Family Therapy, Commission on Accreditation for Marriage and Family Therapy Education. (2003). *Commission of Accreditation for Marriage and Family Therapy site visitor handbook.* Washington, DC: Author.

Aponte, H. J., Powell, F. D., Brooks, S., Watson, M. F., Litzke, C., Lawless, J., et al. (2009). Training the person of the therapist in an academic setting. *Journal of Marital and Family Therapy, 35,* 381–394.

Aponte, H. J., & Winter, J. E. (2000). The person and practice of the therapist: Treatment and training. In M. Baldwin & V. Satir (Eds.), *The use of self in therapy.* New York: Hawthorne.

Barrows, H. S. (1993). An overview of the uses of standardized patients for teaching and evaluating clinical skills. *Academic Medicine, 68,* 443–453.

Berbano, E., Browing, R., Pangaro, L., & Jackson, J. L. (2006). The impact of the Stanford Faculty Development Program on ambulatory teaching behavior. *Journal General Internal Medicine, 21,* 430–434.

Bowers, M. (Executive Director). (2004, June). *The future of clinical competencies.* Symposium at Educators Summit, Reno, NV.

Brooks, S. (2010). *Outcome based education and the quest for competency: Perspectives from couple and family therapy educators.* Unpublished doctoral dissertation, Drexel University, Philadelphia.

Brooks, S., & Allen, A. (2008a). *J[...] Family.* Philadelphia, PA: Couple and Family Therapy Department, Drexel University.

Brooks, S., & Allen, A. (2008b). *S[...] Family.* Philadelphia, PA: Couple and Family Therapy Department, Drexel University.

Cassel, C. K. (2004). Quality of care and quality of training: A shared vision for internal Medicine? *Annals of Internal Medicine, 140,* 927–928.

Commission on Accreditation for Marriage and Family Therapy Education. (2006). *Marriage and family therapy: Manual on accreditation.* Washington, DC: American Association for Marriage and Family Therapy.

Committee on Quality Chasm: Adaption to Mental and Health Addictive Disorders. (2006). *Improving the quality of health care for mental and substance-use conditions.* Washington, D.C: Institute of Medicine, National Academies Press.

Committee on Quality of Health Care in America. (2001). *Crossing the quality chasm: A new health system for the 21st century.* Washington, DC: Institute of Medicine, National Academies Press.

Diekelmann, N. (2002). "Too much content...." Epistemologies' grasp and nursing education. *Journal of Nursing Education, 41,* 469–470.

Freeman, L., Voignier, R. R., & Scott, D. (2002). New curriculum for a new century: Beyond repackaging. *Journal of Nursing Education, 41,* 38–40.

Hale, L. S., Lewis, D. K., Eckert, R. M., Wilson, C. M., & Smith, B. S. (2006). Standardized patients and multidisciplinary classroom instruction for physical therapist students to improve interviewing skills and attitudes about diabetes. *Journal of Physical Therapy Education, 20,* 22–27.

Hamner, J., & Wilder, B. (2001). A new curriculum for a new millennium. *Nursing Outlook, 49,* 127–131.

Hayden, S. R., Dufel, S., & Shih, R. S. (2002). Definitions and competencies for practice-based learning and improvement. *Academic Emergency Medicine, 9,* 1242–1248.

Henry, P., Sprenkle, D. H., & Sheehan, R. (1986). Family therapy training: Student and faculty perceptions. *Journal of Marital and Family Therapy, 12,* 249–258.

Hills, K. J., & Pollard, S. (2003). Focused teaching for focused learning: An approach to teaching clinical medicine using standardized patients. *Perspective on Physician Assistant Education, 14,* 145–148.

Hodgson, J. L., Lamson, A. L., & Feldhousen, E. B. (2007). Use of simulated in marriage and family therapy education. *Journal of Marital and Family Therapy, 33,* 35–50.

Hoge, M. A. (2002). The training gap: An acute crisis in behavioral health education. *Administration and Policy in Mental Health, 29,* 305–317.

Hoge, M. A., & Morris, J. A. (2002). Special issue: Behavioral health workforce education and training. *Administration and Policy in Mental Health, 29*(4/5), 295–439.

Kniskern, D. P., & Gurman, A. S. (1979). Research on training in marriage and family therapy: Status, issues, and directions. *Journal of Marital and Family Therapy, 5,* 83–92.

LaMantia, J., & Panacek, E. (2002). Core competencies conference: Executive summary. *Academic Emergency Medicine, 9,* 1213–1215.

Lee, R., & Everett, C. A. (2004). *The integrative family therapy supervisor: A primer.* New York: Brunner-Routledge.

Lee, R., Nichols, D., Nichols, W., & Odom, T. (2004). Trends in family therapy supervision: The past 25 years and into the future. *Journal of Marital and Family Therapy, 30,* 61–69.

Locke, L., & McCollum, E. (2001). Client's views of live supervision and satisfaction with therapy. *Journal of Marital and Family Therapy, 27,* 129–133.

Lutz, L., & Irizarry, S. S. (2009). Reflections of two trainees: Person of the therapist training for marriage and family therapists. *Journal of Marital and Family Therapy, 35,* 370–380.

McCollum, E., & Wetchler, J. L. (1995). In defense of case consultation: Maybe "dead" supervision isn't dead at all. *Journal of Marital and Family Therapy, 21,* 155–166.

Menanchery, E. P., Knight, A. M., Kolodner, K., & Wright, S. M. (2006). Physician characteristics associated with proficiency in feedback skills. *Journal of General Internal Medicine, 21,* 440–446.

Miller, J. K. (2009). Competency-based training: Objective structured clinical exercises (OSCE) in marriage and family therapy. *Journal of Marital and Family Therapy, 36*(3), 320–332.

Miller, J. K., Linville, D., Todahl, J., & Metcalfe, J. (2009). Using mock trials to teach students forensic core competencies in marriage and family therapy. *Journal of Marital and Family Therapy, 35,* 456–465.

Miller, J. K., Todahl, J. L., & Platt, J. J. (2010). The core competency movement in marriage and family therapy: Key considerations from other disciplines. *Journal of Marital and Family Therapy, 36,* 59–70.

Nichols, W. C. (1979). Doctoral programs in marital and family therapy. *Journal of Nichols,* M. P. & Schwartz, R. C. (1991, 2007). *Family Therapy: Concepts and Methods.* (8th). Needham Heights, MA: Allyn & Bacon.

Nichols, W. C., Nichols, D. P., & Hardy, K. V. (1990). Supervision in family therapy: A decade review. *Journal of Marital and Family Therapy, 16,* 275–285.

Perosa, L. M., & Perosa, S. L. (2010). Assessing competencies in couples and family therapy/counseling: A call to the profession. *Journal of Marital and Family Therapy, 36,* 126–143.

Pew Health Profession Commission. (1993). *Health professions education for the future: Schools in service for a nation.* San Francisco, CA: Author.

President's New Freedom Commission on Mental Health. (2003). *Achieving the promise: Transforming mental health care in America. Final report* (DHHS Pub. No. SMA-03–3832). Rockville, MD: U.S. Department of Health and Human Services.

Roberts, M. C., Borden, K. A., Christiansen, M. D., & Lopez, S. L. (2005). Fostering a culture shift: Assessment of competence in the education and careers of professional psychologists. *Professional Psychology, Research and Practice, 36,* 355–361.

Silverthorn, B. C., Bartle-Haring, S., Meyer, K., & Toviessi, P. (2009). Does live supervision make a difference? A multilevel analysis. *Journal of Marital and Family Therapy, 35,* 406–414.

Whitcomb, M. E. (2004). More on competency-based education. *Academic Medicine, 79,* 493–494.

Yoo, M. S., & Yoo, I. Y. (2003). The effectiveness of standardized patients as a teaching method for nursing fundamentals. *Journal of Nursing Education, 42,* 444–448.

APPENDIX 25.A

Core Competencies	Satisfactory	Fair	Unsatisfactory	Comments
Ability to engage in systemic and relational thinking.				
Ability to recognize, understand, and be sensitive to cultural differences.				
Evolving professionalism and developing a professional identity as an MFT.				
Demonstrates ethical and professional integrity.				

FEEDBACK EVALUATION FORM

Student Name:_____ _____ Date: _____
Strengths:
Concerns: •
Recommendations:
Faculty Signature:_____

APPENDIX 25.B

Dear Student,

This letter will summarize information we discussed on January 5, 2010, at the MFT Feedback Session. I would like to repeat that the feedback sessions are designed to facilitate your development over the next few quarters. The program will be sharing our recommendations with your clinical supervisors and encourage you to discuss them and set appropriate learning goals.

The recommendations are based on your self-evaluation and faculty observation of your simulated laboratory experience. Our recommendations were guided by the following core competencies: (1) ability to engage in systemic and relational thinking; (2) ability to recognize, understand,

and be sensitive to cultural differences; (3) ability to identify and understand how person-of-the-therapist issues interface with the case; (4) evolving professionalism and developing a professional identity as an MFT; and (5) ability to demonstrate ethical and professional integrity.

Faculty identified your areas of strength as attentiveness to clients and including everyone in the process, staying calm in the face of conflict, recognition of systemic interactions such as triangulation intellectual recognition of clinical issues, and self-awareness of your own personal issues such as controlling others, recognizing cultural difference, and questioning how that translates to intervention.

The faculty recommends that you set the following learning goals:

- Engage in the therapeutic process at a more emotional level.
- Become aware of how lack of emotional connection impacts on how others (clients) perceive you.
- Work more on therapeutic presentation.
- Engage more in actively engaging culture in a direct way in therapy.

We wish you continued success in the program.
Sincerely,

APPENDIX 25.C

POTT II S. Case Study Background

Anne S. is a 71-year-old widowed woman of Irish descent. She has been widowed for 5 years. She lives alone and is a practicing Catholic. She has two adult daughters, Maddie (49 years old) and Clare (45 years old).

Clare lives in Chicago and was never married. In the past 2 years, she has come to Philadelphia to visit her mother at least 12 times.

Maddie is married to George (51 years old). They live just outside Philadelphia. They also have one son in college.

Backdrop is that Anne struggles with insulin-dependent diabetes and hypertension. She refuses to follow her diet and continues to eat sweet and rich foods. Over the past 2 years, she seems to be more accident prone. Recently, she fell down the stairs in her home and was hospitalized. She hit her head but did not sustain any other injuries.

Anne married her husband at the age of 21 years. She worked a number of part-time jobs, but he was her rock. Anne's husband died 5 years ago after a massive heart attack. His death was a surprise for the entire family, especially Anne and Maddie.

Maddie and Clare both agree their mother needs closer supervision. However, they have not been able to agree on a solution.

Anne wants to stay in her home. Maddie wants her to move to a small apartment or assisted living community. Clare thinks Maddie should take her in: after all, she has enough room.

Maddie was extremely close to her father and thinks her mother kept him from enjoying life—she hated that her dad never had much time for himself because he took care of their mom. Although she loves her mother, she believes she is needy and will not allow her to move in. "She will suck all of the life out me."

Clare is close to her mother. Because of money, Clare is unable to move back to Philadelphia and cannot afford a larger place in Chicago. She feels very stuck and is angry with her sister.

George wants to support his wife but is concerned about Mrs. S. She has treated him like a son. George's parents died in a car accident when he was 15 years old. He was raised by his maternal uncle and wife. His uncle had seven children, and George never really fit in.

The family is stuck. They fight, and one time Maddie threatened not to speak to Clare if she continued to "bully" her about this decision. They could not work this out, and Clare made an appointment with a family therapist so that they can make the right choice for Mrs. S.

During the course of the treatment, the family was able to design a plan for Mrs. S., which has enabled her to stay in the home. The plan consisted of organizing her medications, purchasing an alert button, and developing an organized support system with her neighbors, church members, and family.

POTT III S. Case Study Background

The sisters were beginning to address some of the conflict between the two of them. They have clearly established the significant changes in their relationship that happened as they approached preadolescent and adolescent years. Each child found themselves aligned and developed a special with one parent. Clare was mom's special child, and Maddie was her father's special child.

The family has agreed to continue with therapy with the expressed purpose of working on the relationship between the sisters. The sisters want to improve their communication so that they are able to better take care of Mrs. S.

Surprisingly, Maddie admits during the first or second session that she wants to fix whatever happened between her and Clare. She misses Clare and is beginning to realize she is confused and really does not understand what happened between the two of them. She tried to accept the distance in their relationship and reasoned that the geographic location and Clare's anger keep her away—but deep down inside she knows this is not completely it.

Mrs. S. seems to be doing well with her medication and medical care. She is going out with friends and has actively resumed going to church. Over the past two weeks, while visiting her mother, Maddie asked Mrs. S. what she thinks was the problem between her and Clare. Maddie also began to ask some questions about her father, which more recently began to bother her.

Maddie admitted that she loved her mother and father but always felt her father needed her more. Her father was a good dad and made sure they did not want anything, but he was sometimes distant and cold. He often retreated in books and in the den, which was a clear sign of not wanting intrusion. Maddie also remembered a sadness about him but was never sure what was wrong, and therefore worked hard to please him.

Mrs. S. told Maddie her father was a good man. Earlier on in their marriage, they had a rough time and her husband never recovered. Mr. S.'s mother died eight months after they were married. She had been sick on and off and was in the hospital several times with severe headaches, but the doctors were not sure what was really wrong with her. They think she may have had a blood clot or tumor. She died after a seizure in the hospital. Mr. S.'s father did not want an autopsy, which was very upsetting to Mr. S. and his siblings.

Shortly after that, they became pregnant. It was a difficult pregnancy. Mrs. S. admits she was sick a lot—but they could not have anticipated any problems with the baby. At the end of the nine months and a difficult labor, they gave birth to a baby boy who died within hours of his birth. They named him Robert Jr.

After these two incidents, Mr. S. seemed different. He worked a lot, had few friends, and sometimes drank too much. He cut himself off from his family of origin. Usually, he was home and rarely drank in public. Mrs. S. states she lost the man she fell in love with—he was never the same. She also said they were never the same.

In the meantime, Maddie shared some of this information with Clare. Clare was surprised to learn they had a brother and this new information about her father. She is much warmer toward Maddie but is not sure how to be with her.

The family is now resuming therapy with this new information, which shifts the focus from Mrs. S.'s health to this new information. This is all new information to George, as Maddie had not shared any of it with him until now. He is in shock and also concerned because Maddie generally tells him everything and she, too, has been very distant (revised September 1, 2010).

CHAPTER 26

Use of Human Simulation in Behavioral Health Counselor Education

Ronald Clay Comer and Robert J. Chapman

Strengthening the effectiveness in preprofessional training of behavioral health counselors continues to be a subject around which much has been written over the past 40 years. Various methods pertaining to specific aspects of counselor training have been described. These methods run a wide gamut ranging from knowledge-building through lecture discussion, to values clarification exercises, to skill-building approaches making use of such methods as role-playing and computer simulations (Kurtz, Marshall, & Banspach, 1985). The focus of this chapter will be on instructional methods involving the use of human simulation in behavioral health counselor training. A historical review of significant developments in the implementation of human simulation in counselor training will be followed by an introduction to the use of a new approach to human simulation involving standardized patients in simulated clinical encounters.

As pointed out by Kurtz et al. (1985) in his literature review over the prior 12 years, a diversity of program models had developed for behavioral health counseling skills training. More recently, a comprehensive review of training approaches common to counselor education programs at undergraduate and graduate levels of training was conducted by Hill and Lent (2006). This latter review includes a useful overview of the three training program models that have received the most empirical attention. The first of these is most often referred to as Integrated Didactic Experiential Training (IDET; Carkuff, 1972). The basis of this training involves learning and applying counseling skills associated with three stages through which therapists are expected to guide their clients: self-exploration, deepening understanding, and taking action (Hill & Lent, 2006).

The second well-investigated approach is Ivey's (1971) microcounseling training program. This differs from Carkuff's approach in that the focus is not on the therapeutic stages through which one would make use of specific counseling skills, but on the mastery of the skills themselves as they are arranged in a hierarchy from fundamental to more advanced therapeutic intervention skills. Such skills development would include the practice of basic attending behavior before moving on to more advanced counselor–client interactions, as in reflection of feelings and use of interpretation (Hill & Lent, 2006).

The third major training approach cited by Hill and Lent (2006) is Kagan's (1984) interpersonal process recall. This approach differs from Carkuff's and Ivey's by focusing not so much on the acquisition of specific counseling skills, but on the ability of the counselor in training to make use of counseling skills in practice sessions. Concern is with the in-session thoughts and feelings experienced by the trainee, such as performance anxiety, that may interfere or otherwise prevent success in fully responding to or addressing the client's needs (Hill & Lent, 2006).

Common to all these approaches is the emphasis placed on the ability of the counselor to make appropriate use of counseling skills. Whether emphasis is placed on the successful acquisition of counseling skills, their use in moving the client through basic stages in the therapeutic process, or on interpersonal process issues arising in the application of counseling skills, the goal of various training models implemented over the past 50 years is to produce competent behavioral health care professionals. In service of achieving this goal, a variety of training or teaching techniques developed over these 50 years have become commonplace in the classroom repertoire of behavioral health care educators.

Among the teaching methods employed in counselor training programs has been the use of instructional reading followed by lecture and discussion, role-playing (Teevan & Gabel, 1978), therapist modeling, response to written client statements, response to videotaped client statements (Hill & Lent, 2006), computerized client simulations (Hummel, Lichtenberg, & Shaffer, 1975), analysis of recorded interview sessions (Gelso, 1974), analysis of videotaped interview sessions (Gelso, 1974; Thayer, 1977), and use of live actors simulating counseling sessions (Klamen & Yudkowsky, 2002; Lane, 1988). All of these teaching approaches have experienced varying degrees of success. In the more recent review of training approaches by Hill and Lent (2006), their general conclusion was that multi-method approaches outperformed single-method training.

It does not take long in reviewing counseling skills syllabuses placed online by various colleges and universities to see that instructional reading, along with lecture and discussion, continues to be a common component of the various teaching approaches otherwise outlined. Class work in the helping professions has historically placed a good deal of emphasis on the teaching of concepts and theories that comprise the knowledge dimension of competency-based counselor training (Anthony et al., 1977). The salient issue in the design of training programs is in determining the relative importance of experiential versus didactic components (Teevan & Gabel, 1978). In one of the earlier studies investigating this issue, Teevan and Gabel (1978) compared two groups: one group exposed only to lecture and discussion on selected topics such as listening skills, crisis theory, and drug counseling, and the other group exposed to modeling by trainers of counseling techniques considered relevant to each topic, followed by participant-involved role-playing. Their finding supported the superiority of the experiential modeling and role-playing methods over lecture and discussion approaches alone.

In an earlier study comparing traditional approaches to counselor training with the IDET model developed by Carkuff, it was found that whereas both groups achieved measurable growth in interpersonal counseling skills, exposure to IDET methods appeared to be most effective (Vander Kolk, 1973). The traditional approach was defined as constituting a didactic approach to knowledge-building as a prerequisite to engagement in experiential learning involving modeling and role-playing. In the IDET method, the experiential components of training are integrated along with the didactic, as the name implies, providing greater emphasis on immediate feedback in a supportive atmosphere, while making use of the trainer as a model of both essential learning attitudes and counseling skills (Vander Kolk, 1973).

The importance of role-playing as an effective means of teaching counseling skills has been demonstrated repeatedly over the years (Hill & Lent, 2006; Kurtz et al., 1985). In the microcounseling method of Ivey, role-play constitutes an essential part in the four basic components of this method: written or video models, role-play practice, observer feedback, and remediation practice (Ivey, 1971). Interestingly, one study (Peters, Cormier, & Cormier, 1978) found no substantial difference in beginning graduate students randomly assigned to each of four conditions: modeling; modeling and practice; modeling, practice, and feedback; and modeling, practice, feedback, and remediation. Admittedly, their subject pool was rather small, but their conclusion was that the lack of significant differences nonetheless demonstrated the ability of subjects to apply to different dialogues in the role-play measure specific counseling skills taught through modeled and modeling with role-play conditions (Peters et al., 1978). Also interesting in their study was the use of a standardized client model across all subjects and conditions.

Probably nowhere have attempts to standardize the client in the training process been more evident than in the early development and repeated uses of computerized training models. The earliest of these client-standardization approaches were developed on mainframe computers before the advent of personalized computers widely used today (Hummel et al., 1975). A common goal was to simulate client behavior in an initial counseling interview making use of programmed cognitive-client variables. One noticeable drawback of these early simulations was the rather restricted grammar that the counselor must use in statement construction to be inputted via the terminal connected to the mainframe (Hummel et al., 1975).

Another common use of computers in training counselors is described by Alpert (1986). She describes using computers to enhance training curricula and practices. Specifically, computers are used to test response choices made by students who select from increasingly complex levels of counseling skills categories ranging from accurate identification of client feelings contained in a client statement appearing on the screen, to more facilitative responses essential in relationship-building, such as clarification, reflection of feeling, and paraphrasing. At each level, the student is presented with examples of client statements accompanied by five verbal response statements from which the student must choose the one in most accord with counseling skills as presented in other components of their classroom learning (Alpert, 1986).

In addition to computerized simulations designed to augment teaching basic counseling skills, applications have also been introduced for training therapists in clinical diagnoses and treatment decision making (Lambert & Meier, 1992). After the presentation of general client information, the student then selects options from various menus leading to additional information necessary to make a clinical diagnosis and construct a treatment plan. This approach initially showed promise largely because of the perceived acceptance of trainees to the use of computerized case presentations in teaching critical aspects associated with diagnoses and treatment planning decision making (Lambert & Meier, 1992). As an adjunctive tool in preprofessional training, other advantages of computerized training appear to be the ability to standardize client simulations without the need for a varied pool of client actors and space in which to conduct in vivo interviews, the ability of the computer to provide immediate feedback along with allowing students to repeat a consistent client–counselor exchange a number of times, and the ability to construct a wider variety of practice case types that may not be otherwise available (Alpert, 1986; Lambert & Meier, 1992).

Although methods of simulations for training in behavioral health care clinical practice have been varied, the most common approaches, as evidenced in the syllabuses of counseling skills classes easily accessed through the Google search engine, continue to be didactic presentation of essential knowledge, theory, and values; use of videotaped role-play counseling sessions either in-class or outside class; modeling through either live, taped demonstration, or written handouts; and in-class role-playing in which students exchange roles, playing both the client and then the counselor.

Defining the specific counseling skills to be taught has been as varied as the methods used to teach counseling skills. There are dozens of texts on behavioral health care counseling in use in college classrooms, each one with its own particular subject of interest. In part, this is a result of the fact that the targets of service attended to by behavioral health care professionals are so varied. Counselors may be working with child, adolescent, adult, or elderly individuals, with issues ranging from situational or relationship disruptions to drug and alcohol disorders and severe psychiatric disturbances. Counseling interventions may be called on in situations ranging from immediate crises to process interventions as part of long-term recovery and rehabilitation programs. Counselors work not only with individuals, but with couples and families, often confronting multicultural variables. Counselors also work with groups in inpatient, outpatient, school, and prison settings. The list could go on, but suffice it to say that little is standard with respect to the areas in which behavioral health care professionals work.

Obviously, the skill-oriented approach to teaching behavioral health counseling skills is challenging, considering the varied dimensions within which counselor–client interactions occur. Doyle's (1982) conceptual model, referred to as the role communication skill model, proposes a framework for considering the varied dimensions possible in the counseling process. Because counselors engage in different behaviors with respect to the various stages of their work with clients, such distinctive ways of behaving gain clarity best in terms of the major roles that counselors play, including (a) attendee, (b) clarifier, (c) informer or describer, (d) prober or inquirer, (e) supporter or reassurer, (f) motivator or prescriber, (g) evaluator or analyzer, and (h) problem solver (Doyle, 1982). He also labeled these roles as second-order behaviors, whereas the actual verbal responses that counselors make while interacting with clients are considered as first-order behaviors. Thus, the actual interpersonal counseling skills employed can be viewed as appropriately or inappropriately used within the context of the role dimension in which their use is intended. Furthermore, Doyle proposes that the evaluation of a counselor's first-order skills within the active roles that counselors play can be divided into the following communication channels: nonverbal, paraverbal, and verbal communication.

The return to a focus on basic interpersonal communication skills appears to be an inevitable feature of nearly all behavioral health counselor education programs. And not much has really changed in the manner in which counselor education is conducted in undergraduate or graduate training programs. What has changed is the increasing number of ways in which basic counseling skills are made use of in the behavioral health care field.

Within the last 10 years, the call for a "transformation" of behavioral health care services (Power, 2005) has led to the recognition that former paradigms of professional practice within which counselor training was to be directed have begun shifting. In large part, the transformation of behavioral health care services has been understood to include movement away from what may have been an overreliance on a medical model of care for people who have severe and persistent behavioral disorders to a model that encompasses a psychosocial rehabilitation approach to care. The distinction being that of the need to expand beyond a focus primarily on disorder diagnosis and symptom alleviation through biomedical treatment, to one that fully encompasses a recovery-oriented approach in responding to major psychiatric and substance use disorders.

Although the roles of counselors in this paradigm shift are increasingly different from the traditional roles played by counselors in psychotherapeutic work, the fundamental interpersonal counseling skills required to carry out these new roles look a lot like the same kinds of initial counseling skills that have been part of training programs for the past 50 years. Within the evolving psychosocial rehabilitation model, the behavioral health care professional's role is now seen as more of a collaborator; working with the consumer of behavioral health care services in both assessing needs and participating with the consumer in the organization of community-based resources considered useful in the recovery process (Anthony, 1993). An emphasis is placed on supporting consumers in the identification of functional skill deficits and in the acquisition of functional skills that promote the consumer's ability to live, to learn, and to work in the community (Anthony et al., 1977). To effectively interact within this new paradigm of recovery and rehabilitation, the effective use of core counseling skills oriented toward establishing a therapeutic relationship between the counselor and the consumer are required.

As the importance of effective training in the preparation of future behavioral health care professionals continues to be emphasized across disciplines, and at all levels of the behavioral health care system, emphasis on the exploration and implementation of new technologies in teaching methods continues (Hoge et al., 2005). An example of one such technology is the emerging use of "standardized patients" in the training of psychotherapists. Although the use of standardized patients has been achieving growing acceptance and implementation in the training of medical students, little appears in the literature describing the application of this new approach in training behavioral health care professionals.

The fundamental idea behind the use of standardized patients is not dissimilar to the long-standing use of role-play to simulate aspects of an actual clinical counseling session. Actors are recruited to play the roles of clients, allowing trainees in vivo opportunities to practice assigned skills. Use of trainees to play both counselor and client roles is the traditional way in which role-play exercises are conducted in counselor training. However, this has presented a major disadvantage to achieving realism in the encounter because trainees in the same classroom often know each other already and are both aware of the techniques and purposes of the interview (Lane, 1988).

The desire to provide training to second-year psychiatry residents that allows for sequential learning of counseling skills in a controlled and structured environment and that also realistically portrays clinical encounters is what motivated Coyle, Miller, and McGowen (1998) to develop one of the first described uses of standardized patients to teach psychotherapy. They developed scripts based on realistic clinical scenarios that were structured to elicit the use of specific counseling skills. Instead of relying on trained standardized patient (SP) actors to portray mental health clients, they recruited experienced mental health counselors, reasoning that such actors would have "the expertise necessary to respond appropriately to both the spontaneous behaviors of the resident and the realistic clinical expectations" (Coyle et al., 1998).

Klaymen and Yudkowsky (2002) describe the use of SPs in the now more commonly understood usage of the term: actors trained and paid to portray persons with various ailments or disorders. Their use of SPs for training first-year psychiatry residents involved the use of rooms with built-in, unobtrusive cameras and microphones to record the sessions for later review. The SPs were unscripted and encouraged to come in with a problem either real or concocted and to interact with the residents using their own discretion. The residents were only told that they could "assume that these 'patients' had been prescreened and had been deemed appropriate for psychotherapy" (Klamen & Yudkowsky, 2002). Sessions were evaluated in part through the use of the session evaluation questionnaire (Stiles & Snow, 1984).

Among the advantages identified by Klamen and Yudkowsky (2002), in addition to the increased realism for the sessions provided by use of SPs, was the ability after the sessions to get feedback from both SPs and from other residents and trainers through review of videotapes made during the sessions.

Again, the relevance of incorporating the use of SPs in training counselors is thought to be the increased level of authenticity in the training sessions over more traditional role-play exercises in which trainees simply exchange counselor–client roles. One would imagine then that to achieve a higher level of realism, particularly in the portrayal of persons who have a mental illness of substance use disorder, it is imperative that adequate pretraining of the SPs be provided. In only one previously published article has the issue of emotional realism been substantially raised in the use of SPs to train psychotherapists (Krahn, Sutor, & Bostwick, 2001). In their report, Krahn et al. (2001) observed that although SPs offered a clear presentation of symptoms, direct answers, and cooperative interactions, they, along with their students, found it harder to experience empathy for an SP. Their concern over the degree of emotional realism present in the use of SPs for experiential training has not been shared in other published sources reviewed for this chapter.

Within the undergraduate Behavioral Health Counseling (BHC) program in the College of Nursing and Health Professionals at Drexel University, use of human simulation in the form of standardized patients has been a recent addition to the ongoing use of traditional methods of teaching counseling skills. The BHC curriculum is designed to prepare undergraduates for careers as direct-care behavioral health care professionals. Students receive coursework training in basic counseling skills similar to that taught in many traditional undergraduate and graduate counseling and psychology programs. In addition, they also received more advanced training in group counseling, crisis counseling, and cognitive-behavioral therapy. Students may also enroll in a counseling class in which skills specifically associated with the practice of motivational interviewing (Miller & Rollnick, 2002) are taught. Because a central focus of the BHC program is on preprofessional training for actual clinical practice, assessment and treatment planning skills are also taught in conjunction with two courses in psychiatric rehabilitation: one covering principals and one on competencies, as well as courses in addiction and dual-diagnosis treatment and recovery.

First use of SPs by the BHC program was made in 2009, by Robert Chapman, Ph.D., Clinical Associate Professor and an Associate Director of the BHC program. The training sessions took place in the College of Nursing and Health Profession's Center for Interdisciplinary Clinical Simulation and Practice (CICSP) Standardized Patient Laboratory. The SP laboratory consists of 10 simulation rooms along with a reception area. In addition, the CICSP contains a student class and debriefing room, student check-in room, observation room, actor's lounge, and control room. Each simulation room is equipped with wall-mounted computer stations and digital cameras that record audio and digitized video of the simulation. The simulation suites also contain computer stations with Internet access for both the student and standardized patient to access evaluation material and other interactive software. A state-of-the-art digital recording system from Education Management Solutions is used to record all SP encounters. Students, as well as faculty, are then able to observe their SP encounters at a later date from their own computers at home or office as a form of follow-up evaluation.

In addition to the state-of-the-art resources for training provided through use of the CICSP, students are also encouraged to download and save their personal SP counseling session encounters onto a compact disk that they may then choose to include in their student portfolios. These portfolios, developed throughout the four-year undergraduate program, will contain evidence of all learning in which the student was engaged and may be of use upon graduation in application to graduate schools or professional work settings.

Dr. Chapman's use of the CICSP with BHC students was for the class he teaches on Motivational Interviewing (MI). Basic skills to be mastered in MI include what has become known as OARS: (1) open-ended questions, (2) affirmations, (3) reflective listening, and (4) summaries (Miller & Rollnick, 2002). It is a suitable acronym in that these basic skills are considered essential in helping to move initial counseling sessions forward. Also, it should be noted that with the possible exception of "affirmations," these are the same types of basic counseling skills that have traditionally been taught. Other common counseling skills include nonverbal attending skills (good eye contact, body posture, etc.) and verbal skills such as paraphrasing, perception checking, and confrontation.

There are few instances of the use of SPs in the training of MI counseling techniques. Baer et al. (2004) reported on the use of SPs in training clinicians working in addictions treatment. Their observation was consistent with others who note that SPs provide a level of consistency across trainees that allow changes in observed behavior to be more confidently attributed to changes in trainee application of MI skills. However, it was also noted that differences in SP styles in portraying the case example may also be a contributing factor to brief training session encounters (Baer et al., 2004).

In the training sessions administered by Dr. Chapman, the SPs were three female actors who had much previous experience serving as SPs for other departments within the college. After brief orientations, each SP was told to wait in separate CICSP rooms set up for the interview sessions. All three SPs were given the following case and instructed to stay as close to character as possible in all their interactions with student trainees:

The Case of Karen K. is an "X"-year-old woman who started drinking regularly in high school. She has a family history of alcoholism, and Karen's paternal grandfather was killed when he fell off a ladder, which her family believes was likely because of his drinking. Karen's adult life revolved around drinking, as her husband, her family, and several of their friends also drank heavily. For Karen, alcohol was "performance-enhancing" because she was usually shy, and alcohol allowed her to socialize better, a trait that helped her work in sales. Her ability to drink large amounts—a 12-pack of beer a night, or three to four bottles of wine, or beer plus six to seven mixed drinks—became almost a "source of pride." About 4 years ago, Karen's employer suspected she had a drinking problem and voiced concern to her. Subsequently, Karen tried to stop drinking on her own but became very sick. She returned to drinking but was embarrassed, as indicated by her special efforts to "get rid of the evidence" of her drinking. But when she passed out one afternoon and forgot to pick up her daughter after soccer practice, Karen believed she had hit bottom. Karen had become so tolerant of alcohol that when she drove to the treatment center the day after a night of heavy drinking, her blood alcohol level was 0.3%. She underwent detoxification and began outpatient counseling, which consisted of group therapy 3 to 4 times a week, and individual therapy was recommended as well. Because of maternity leave, the individual counselor Karen had been seeing is unavailable to continue her counseling, and you are continuing as her replacement (Karen knows that you are coming in as a replacement counselor and is fine with this). In addition, she had started attending 12-step groups (AA), initially 5 to 6 times a week, but this has become once per week recently.

In addition to students also receiving the same case, their instructions included the following:

You will have 20 minutes to conduct your interview. You will enter the counseling office where your "client" is already seated and introduce yourself, and then you may begin your interview. At about 15 minutes, you will get a reminder that you have 5 minutes remaining. The focus of the session is not on "solving the problem," rather it is on establishing a therapeutic relationship that increases the likelihood that your client will return.

Rating sheets were given to students observing the interviews in an observation room that features a large, flat-screen monitor for viewing the interactions within the simulation rooms. SPs were also given the same rating sheet to be used in providing immediate postsession feedback. Each of the following rating sheet items were evaluated as either (1) minimally accomplished, (2) accomplished, or (3) accomplished to a significant extent:

1. Ability to establish a warm, open, inviting interaction with you
2. Created a safe, comfortable environment in which to consider change
3. Asked open-ended questions that invited you to share your story
4. Affirmed your strengths/ability to address the identified issue
5. Reinforced your sense of self-efficacy ("I can do this")
6. Motivated you to consider movement along the continuum of personal change
7. Helped you look at change as a personal choice rather than a counseling mandate
8. Helped you reduce ambivalence about change (less resistance to change/greater incentive to change)
9. Increased the likelihood that you would consent to and actually return for another session
10. Provided you with a different perspective from which to look at your drinking or other drug use

Although all students initially reported varying degrees of nervousness before participating in the laboratory exercise, the consensus at the conclusion was that each wanted more training experiences like this. Their feeling was that the SPs presented highly realistic portrayals of actual clients with alcohol abuse problems. One of the concerns that both students and faculty shared was the possible inhibitory effects of sessions being recorded, as well as being simultaneously viewed by other students in the observation room. Concern regarding the effects of recording on counselors and clients is not new. Gelso (1974) provided a number of observations on the subject based on his own research and the research of others who had been experimenting with both audio and video recording in actual client–counselor sessions throughout the previous decade. One of the concerns raised by Gelso was the often inhibiting factor session recording seemed to play (Gelso, 1974). Clearly, the use of trained SPs renders this concern insignificant because being recorded is a routine part of their work. As for the students, each reported that although they were aware before entering the simulation room that they would be recorded, this fact quickly grew irrelevant as they became immersed in the immediacy of the counseling session. It is also significant to note that although all students were given the option of having the monitor in the observation room turned off during their interview, none chose to take this option, trusting instead in the educational value of having fellow students observe their sessions and provide feedback.

The usefulness of student practice of counseling skills in the CICSP has certainly not been lost on the students themselves. Given the familiarity that students today have with a wide variety of computerized technologies, working in a computerized laboratory with digital recording equipment that links up directly with personal computers for later review and study offers a perfect fit for what today's students increasingly expect in educational experiences. The challenge for the BHC program is now in expanding this human simulation resource to other areas of the curriculum. Plans are already underway to use SPs in training students to do functional assessments as part of the psychiatric rehabilitation curriculum. Case applications are also being prepared for training with SPs in the cognitive-behavioral counseling class as well. Because one of the rooms in the CICSP can accommodate small group therapy sessions, there are plans to make use of this as well, particularly because of the ease this resource presents for allowing students and faculty to review sessions later through digital retrieval of files stored in the CICSP.

This past summer, the BHC faculty hosted 10 high school students in a week-long program entitled "Explorations in Behavioral Health Care Careers." Field trips to agencies serving people with addiction and mental health disorders, along with seminars featuring invited speakers and various workshops comprised the week's activities. The purpose was to give the students an opportunity to learn more about the behavioral health professions. Participants were all either high school juniors or seniors who were considering pursuing majors in college relevant to the helping professions. Among the workshops in which they participated was an opportunity to gain exposure through the use of modeling and role-play to an introductory experience with the basic counseling skills of attending and reflective listening. The very next day, these students were able to practice these same skills in the CICSP, with current BHC seniors serving as volunteer SPs. The reaction of the students to this experience was highly positive, with all stating that they felt this form of learning provided an exciting and realistic atmosphere in which to receive counseling skills training. Each was also thrilled to be handed a CD recording of their session delivered immediately after their sessions by the CICSP technical staff.

Clearly, this technology represents the most current approach in the decades-long history of counseling skills training innovations. Beyond the initial steps in making use of this technology that have already been taken, faculty within the

BHC program expect to now begin gathering data regarding the varied uses of this training resource and ultimately its impact on the future performance of its students.

REFERENCES

Alpert, D. (1986). A preliminary investigation of computer-enhanced counselor training. *Computers in Human Behavior, 2*(1), 63–70.

Anthony, W. A. (1993). Recovery from mental illness: The guiding vision of the mental health service system in the 1990s. *Psychosocial Rehabilitation Journal, 16*(4), 11–23.

Anthony, W. A., Dell Orto, A. E., Lasky, R. G., Marinelli, R. P., Power, P. W., & Spaniol, L. J. (1977). A training model for rehabilitation counseling education. *Rehabilitation Counseling Bulletin, 20*(3), 218–235.

Baer, J. S., Rosengren, D. B., Dunn, C. W., Wells, E. A., Ogle, R. L., & Hartzler, B. (2004). An evaluation of workshop training in motivational interviewing for addiction and mental health clinicians. *Drug and Alcohol Dependence, 73*(1), 99–106.

Carkuff, R. R. (1972). *The art of helping.* Amherst, MA: Human Resource Development.

Coyle, B., Miller, M., & McGowen, K. R. (1998). Using standardized patients to teach and learn psychotherapy. *Academic Medicine, 73*(5), 591–592.

Doyle, R. E. (1982). The counselor's role, communication skills, or the roles counselors play: A conceptual model. *Counselor Education and Supervision, 22*(2), 123–131.

Gelso, C. J. (1974). Effects of recording on counselors and clients. *Counselor Education and Supervision, 14*(1), 5–12.

Hill, C. E., & Lent, R. W. (2006). A narrative and meta-analytic review of helping skills training: Time to revive a dormant area of inquiry. *Psychotherapy: Theory, Research, Practice, Training, 43*(2), 154–172.

Hoge, M. A., Paris, M., Adger, H., Collins, F. L., Finn, C. V., Fricks, L., et al. (2005). Workforce compentencies in behavioral health: An overview. *Adminstration and Policy in Mental Health, 32*(5/6), 593–631.

Hummel, T. J., Lichtenberg, J. W., & Shaffer, W. F. (1975). CLIENT 1: A computer program which simulates client behavior in an initial interview. *Journal of Counseling Psychology, 22*(2), 164–169.

Ivey, A. E. (1971). *Microcounseling: Innovations in interviewing training.* Springfield, IL: Charles C. Thomas.

Klamen, D. L., & Yudkowsky, R. (2002). Using standardized patients for formative feedback in an introduction to psychotherapy course. *Academic Psychiatry, 26*(3), 168–172.

Krahn, L. E., Sutor, B., & Bostwick, J. M. (2001). Conveying emotional realism: A challenge to using standardized patients. *Academic Medicine, 76*(3), 216–217.

Kurtz, P. D., Marshall, E. K., & Banspach, S. W. (1985). Interpersonal skill-training research: A 12-year review and analysis. *Counselor Education and Supervision, 24*(3), 249–263.

Lambert, M. E., & Meier, S. T. (1992). Utility of computerized case simulations in therapist training and evaluation. *Journal of Behavioral Education, 2*(1), 73–84.

Lane, K. (1988). Using actors as "clients" for an interviewing simulation in an undergraduate clinical psychology course. *Teaching of Psychology, 15*(3), 162–164.

Miller, W. R., & Rollnick, S. (2002). *Motivational interviewing, second edition: Preparing people for change.* New York: Guilford Press.

Peters, G. A., Cormier, L. S., & Cormier, W. H. (1978). Effects of modeling, rehearsal, feedback, and remediation on acquisition of a counseling strategy. *Journal of Counseling Psychology, 25*(3), 231–237.

Power, K. A. (2005). Achieving the promise through workforce transformation: A view from the Center for Mental Health Services. *Administration and Policy in Mental Health, 32*(5/6), 489–495.

Stiles, W. B., & Snow, J. S. (1984). Counseling session impact as viewed by novice counselors and their clients. *Journal of Counseling Psychology, 31*(1), 3–12.

Teevan, K. G., & Gabel, H. (1978). Evaluation of modeling—Role-playing and lecture—Discussion training techniques for college student. *Journal of Counseling Psychology, 25*(2), 169–171.

Thayer, L. (1977). Video packaging: Integrating simulation techniques and systematic skill training. *Counselor Education and Supervision, 16*(3), 217–222.

Vander Kolk, C. J. (1973). Comparison of two mental health counselor training programs. *Community Mental Health Journal, 9*(3), 260–269.

CHAPTER 27

Interdisciplinary Human Simulation

Jose M. Maestre and Alberto Alonso Felpete

OBJECTIVE

*T*his chapter provides an overview of the development and implementation of inter-disciplinary human simulation. Included is a sample scenario.

HEALTH CARE ENVIRONMENTS AND SYSTEMS TRANSFORMATION: THE TEAM APPROACH

In the rapidly changing health care industry, clinical developments and technological advances in combination with cost-effectiveness and containment measures are shaping organizations. One of the most significant trends in hospital care over the past decade has been the proliferation of outpatient departments. Technological advances in surgery and anesthesia have enabled great numbers of procedures to be performed safely on an ambulatory basis (Fraser, Lane, Linne, & Jones, 1993).

As the emphasis on providing services on an outpatient basis increases, there is a growing complexity in hospital care. Patients admitted to hospitals have more severe diseases and undergo a wide range of diagnostic and therapeutic procedures performed by a diverse workforce in a constantly dynamic organizational system. This is especially relevant in the high-acuity clinical areas such as perioperative care, anesthesia, intensive care, and emergency departments, where patients are physiologically vulnerable and less likely to recover from mistakes. In these areas, nurses and faculty from different disciplines interact around patients in an environment characterized by multiple concurrent tasks, times of high workload, dynamism, major time pressure, rapidly evolving and changing information, data ambiguity, and high risk with regard to patient safety and clinical errors (Østergaard, Østergaard, & Lippert, 2004).

In addition, this complexity coupled with inherent human performance limitations, even in skilled, experienced, highly motivated individuals, has lead to an increase in the number of complications and in classifying hospital-based health care as a high-hazard industry (Hicks, Bandiera, & Denny, 2008).

In consequence, quality and safety have been at the forefront of the worldwide health care agenda. This was accelerated after the Institute of Medicine report in 1999 describing errors as a leading cause of death in the United States, recommending the development of newer ways to provide care for increasingly acute and complicated problems in a variety of settings (Kohn, Corrigan, & Donaldson, 1999).

This and subsequent reports have uncovered human factors as a key component of errors in health care, with insufficient or ineffective communication between professionals as a contributing factor in 60% to 80% of adverse events worldwide. Reflecting the seriousness of these occurrences, approximately 75% of the patients involved died. Human factors are the study of how interactions between organizations, tasks, and the individual provider influence human behavior and affect organizations or systems performance.

Although health care is delivered by multiple providers, clinical quality and safety have historically been structured on the performance of expert, individual practitioners. Therefore, the focus is now shifting onto the performance of teams and human factors analysis to provide insight into how interactions affect systems reliability. Moreover, most teaching hospitals use nurses and physicians in training in the high-acuity clinical areas and may expose patients to harm because of lack of experience, knowledge, and technical and behavioral skills while working with limited resources and supervision (Rodriguez-Paz et al., 2009).

As a consequence, numerous calls to reexamine and redesign care environments for ensuring competency and safety have come from both within and outside health care. The creation of new connections between individuals and groups of providers and new synergies among concepts, ideas, and innovations toward a unified vision of patient care through interdisciplinary teamwork is one of the main challenges to revolutionize health care organizations (Taft & Seitz, 1994).

WHAT IS A HEALTH CARE TEAM?

As health care providers, we have the opportunity to be observers and participants during numerous clinical situations. How can we ensure that the right people are working together in the right way at the right time? We like to think that all professionals are highly skilled and highly trained to perform their individual jobs, but it is known that team performance varies greatly among members (Sexton, Thomas, & Helmreich, 2000). What makes some providers work together better than others?

A critically important element is to dissociate the issue of clinical competency from the inevitable errors associated with human factors. It is now clear that success depends not only on individual performance, but also on the ability of the components to function in a coordinated, effective manner (Fernández et al., 2008).

A team is a group of two or more individuals who have each been assigned specific roles or functions, who interact dynamically and interdependently, and who adapt to achieve specific shared, valued objectives. Unlike a group that shares ideas and discussions but produces individual work products, a team produces a work product that is a joint result of contributions from all of its members (Raemer, 2004).

Several taxonomies of teamwork competencies and processes have been outlined. Two aspects are especially important: the individual's ability to function as a member of the team and the entire team's ability to function as an efficient collective entity (Fernández, Kozlowski, Saphiro, & Salas, 2008).

The main components to focus on are role clarity, communication, cooperation and support, resource utilization, and global assessment. It is necessary to emphasize the importance of leadership and followership and defining roles in an explicit way. All members should share information in an efficient and reliable manner and use all available resources. Equally important is achieving situational awareness and avoiding fixation on an incorrect diagnosis to maintain perspective on the problem (Rudolph & Raemer, 2004).

Several factors, such as task demands, team composition, and organizational context influence team performance. Health care teams have a variety of tasks and are made up of many different members that change from task to task and from day to day. This implies that each of the team members should possess general team competencies or generic team skills (Østergaard et al., 2004).

INTERDISCIPLINARY HEALTH CARE TEAMS

High-quality health care should be characterized by multisector, multiprofessional care delivered in an integrated way so that it would enable patients to receive a coordinated, comprehensive plan of care. This is of particular relevance when emergent situations mandate that we work with members from other departments or services that we rarely interact with. In these situations, effective teamwork can help prevent mistakes from becoming consequential and harming patients and providers.

Terms such as *multiprofessional, interprofessional, multidisciplinary*, and *interdisciplinary* are being used interchangeably without careful consideration or agreement as to their meaning (Craddock, O'Halloran, Borthwick, & McPherson, 2006). In this chapter, we will use the "interdisciplinary health care team" concept defined as a group of individuals with diverse training and backgrounds who work together as an identified unit or system. Team members consistently collaborate to solve patient problems that are too complex to be solved by one discipline or many disciplines in sequence (Drinka & Clark, 2000).

To accomplish this common goal, mutual respect for the expertise of all members of the team is the norm. Shared responsibility suggests joint decision making for patient care and practice issues within the organization. They also share leadership that is appropriate to the presenting problem and promote the use of differences for confrontation and collaboration. For an interdisciplinary team to function well, it must have the capacity to adapt to changing and complex situations. Cooperation and coordination promote the use of skills of all team members, prevent duplication, and enhance productivity in practice. Communication that is not hierarchic, but rather two way, also facilitates sharing of patient information and knowledge. Questioning the approach to care of either partner cannot be delivered in a manner that is construed as criticism, but as a method to enhance knowledge and improve patient care. It is also a method to enhance personal confidence and professional development. Finally, it provides an opportunity for establishing mutual understanding and respect between health and social care practitioners (Milligan, Gilroy, Katz, Rodan, & Subramanian).

Although the family is ostensibly a part of the team, the fact remains that the family is often relegated to the periphery of actual in-patient care. The traditional argument is that they might get in the way of the professionals' work, and they might violate the privacy of other patients. During the last several years, however, family members (or designated loved ones) are being involved as team members in the care and treatment of patients. This approach not only creates a more conducive environment for holistic healing but also contributes to a more efficient process. Furthermore, family members become essential and valuable advisors and partners in improving care practices and systems of care.

In this regard, some programs allow patient and family activation of the rapid response team. The most frequent reason for calls identified by the patient or family member was "something just doesn't feel right." Other leading reasons for calls were similar to criteria that are used by staff-initiated calls, such as shortness of breath and pain issues (Gerdik et al., 2010).

DEVELOPING EXPERT INTERDISCIPLINARY TEAMS

Appreciation that the clinical care environment has become progressively more complex, combined with the inherent limitations of human performance, has spurred interest in applying the lessons learned over the last few decades in other high-reliability industries to medicine. The experience to date has shown us the value of embedding standardized tools and behaviors into the care process to improve safety. Approaching improvement from the perspective of correcting system flaws and using standardized communication tools to make the day go more smoothly and keep everyone safe is effective. The message of "good people are set up to fail in bad systems—let's figure out how to keep everyone safe" is readily accepted (Leonard, Graham, & Bonacum, 2004).

All too often, clinicians providing care had very divergent perceptions of what was supposed to happen. Effective communication and teamwork is aimed at creating a common mental model or "getting everyone in the same movie." This work has been approached from the perspective of defining the practical successful elements that can be spread across disciplines in our larger care system.

Advancing care delivery systems toward these goals involves the articulation of a variety of initiatives. The creation of new connections between individuals and groups and new synergies among concepts, ideas, and innovations will be a key component in revolutionizing health care organizations. A current model involves merging institutional efforts to facilitate articulation of a professional collaborative practice model that can be defined as interlocking pieces, with all such pieces inherently related. In effect, all elements are grounded in a common vision and values toward the provision of patient-centered care based on defined standards.

Two absolute requirements for successful clinical change include (1) visible support from senior leadership and (2) strong clinical leadership. In health care culture, physicians and nurses who stand up and say, "This is the right thing to do, I support it and you need to also," have great influence. It is essential to approach medical culture from a "bottom-up" perspective. Traditional improvement efforts have been seen as "top-down"—that is, "you have a problem that needs to be corrected."

In addition, the model calls for developing, implementing, and evaluating organizational, educational, and training initiatives and support research.

All of the components build to promote clinical inquiry and experiential and team learning that impact staff development toward safe, effective, and evidenced-based care (Erickson, Ditomassi, & Jones, 2008).

Embedding such changes in clinical work is essential. Equally important is making such changes viable. They must be perceived as making the day simpler, safer, and easier for everyone. Once the case has been made for change, then having a very clear focus, taking "one bite of the elephant at a time," getting finite time commitments from the people involved, and measuring and celebrating success are all important components.

These elements may evolve into multiple numerous interdisciplinary programs and initiatives that will help facilitate innovations in practice. Training, which becomes a key element in this model, facilitates promotion of teamwork throughout all clinical disciplines, a commitment to collaborative decision making, and clinical recognition and advancement that will enable moving the vision forward.

SIMULATION AS AN EDUCATIONAL STRATEGY FOR INTERDISCIPLINARY TEAM TRAINING

Although the importance of developing team skills and effective communication is now well-recognized, there are currently no clear guidelines for designing and implementing interdisciplinary team training programs. In fact, teamwork is generally not encouraged in health care.

For decades, clinical education followed a model toward independence of the caregiver rather than dependence on others. Most content was delivered passively to the individual learner through lectures, and clinical training was done on the job around acutely ill, hospitalized patients as events occur. The principle behind this construct ("learning by doing") is that experience facilitates learning while simultaneously promoting trainee education and competency. However, such events are rarely followed by debriefing for learning and patient safety improvement.

In this process, physicians and nurses in training may expose patients to harm because they lack the required knowledge, skills, or attitudes. There is dependence on time and chance rather than on competence-based standards. Delivering patient-centered care as members of an interdisciplinary team in the intense clinical environment has traditionally left little time for interdisciplinary dialogue regarding health delivery systems and potential process improvement. In addition, there is a lack of practice on a regular basis, especially with uncommon events, procedures, or complications, and a lack of standardization and rigorous evaluation (Rodriguez-Paz et al., 2009).

The best way to cope with these limitations is not completely clear. Many aspects resemble those in hazardous industries, such as aviation and nuclear power industries, which became aware of problems years ago and made safety a priority. In such organizations, routine training has become a cornerstone to prepare for complex and urgent situations, with simulation the tool of choice.

As a result, during the past decade, simulation experiences have been gradually incorporated into health care agendas to provide a platform for clinicians to develop and to study effective teamwork in an environment that resembles real-life team situations and is safe for patients and providers. The use of simulation facilities set an environment for reflecting deeply about performance, providing skills training outside the production environment, discussing error without punishment, and testing new procedures for safety (Cooper, 2004).

Interprofessional simulation can be beneficial in preventing barriers from rising between different professional groups—through sharing knowledge and engendering respect for each others' roles. Current practice also recognizes shifting boundaries in relation to roles and responsibilities between health care professionals in the delivery of care, which must be considered when developing new shared learning programs.

Simulation allows clinicians to spend time in clarifying system error and the inherent limitations of human performance while helping to dissociate error from the common perception of mistakes as episodes of personal failure (Reader, Flin, Mearns, & Cuthbertson, 2007).

In addition, as complex organizational structures present unique challenges to teamwork, communication, interdisciplinary collaboration, and dissemination of new knowledge, simulation enables health care professionals to focus on systems-based practice competencies (Ker, Mole, & Bradley, 2003).

The effectiveness of interdisciplinary teamwork training in a simulation setting has been reported in acute obstetric emergencies. Clinical data showed an improved perinatal outcome in terms of five-minute Apgar scores and hypoxic-ischemic encephalopathy (Draycott et al., 2006). Many studies resulted in improvement of knowledge, practical skills, communication, and team performance (Merién, Van de Ven, Mol, Houterman, & Oei, 2010).

In malpractice cases, causative themes can often be grouped into the following categories: lack of reliable processes, delayed or inadequate crisis response, failure to develop differential diagnoses, inconsistent technical performance, and poor communication. All such themes can be directly addressed by well-developed simulation and team-training programs, including those offered by risk insurance companies. To improve patient safety and to reduce (even eliminate) preventable events that result in patient injury, some companies have developed premium incentive plans that incorporate simulation-based training and teamwork training. The first plan, introduced in 2000, incentivized anesthesiologists to go through crisis response simulation training at the Center for Medical Simulation, Cambridge, Massachusetts (Hanscom, 2008).

DEVELOPING A SIMULATION AGENDA

Comprehensive Needs Analysis

A comprehensive needs assessment is a key initial step in designing a simulation-based training program. Simulation experiences designed around specific goals and objectives will provide maximally effective learning experiences and outcomes.

Undergraduate and graduate education is changing from process and structure-oriented education to competency-based teaching and outcomes assessment. Various areas of competencies have been identified in relation with interpersonal and communication skills, systems-based practice, professionalism, patient care, and patient-based learning and improvement. Moreover, educators now design curricula that incorporate team projects to teach collaboration, sharing of knowledge, and effective communication. Although a challenge to health care educators, acquisition and assessment of these skills can now be addressed by designing independent simulation programs. Interpretation of the appropriate subject matter to teach may vary among schools and departments, may be adapted to the needs of each specific teaching program, and may be integrated into other preexisting teaching models (Delphin & Davidson, 2008).

Determining objectives for postgraduate education involves a more difficult approach, given its focus on interfacing with health care systems. It should include analysis at organizational, personnel, and task levels. Analysis at the organizational level will detect systems practice and team performance. Personnel analysis involves identifying experience and knowledge, skills, or attitudes deficiencies of team members. In addition, task analysis helps shaping specific objectives. It is essential to stress the relevance of conducting a multidisciplinary and multilevel needs analysis. What works well in one institution may fail in another and may be viewed as unsuccessful if the objectives are not aligned with the expectation of the individuals and organization (Fernández et al., 2008).

Examples of key learning points matched to the level of the participant and objectives of the training are listed on Table 27.1.

Defining the Interdisciplinary Team Training Program

There are many different articulations of teamwork training. Some are adaptations and developments of the paradigm training in aviation (crew resource management) to health care. Here the principles of individual and crew behavior in ordinary and crisis situations enhance focus on the skills of dynamic decision making, interpersonal behavior, and team management, traditionally grouped into the term *behavioral skills*.

Behavioral skills can be defined as the cognitive, social, and personal resource skills that complement technical skills and contribute to superior or substandard task performance of teams or individuals. They typically include four categories of behaviors for training and evaluation: cooperation and communication, leadership and management, situation awareness, and decision making.

Anesthesiologists share with pilots an analogous work process, their special concern for patient safety, and were the first to adapt crew resource management and to develop a crisis resource management course in 1990 (Table 27.2; Gaba, Howard, Fish, Smith, & Sowb, 2001). Currently, this method has spread to analogous specialties, such as critical care, emergency medicine, surgical teams, obstetrics, pediatrics, and neonatology, as

Table 27.1 *Examples of Interdisciplinary Teamwork Learning Objectives*

Undergraduate
Communication models and its functions within the context of clinical practice; recognize communication as a defense or barrier against error within the organization
Team coordination training, with clear identification of the team leader and role clarity among the other team members
Address professional boundaries early in their careers
Graduate
Identify areas or gaps in teamwork that are relevant to clinical practice
Implement preoperative briefing to improve safety processes and attitudes; introduce the surgical safety checklist in the operating room to maintain a team shared mental model
Postgraduate
Standardize the approach to hands-off communication when passing information and responsibility from one health care provider to another to ensure the continuity of care
Identify and analyze significant errors and sentinel events

Table 27.2 *Key Points of Anesthesia Crisis Resource Management*

Points Regarding Decision Making and Cognition
Know the environment
Anticipate and plan
Use all available information and cross check
Prevent or manage fixation errors
Use cognitive aids
Points Regarding Teamwork and Resource Management
Exercise leadership and followership
Call for help early
Communicate effectively
Distribute the workload
Mobilize all available resources for optimum management

well as to less acute settings as medical and surgical wards. This has resulted in numerous descriptions of team taxonomy and performance models that will help to guide design, implement, and assess simulation-based interdisciplinary teamwork training programs in undergraduate and graduate education (Clark, Fisher, Arafeh, & Druzin, 2010; Eppich, Brannen, & Hunt, 2008; Fernández et al., 2008; Morrison, Goldfarb, & Lanken, 2010; Walrath et al., 2006).

Other standardized teamwork training curricula have been developed over the last decade: for example, MedTeams® (adapted from the U.S. Army safety experience), TeamSTEPPS® (developed by the Department of Defense's Patient safety program in collaboration with the Agency for Healthcare Research and Quality), or the Medical Team Training Program (developed by the U.S. Department of Veterans Affairs). Either of them focuses on single-discipline or interdisciplinary teams (Fernández et al., 2008).

There are similarities and differences between these approaches; all of them have advantages and disadvantages, but there is no evidence that any of them are better than the other. They can be viewed as different paths to the same destination. Health care organizations should choose the interdisciplinary teamwork training that best meets their needs, resource availability, and preferences. They can outsource one of those mentioned above or develop their own expertise.

In general, all training programs focus on principles of teamwork and tend to highlight specific techniques of improving communication. Embedding standardized tools and behaviors such as the "I SBAR situational briefing model" (Table 27.3), the "I PASS the BATON" mnemonic for handing off patients care to another provider (Table 27.4), the "5 Ps" for patient transfers or provider shifts change (Table 27.5), appropriate assertion, or critical language can greatly enhance safety. These tools can effectively bridge the differences in communication style between nurses, physicians, and others that result from the current health care process (Gaba, 2010).

The need for interdependence and collaboration among members of the interdisciplinary team to solve patient problems is the trigger that determines the method of team practice and how particular problems are encountered, whether related to patient care or to the operation of the health care system. Team members work interdependently to

Table 27.3 *"I SBAR" Technique of Structuring Communication*

I—introduction: state your name and unit and the patient's name
S—situation (the current issue): e.g., patient age, gender, diagnosis, procedure, mental status preprocedure, patient stable/unstable
B—background (brief, related to the point): e.g., pertinent medical history, allergies, family location, medicines given, blood given, units available, tubes/drains/catheters, dressings/cast/splints, and laboratory/path pending
A—assessment (what you found/think): e.g., vitals, isolation required, risk factors, issues you are concerned about
R—recommendation/request (what you want next): e.g., specific care required immediately or soon, priority areas, pain control, intravenous pump, family communication

Table 27.4 *"I PASS the BATON" Mnemonic for Handling Off Care to Another Provider*

I—introduction: introduce yourself
P—patient name: identifiers, age, sex, location
A—assessment: the problem or the procedure in the process
S—situation: current status/circumstances, uncertainty, recent changes
S—safety concerns: critical laboratory values/reports, threats, pitfalls, and alerts
B—background: comorbidities, previous episodes, current meds, family
A—actions: what are the actions to be taken
T—timing: level of urgency, explicit timing, prioritization of actions
O—ownership: who is responsible (person/team) including patient/family
N—next: what happens next, anticipated changes, contingencies

Table 27.5 *The "5 Ps" to Ensure Proper Information Is Passed During Patient Transfers or Provider Shifts Change*

Patient
Plan
Purpose
Problems
Precautions

define and treat patient problems and learn to accept and capitalize on disciplinary differences, differential power, and overlapping roles.

Following this model is a description of the interdisciplinary teamwork skills we train at in our Center in Santander (Del Moral, Rabanal, & Díaz de Terán, 2001; González et al., 2005).

Role clarity is defined as the ability to establish and maintain clear responsibilities of team members, especially if equal-rank team members are present. Commonly, teams have an implicit structure to define roles and they become blurred when changes occur through task overload or distraction. Also, there is often some overlap in the skills of the various providers. This can be elicited in a number of ways: for example, creating scenarios where plans vary upon time or creating leadership conflicts with confederated actors. The team has first the opportunity to organize themselves during the simulation and then to reflect about the importance of establishing leadership and clarifying roles in an explicit way.

The leader is expected to maintain an overview of the clinical case, to articulate the goals in advance, to recognize changes in the situation balance and allocate resources, and to function as the communication or coordination center.

There are several approaches to the leadership of an interdisciplinary collaborative team. Historically, physicians have had the role of a team leader because of various cultural factors and the issue of legal responsibility for patient care. An emerging pattern involves equal participation and responsibility of team members determined by the nature of the problem to be solved. Emphasis by the team on "health care" rather than the more narrow focus of "medical care" broadens the roles and responsibilities on non-physician providers. For example, nurses coordinate central-line insertion procedures and are empowered to question doctors who do not follow the safety checklist on how to best prevent bloodstream infections.

It is better to emphasize on tasks instead of roles because it tends to diminish issues of professional territoriality and ownership. The decisions of who does what can be guided by provider availability, level of training, or member preferences. As with the setting of goals, it is important to periodically review and revise member roles as necessary (Raemer, 2004).

Communication is defined as the ability of the team to exchange information in an efficient and reliable manner. Everyone is expected to share his or her findings, concerns, and decisions to the leader.

It can be elicited by introducing data to individual participants into the scenario from various sources or incorporating help as the case develops to see how much data flow among the team.

Communication is much more than delivering a message from one individual to another. It has important functions in a high-stakes health care environment. It serves to build and maintain team structure, determined partly by explicitly allocating and coordinating responsibilities. From an operational point of view, it serves as an enabling tool for achieving task execution and for coordinating team efforts. It also enables information exchange and facilitates relationships among team members.

Communication differs from everyday conversations, as it should be explicit and direct. It is also not hierarchical but rather two way and, hence, may facilitate sharing of patient information and knowledge. It is necessary to close the loop to confirm what was meant by each part involved. Questioning of the approach to care of either partner cannot be delivered in a manner that is construed as criticism but as a mechanism for evaluating outcomes and making adjustments to the team.

We also transmit messages through nonverbal (gesture, eye contact) and paraverbal (tone and pace of voice) communication. It is like a commentary for the spoken language, and its interpretation takes place subconsciously. If we feel they both are at odds, we will place greater importance on the nonverbal and paraverbal cues rather than the spoken word (Pierre, Hofinger, & Buerschaper, 2008).

Support is defined as the ability to enlist and apply appropriate help in a timely and effective manner. New members are frequently confused regarding what is expected of them and what they can expect from others. It can be assessed creating scenarios with task overload or critically ill patients.

The team should seek for help early, share information to effectively orient the new members, and clearly make their roles. Given the mixture of skills and professional backgrounds and the complexity of interdisciplinary collaboration, a diversity of views and differences of opinion are inevitable. The team must be ready to discuss patient-management issues. It is important to recognize that conflict is both neces- sary and desirable for the team to grow and thereby develop greater efficiency and effectiveness.

Global assessment is the ability of the team to maintain perspective on the problem. Frequently, team members are absorbed by tasks, and no one is considering the problem as a whole, especially in critical situations. Once a situation assessment is made, it is easy to lose situational awareness, and people tend to become fixated. This is character- ized by a tendency to search for confirming information and to distort data to fit the current mental model.

It can be studied in a simulated scenario, providing data to evoke a mental model that does not correct the actual situation. The team has to take notice of other data, indi- cating that there is another explanation for the ongoing problem.

The leader has to gather all the information available, ask for other ideas among the team members, and promote reevaluation of the situation, seeking anything that can be missed and call for help.

Task management is defined as the skill for organizing resources and activities with the goal of satisfying the health care needs of the patient. In high-acuity areas, it is common to experience multiple tasks, stress, and time pressure while treating patients, which may result in failure to adapt to changing clinical situations, to use available resources, or to adhere to protocols or guidelines. It may be elicited by designing a case scenario with work overload. Managing this situation has four elements.

- Planning and preparing—developing in advance strategies and making necessary arrangements to ensure plans can be achieved.
- Prioritizing—being able to identify key issues and schedule tasks, activities, or infor- mation channels according to clinical relevance.
- Resource utilization—ability to anticipate, acquire, and use all available equipment and system resources. Membership on a health care team should ideally be deter- mined by the disciplines and skills that are required for the effective realization of the goals of the team.
- Providing and maintaining standards—adhering to evidence-based protocols, guidelines, or codes of good practice.

Educational Methodologies

Learning is facilitated through experience, but experience is not sufficient to learn. It is necessary to reflect on the experience to make generalizations and formulate concepts that can then be applied to new situations. Kolb developed this theory, called the experiential learning cycle, that gives us a useful model by which to develop our simulation program.

For successful learning, the participant should be able to enter this cycle at any point because people naturally prefer a different learning style or preference, but all stages must be followed in sequence (Kolb, 1984).

Interdisciplinary simulation needs to have all these components to create meaning- ful learning experiences and opportunities for the professionals to become more aware of their relationships with other individual groups and organizations.

Furthermore, health care providers could pursue a cycle of learning of interdisci- plinary skills to be applied in real-life clinical settings, reflect with other caregivers on their experiences, and redefine how these skills may be adapted and reapplied to other settings (Craddock et al., 2006).

The learning cycle suggests we need to articulate our reflections in some systematic way so that we remember what we thought and build for next time. "Reflective practice" is a method used to scrutinize one's own taken-for-granted assumptions and professional work practices. Those who learned to scrutinize their assumptions and mental routines were able to self-correct and improve their professional skills. On the other hand, those without skill in this self-scrutiny tended to seal out or ignore disconfirming data and maintained ineffective habits of practice.

However, how can we deliver critical messages and share our expertise with the caregivers while avoiding negative emotions, preserving social "face," and maintaining our relationship with the trainees?

The "debriefing with good judgment" as described by Jenny Rudolph et al. offers an approach to address this dilemma. This model guides the instructor on how to elicit the mental models that influenced trainees' actions during the simulation. The instructor has an underlying debriefing "stance" that unites the apparently contradictory values of curiosity about and respect for the trainee and the value of clear, evaluative judgments about trainee performance. Using a style of debriefing speech that combines advocacy (observation or statement) and inquiry (question) can be very effective (Rudolph, Simon, Dufresne, & Raemer, 2006).

One option for debriefing is to incorporate instructors from different disciplines to facilitate a balanced, multifaceted discussion after the scenario. For example, when an emergency team is undergoing the training, the debriefing may be handled by an experienced instructor from the anesthesia, surgical, or medical department in concert with a nursing or allied health disciplines instructor. Such multidisciplinary approach further reinforces the teamwork concepts required.

Scenario Design

Creating simulations for successful interdisciplinary team training is more reliant on creativity than on technology. Scenarios should be designed to reproduce some aspect of the working environment. This may vary from the replication of a few aspects of a clinical setting to the recreation of an entire clinical environment, such as an emergency room, an operating theater, an intensive care unit (ICU), or a ward. Any real-life situation is multifaceted, and only some characteristics are reproduced during the development of the scenario. The goal is to create an atmosphere where the participants can achieve a "fiction contract" to allow themselves to fully immerse in the simulation.

Full-body human patient simulators, standardized patients, and hybrids have all been successfully used to train interdisciplinary teams. However, for particular skills sets, such as managing a difficult airway event or advanced life support, mannequins hold advantages, as they allow the performance of invasive maneuvers. Actors better interact with the trainees when it is necessary to take a history or to perform some portion of a physical examination, providing counseling or patient education.

Simulation may occur off site in a simulation laboratory or on site at the organization. Regardless of its physical location, the most important element to impact training effectiveness is to create an environment in which trainees feel simultaneously challenged and psychologically safe enough to engage in rigorous reflection.

Measurement and Evaluation Tools

There are different rating scales for assessing high-performance teamwork skills in simulation settings. There is general agreement that behavioral rating tools are most appropriate, although standardized and widely accepted methods for measuring the outcomes in health care are not presently available.

On the basis of the categories of behavioral skills, Fletcher's group developed the Anesthetists' Nontechnical Skills (ANTS) evaluation method to rate individual team member performance using clearly specified behavioral markers (Table 27.6; Fin, Patey, Glavin, & Maran, 2010).

Kim et al. have reported the Ottawa Global Rating Scale. It uses global rating scales of eight important aspects of medical teamwork: problem-solving, situational awareness, anticipation and planning, leadership, resource utilization, communication output, communication input, and clinical management as well as an overall rating of team performance.

The Mayo High-Performance Teamwork Scale provides a brief measure that is the target of crisis resource management training in medical settings (Malec et al., 2007).

All present satisfactory construct validity, internal consistency, and interrater reliability for a measure of team functioning in high-acuity settings. The advantage of using a skills framework is that by identifying specific behavioral performance with illustration of the positive and negative impact of those actions on patient care, course participants rapidly build their understanding.

Remaining Challenges

Simulation training is being increasingly used, but the penetration is still relatively small. There are substantial culture barriers to adopt this vision and barriers to openly

Table 27.6 *Anesthetists' Nontechnical Skills Taxonomy*

Categories	Elements
Task management	Planning and preparing
	Prioritizing
	Providing and maintaining standards
	Identifying and utilizing resources
Team working	Coordinating activities with team members
	Exchanging information
	Using authority and assertiveness
	Assessing capabilities
	Supporting others
Situation awareness	Gathering information
	Recognizing and understanding
	Anticipating
Decision making	Identifying options
	Balancing risks and selecting options
	Reevaluating

recognize safety issues and to discuss interdisciplinary team process and dynamics. The need of training and the need to develop faculty expertise in systems thinking and quality improvement are not equally accepted throughout all health care providers (Walrath et al., 2006).

On the other hand, some stakeholders want to focus only on cost containment and make it difficult to endorse simulation efforts. In our experience, interdisciplinary training is difficult to coordinate, as participants find difficulties in balancing competing academic, personal, and clinical responsibilities. In addition, we have found difficulties in expanding our simulation efforts as required to motivate and to train capable instructors-clinicians in reflective practice and debriefing. Involvement of leadership at all levels is a key element to foster simulation and patient safety initiatives.

CONCLUSIONS

Health care providers do not want patients to be injured because of their actions. We expect our health care system to become a high-reliability organization. Interdisciplinary simulation is an innovative tool that is contributing to make patient care safer. It sets an environment for reflecting deeply about the inherent limitations of human performance and the prevalence of system error. It provides the opportunity to train skills outside the production environment, discussing error without punishment and testing new procedures for safety.

Nevertheless, only a tiny fraction of health care practitioners have had a meaningful exposure to a high-fidelity and fully interactive interdisciplinary simulation. Much remains to be done to fully integrate simulation into education and training in health care.

EXAMPLE SCENARIO OF INTERDISCIPLINARY TEAMWORK AT VALDECILLA VIRTUAL HOSPITAL

Case title: acute pulmonary embolism

OBJECTIVES (HUMAN FACTORS INFLUENCING PERFORMANCE)
Team work
Call for help early (nurse→faculty→intensive care)
Exchange of information among team members
Task management

Prioritizing: identify key diagnostic issues, schedule diagnostic tasks, and request information from specialists

Providing and maintaining standards: use of empiric anticoagulant therapy

PARTICIPANTS AND ACTORS

PARTICIPANTS: two nurses, one surgical resident, and one faculty from general surgery

Actors: one nurse assistant and one relative of the patient

CASE STEM TO BE READ TO PARTICIPANTS: "You are the health care team in charge of the general surgery ward today. You will be called to assist a 62-year-old man admitted 2 days ago from the ICU after open splenectomy due to blunt traumatic injury to the spleen. He is now complaining of chest pain and dyspnea. With respect to his past medical history he suffers from chronic obstructive pulmonary disease and does not have any known drug allergies."

Scenario setup

ROOM: general surgery ward

High-fidelity human patient simulator lying supine on a hospital bed

Prop

Patient with large bore peripheral intravenous access and lumbar epidural catheter connected to a patient-controlled analgesia pump (morphine)

Occlusive dressings on the splenic incision

Right leg in plaster due to a fracture of the tibia

Standard monitors (electrocardiogram, noninvasive blood pressure [BP], and pulse oximeter) and emergency crash cart are available but are not in place until the participants ask for them

The relative of the patient is in the room, and the nursing assistant will be throughout the scenario to help the participants

Medical record

Personal history: heavy smoker, chronic obstructive pulmonary disease, occasional aerosol bronchodilator therapy, acute angina 3 years ago, aspirin 325 mg once daily, hypertension, unknown drug allergies

Emergency unit record: male, 62 years old, 220 pounds, 8 feet, fell while working, presents fracture of his right tibia, loss of consciousness for a few minutes, and severe pain. Vitals: BP, 80/55 mm Hg; HR, 129 bpm. Laboratories: hematocrit, 28.5%. Ultrasound: splenic rupture and bleeding into the abdominal cavity. Emergent splenectomy indicated. Trauma surgeon indicated right leg in plaster

Anesthesia, surgical, and ICU records without complications

Evolution in the ward had been uneventful over the 48 postoperative hours. The actual symptoms began only a few minutes before the family called

INSTRUCTIONS FOR THE SIMULATOR TECHNICIAN

Baseline: patient initially awake, alert, with chest pain and dyspnea, will become anxious during the scenario, with cold sweaty skin, severe chest pain, and progressive dyspnea

Vital signs evolution throughout the scenario: temperature, 36°C; heart rate, from 100 to 140 bpm; systolic BP, from 100 to 70 mm Hg; respiratory rate, 18 to 24 breaths/min; oxygen saturation, from 97% to 80%

SCENARIO SCRIPT

After the nurse has examined the patient, she is expected to call for help and convey the diagnostic actions that might be expected. Another nurse will come to help with monitoring, laboratory tests, and electrocardiogram. The patient will become nervous, tachypneic, and hemodynamically unstable.

The nurses should begin initial treatment measures (oxygen and intravenous fluids). The patient will complain of increasing dyspnea, and the relative will ask if it might be an acute angina again. The physician in charge should be paged, if not done before.

Upon resident/faculty arrival, information has to be exchanged in a clear and structured way. Team members ideally should share their mental models, reevaluate the current situation, and prioritize the tasks to be done. Faculty are expected to continue or initiate differential diagnosis and treatment.

Soon oxygen saturation will drop and the patient should be ventilated with a face mask or intubated (depending on the expertise of participants), which will stabilize his vitals.

From the clinical perspective, angina should be ruled out because of the pleuritic characteristics of the pain and the electrocardiogram. Pulmonary embolism might be suspected because of the sudden onset of symptoms and the presence of the fracture in an immobilized patient.

Ideally, ICU should be consulted and anticoagulant therapy initiated.

Debriefing guide: Usually, we prepare some questions to help us explore the trainee's perspective on scenario events. We use the theory and method for debriefing with good judgment described by Jenny Rudolph et al.

REFERENCES

Clark, E. A. S., Fisher, J., Arafeh, J., & Druzin, M. (2010). Team training/simulation. *Clinical Obstetrics and Gynecology, 53*(1), 265–277.

Cooper, J. B. (2004). The role of simulation in patient safety. In W. F. Dun (Ed.), *Simulators in critical care and beyond* (pp. 20–24). Des Plaines, IL: Society of Critical Care Medicine.

Craddock, D., O'Halloran, C., Borthwick, A., & McPherson, K. (2006). Interprofessional education in health and social care: Fashion or informed practice? *Learning in Health and Social Care, 5*(4), 220–242.

Del Moral, I., Rabanal, J. M., & Díaz de Terán, J. C. (2001). Simuladores en anestesia. *Revista Española de Anestesiologia y Reanimacion, 48,* 423–433.

Delphin, E., & Davidson, M. (2008). Teaching and evaluating group competency in systems-based practice in anesthesiology. *Anesthesia and Analgesia, 106,* 1837–1843.

Draycott, T., Sibanda, T., Owen, L., Akande, V., Winter, C., Reading, S., et al. (2006). Does training in obstetric emergencies improve neonatal outcome? *BJOG, 113,* 177–182.

Drinka, T. J. K., & Clark, P. G. (2000). *Health care teamwork: Interdisciplinary practice & teaching.* Westport, CT: Greenwood Publishing Group.

Eppich, W. J., Brannen, M., & Hunt, E. A. (2008). Team training: Implications for emergency and critical care pediatrics. *Current Opinion in Pediatrics, 20,* 255–260.

Erickson, J. I., Ditomassi, M. O., & Jones, D. A. (2008). Interdisciplinary institute for patient care. *JONA, 38*(6), 308–314.

Fernández, R., Kozlowski, S. W. J., Saphiro, M., & Salas, E. (2008). Towards a definition of teamwork in emergency medicine. *Academic Emergency Medicine, 15,* 1104–1112.

Fernández, R., Vozenilek, J. A., Hegarty, C. B., Motola, I., Reznek, M., Phrampus, P. E., et al. (2008). Developing expert medical teams: Toward an evidence-based approach. *Academic Emergency Medicine, 15*(11), 1025–1036.

Fin, R., Patey, R., Glavin, R., & Maran, N. (2010). Anaesthetists' non-technical skills. *British Journal of Anesthesia, 105*(1), 38–44.

Fraser, I., Lane, L., Linne, E., & Jones, L. (1993). Ambulatory care: A decade of change in health care delivery. *Journal of Ambulatory Care Management, 16*(4), 1–8.

Gaba, D. (2010). Crisis resource management and teamwork training in anaesthesia. *British Journal of Anaesthesia, 105*(1), 3–6.

Gaba, D. M., Howard, S. K., Fish, K. J., Smith, B. E., & Sowb, Y. A. (2001). Simulation-based training in anesthesia crisis resource management (ACRM): A decade of experience. *Simulation & Gaming, 32*(2), 175–193.

Gerdik, C., Vallish, R. O., Miles, K., Godwin, S. A., Wludyka, P. S., & Panni, M. K. (2010). Successful implementation of a family and patient activated rapid response team in an adult level 1 trauma center. *Resuscitation, 81*(12), 1676–1681.

González, A. M., Díaz de Terán, C., Rabanal, J. M., Maestre, J. M., Placer, J., & Del Moral, I. (2005). Eficacia de los sistemas de simulación en el aprendizaje de la utilización de recursos en crisis anestésicas. *Revista Española de Anestesiologia y Reanimacion, 52,* 481.

Hanscom, R. (2008). Medical simulation from an insurer's perspective. *Academic Emergency Medicine, 15*(11), 984–987.

Hicks, C. M., Bandiera, G. W., & Denny, C. J. (2008). Building a simulation-based crisis resource management course for emergency medicine: Phase 1. Results from an Interdisciplinary Needs Assessment Survey. *Academic Emergency Medicine, 15,* 1136–1143.

Ker, J., Mole, L., & Bradley, P. (2003). Early introduction to interprofessional learning: A simulated ward environment. *Medical Education, 37,* 248–255.

Kohn, K. T., Corrigan, J. M., & Donaldson, M. S. (1999). *To err is human: Building a safer health system.* Washington, DC: National Academies Press.

Kolb, D. A. (1984). *Experiential learning: Experience as the source of learning and development.* Englewood Cliffs, NJ: Prentice Hall.

Leonard, M., Graham, S., & Bonacum, D. (2004). The human factor: The critical importance of effective teamwork and communication in providing safe care. *Quality and Safety in Health Care, 13*(Suppl. 1), i85–i90.

Malec, J. F., Torsher, L. C., Dunn, W. F., Wiegmann, D. A., Arnold, J. J., Brown, D. A., et al. (2007). The Mayo High Performance Teamwork Scale: Reliability and validity for evaluating key crew resource management skills. *Simulation in Healthcare, 2*, 4–10.

Merién, A. E. R., Van de Ven, J., Mol, B. W., Houterman, S., & Oei, S. G. (2010). Multidisciplinary team training in a simulation setting for acute obstetric emergencies: A systematic review. *Obstetrics & Gynecology, 115*, 5, 1021–1031.

Milligan, R. A., Gilroy, J., Katz, K., Rodan, M., & Subramanian, L. N. S. (1999). Developing a shared language: Interdisciplinary communication among diverse health care professionals. *Holistic Nursing Practice, 13*(2), 47–53.

Morrison, G., Goldfarb, S., & Lanken, P. N. (2010). Team training of medical students in the 21st century: Would Flexner approve? *Academic Medicine, 85*(2), 254–259.

Østergaard, H. T., Østergaard, D., & Lippert, A. (2004). Implementation of team training in medical education in Denmark. *Quality and Safety in Health Care, 13*(Suppl. 1), i91–i95.

Pierre, M., St., Hofinger, G., & Buerschaper, C. (2008). *Crisis management in acute care settings.* Heidelberg, Germany: Springer Publishing.

Raemer, D. (2004). Team-oriented medical simulation. In W. F. Dunn (Ed.), *Simulators in critical care and beyond* (pp. 42–46). Des Plaines, IL: Society of Critical Care Medicine.

Reader, T. W., Flin, R., Mearns, K., & Cuthbertson, B. H. (2007). Interdisciplinary communication in the intensive care unit. *British Journal of Anaesthesia, 98*(3), 347–352.

Rodriguez-Paz, J. M., Kennedy, M., Salas, E., Wu, A. W., Sexton, J. B., Hunt, E. A., et al. (2009). Beyond "see one, do one, teach one": Toward a different training paradigm. *Postgraduate Medical Journal, 85*, 244–249.

Rudolph, J., & Raemer, D. (2004). Diagnostic problem solving during simulated crises in the OR. *Anesthesia and Analgesia, 98*, S34.

Rudolph, J. W., Simon, R., Dufresne, R. L., & Raemer, D. B. (2006). There's no such thing as "non-judgmental" debriefing: A theory and method for debriefing with good judgment. *Simulation in Healthcare, 1*, 49–55.

Sexton, J., Thomas, E., & Helmreich, R. (2000). Error, stress, and teamwork in medicine and aviation: Cross sectional surveys. *British Medical Journal, 320*, 745–749.

Taft, S. H., & Seitz, P. (1994). Innovations in human service technologies. Strengthening health care delivery systems. *International Journal of Technology Assessment in Health Care, 10*(2), 214–226.

Walrath, J. M., Muganlinskaya, N., Shepherd, M., Awad, M., Reuland, C., Makary, M. A., et al. (2006). Interdisciplinary medical, nursing, and administrator education in practice: The Johns Hopkins experience. *Academic Medicine, 81*(8), 744–748.

CHAPTER 28

Human Simulation for Medicine

Kathleen F. Ryan

INTRODUCTION

As many patients are becoming more active in their medical care, others have become active in the training of future doctors. Supplementing traditional medical education with exposing learners to patients very early in their training has become standard at most medical schools. Using patients as "experts" in their own illnesses can infuse reality into an otherwise monotonous one to two years of textbooks and testing. Taking this one step further is training lay people to portray illnesses that they may not have or situations they may not have experienced, allowing medical learners and resident doctors to improve their communication, examination, and diagnostic skills. The focus on prevention of medical errors and the move to competency-based medical education with measurable outcomes has increased the use of standardized patients and simulation in medical education, as it has in nursing education. Many programs are being developed in this regard, such as the Expert Patients Program (Department of Health, 2001) in Britain, which recognizes the value of these types of learning encounters to enhance learners' experiences and reinforce the relevance of basic science by showing how it applies in real-life practice.

A Brief Introduction to Medical School Curricula in the United States

Since the Flexner' (1910) report, traditionally allopathic and osteopathic medical schools in the United States have used a 4-year curriculum—with the first 2 years dedicated to acquiring a basic science foundation and the last 2 years in an apprentice capacity caring for patients in clinical settings. To successfully complete medical training, in addition to completing the doctor of medicine degree, the learner must also pass National Board examinations: United States Medical Licensing Examination Step 1, USMLE Step 2 clinical knowledge, and USMLE Step 2 clinical skills (http://www.usmle.org/). Learners then take the last installment, USMLE Step 3, during residency training. For their part, osteopathic schools have a similar examination structure called the Comprehensive Osteopathic Medical Licensing Examination (http://www.nbome.org/). Failure to successfully pass these examinations will restrict learners from practicing medicine in the United States. Since June 2004, the addition of the Step 2 Clinical Skills examination requires learners to pass a 10-station standardized patient encounter. Learners are graded on their ability to take a history, perform a physical examination, and write up their findings. The encounters are typical issues encountered in the practice of medicine. As such, many schools started to expose learners to patient encounters earlier in their training, which helped them to practice communication skills and begin to develop physical examination skills. Some schools have offered a problem-based medical experience, which replaced the traditional lecture and laboratory format with small group-learning experiences—where learning engages more active and interactive processes.

INTEGRATION OF STANDARDIZED PATIENT INTO YOUR MEDICAL SCHOOL

Teaching Communication Skills

Difficult Patients

In 1993, Novack et al. showed by questionnaire that virtually all medical schools were teaching interviewing and interpersonal skills (Coulehan et al., 2001). Most were using standardized patients, which gave learners direct feedback on their performance while providing learners with a wide variety of patient personality types in a controlled environment. Table 28.1 shows examples of common personality types followed by several sample scenarios.

Example:

George J. is a 59-year-old man with a history of hypertension who is coming to see his physician for a routine check-up. Due to the fact that an earlier patient needed to be transferred to the hospital because they were having chest pain, Mr. J. has been waiting for over an hour. The medical learner walks in and comes face to face with a very angry patient.

This basic scenario allows the learner to reflect on the patient's anger and their own response to that anger. They can try different techniques such as reflection or validation (Coulehan et al., 2001) to attempt to improve the situation and hopefully deal with the patient's concerns in a professional manner.

Example:

Charlie T. is a 49-year-old man who was injured when he fell off a ladder and broke his leg. He has done very well healing but still has pain, which he feels requires narcotic pain medication. When the learner starts the encounter, he finds Mr. T. to be very manipulative and insisting on his pain medication not being changed in any way.

Dealing with persons afflicted with substance abuse is a common situation in medical practices today. In 2008, an estimated 20.1 million Americans aged 12 or older were

Table 28.1 *Patient Personality Types*

Angry
Talkative
Vague
Anxious
Manipulative

current (past-month) illicit drug users (8.0% of the population) (Substance Abuse and Mental Health Services Administration, 2008). Here, the student can learn how to start the process of negotiating decreases in pain medication with a patient who may not be aware he is addicted to that medication.

Breaking the Bad News

One of the most difficult things for physicians to do is breaking the bad news to patients and family, from informing them of the death of a loved one to admitting an error in the treatment plan (medication or procedural). As this requires more advanced communication skills, it is usually integrated into the senior year. Oftentimes, it can be found as part of a transition course to prepare learners for their internship year. Scenarios of this sort can be very helpful and can be done in many ways. Again, program size is important and, although it would be optimal to have this done one-on-one with a standardized patient, schools with larger classes can find this challenging. Thus, for larger classes, one can take a group approach with a facilitator, allowing 1 or 2 learner interviews of the patient, and then debriefing with the entire group and standardized patient. If this model fits best, care in managing group size is important, as more than 15 will be very difficult to moderate. Optimum size allows for 10 learners or less. A sample scenario follows.

Example:

> Mrs. S. is a 30-year-old woman with a husband and 2 small children. She had noticed a lump in her neck and came to see you in your continuity clinic. You had investigated the lump and it was surgically removed 1 week ago. She is following up with you for her postoperative check and you must let her know that the biopsy was positive for Hodgkin's lymphoma.

The simple statement "I am sorry" has created much discussion, including the assumption that saying this is a direct admission of error. Others consider it differently, as a brief communication by another human being. For novice and expert alike, however, this situation can provoke considerable discomfort. Quill, Arnold, and Platt (2001) made a special point by distinguishing between sympathy and pity. Although this scenario seems short and simple, it can be developed into several different outcomes. As these scenarios also can branch in different ways, they should be kept simple. It may not be necessary to develop a long, complex past medical history for the standardized patient to learn either. In addition, as this type of scenario can trigger repressed memories in the learner, the facilitator needs to be prepared. This is especially tricky in larger groups. In this author's course, in which scenarios like this are used, the time allocation is from 60 to 90 minutes with the entire role-play being no longer than 10 minutes. One of the benefits of using SPs in this case is the ability to teach learners how to interpret nonverbal clues that the patient is sending as well as the dialogue itself.

Example:

> Mrs. H. is a 90-year-old retired school teacher with 5 children. She was admitted to the medical ICU with multilobar pneumonia. Her condition is grave and she is not expected to survive. The learner is meeting with 2 of Mrs. H.'s children to discuss withdrawal of care.

Here, the learner may be dealing with decision makers who are at odds with what to do. Mediating this type of discussion is commonplace and usually the medical resident—or worse, the intern—is the one conducting this discussion. This would be beneficial as part of the senior year curriculum, again toward the end of the year. The list of communication scenarios can expand into many common situations, including obtaining informed consent.

TEACHING CLINICAL SKILLS

Clinical skills scenarios are a bit more complex and require SPs with excellent memories. They also require more training so that there is consistency between SPs participating in the same scenario. These scenarios can be introduced as early as the first year of medical school. As learners will not have had much formal physical diagnosis training, the goals will be modest. In fact, interviewing may be the main focus with physical examination skills taken as tasks, such as obtaining vital signs and properly positioning the stethoscope on the patient's chest. As learners progress through their first two years, the complexity of the examination will increase. Here is also where standardized patients pose a problem. They may not be able to simulate many of the physical findings associated with certain conditions. Findings such as pulmonary congestion, edema, or heart murmurs are usually absent findings. The learner can be observed to be technically proficient in the technique, but one does not know if they can actually identify abnormal physical findings. In response, many schools have started to employ hybrid simulations using the SP for the interview and the high-fidelity simulator for the physical examination. Having the SP speak through the simulator as the learner examines the mannequin sometimes helps to maintain the suspended reality. Be that as it may, this author still feels the benefit of using the SP for the interview is more powerful than having the entire encounter occur with the SP voicing through the mannequin—the latter does not allow for nonverbal communication. In the hybrid simulation scenario, the learner can also be observed for accuracy and identification of abnormal findings.

Example:
Ms. H. is a 32-year-old with a past history of asthma. She presents to the ER after using her inhaler every 2 hours at home without relief. She also had a prior history of pulmonary embolism while on oral contraceptives when she was 21 years old.

Here, depending on which diagnosis you wish to have as the actual diagnosis, you could either use the SP alone (in the case of the PE) as they would not need to have physical findings and they could fake leg pain if needed. If asthma is what you wish to be the main diagnosis, a hybrid simulation with the SP interviewing short of breath and the mannequin wheezing could be employed.

The evaluation of this case can focus on communication, technical skills, and professional conduct. Learners can be evaluated on their concern for the patient: do they wash their hands and drape the patient properly for modesty, as well as their technical skills.

THE CLINICAL YEARS AND THE SHIFT TO ASSESSMENT OF COMPETENCY

As learners transition into their clinical years, they are faced for the first time with the need to pass the National Board examinations. Before starting third year, most medical students take Step 1 of the USMLE. This consists of a computerized test of basic science knowledge. Before or early in their fourth year, Step 2 of the USMLE is taken.

Step 2 consists of 2 separate examinations: clinical knowledge and clinical skills. Many schools have instituted their own versions of the clinical skills examinations using standardized patients. This is usually done as early as possible before learners sit for the actual examination. As there are limited slots and testing centers available, this can be challenging for schools with large class sizes.

The assessment of the SP is as important as the assessment from the facilitator. As SPs are regular people, things that the facilitator may not pick up on, such as the use of medical terms and the inability to let the patient fully expand on what brought them into the office that day, may be otherwise missed.

CONCLUSIONS

The use of standardized patients in medical school education has greatly expanded over the past decade. This modality of education and assessment allows learners to experience situations that may be difficult for them to process before ever starting clinical rotations. Learners can practice communication and diagnostic skills before being put in a clinical situation where they encounter a truly vulnerable patient. The words of William Osler sum this up the best:

> He who studies medicine without books sails an uncharted sea, but he who studies medicine without patients does not go to sea at all.
>
> William Osler 1849–1919

REFERENCES

Coulehan, J., Platt, F. W., Egener, B., Frankel, R., Lin, C. T., Lown, B., et al. (2001). "Let me see if I have this right...": Words that help build empathy. *Annals of Internal Medicine, 135,* 221–227.

Department of Health. (2001). *The expert patient: A new approach to chronic disease management for the 21st century.* London: Author.

Flexner, A. (1910). *Medical education in the United States and Canada: A report to the Carnegie Foundation for the Advancement of Teaching* (Bulletin No. 4, pp. 346). New York City: The Carnegie Foundation for the Advancement of Teaching.

Quill, T., Arnold, R., & Platt, F. (2001). "I wish things were different": Expressing wishes in response to loss, futility, and unrealistic hopes. *Annals of Internal Medicine, 135*(7), 551–555.

Substance Abuse and Mental Health Services Administration. (2008). *Results from the 2008 National Survey on Drug Use and Health: National findings.* Retrieved from http://www.drugabusestatistics.samhsa.gov/nsduh/2k8nsduh/2k8Results.cfm#Ch2

CHAPTER 29

The Future of Human Simulation

Linda Wilson, Leland Rockstraw, and Gloria F. Donnelly

Simulation in health care is an ever-growing field, and its use is a definite asset in the evolution and improvement of safe, effective patient care, treatment, and integrity. With today's technology, simulation has taken an abrupt turn toward a better and safer future. Through the lens of simulation, we can change the culture of safety by improving the way we operate, practice, and, most importantly, think. The Nurse Services Organization reports that the top reasons that claims are brought against nurses are medication administration errors and failure to monitor (CAN Insurance Company, 2009). The conditions that lead to adverse events can be significantly diminished as simulation is used in educating nurses to process crucial cues that, when accordingly addressed, will prevent adverse events in patient care. Simulation promotes increased interprofessional communication and interdisciplinary problem solving. There is nothing more powerful than a group of faculty members gathering after a simulation session and sharing constructive criticism and problem solving to enhance teaching techniques as well as student learning experiences. Simulation and its concomitant debriefing not only influence the way students learn, but also how faculty teach. Nursing practice can also be positively altered through simulation by creating safe practice environments (simulation laboratories, examination rooms, emergency room, operating room, etc.) where health care practitioners can freely perform and enhance their daily skills.

There are multiple types of simulations available to health care training today, including the human patient simulator, standardized patients or actors, hybrid simulation, task trainers, simulation interactive software programs, virtual patient assessment and intervention interactive software programs, Second Life, and many others. It is essential for all faculty members to be familiar with these types of simulations and be able to incorporate them in a multitude of learning arenas, including live classroom, laboratory, and online distance education.

It would not be surprising for the nursing state board licensing examination to include some sort of required video simulation or objective structured clinical examination with a standardized patient in the next several years. The possibility of NCLEX simulations is a compelling reason for faculty to incorporate simulation so that students are prepared to demonstrate their knowledge and competencies through simulation.

What does the future hold for simulation? We may see a focus on improving the "look and feel" of the simulation environment to replicate actual patient interactions such as the following: (1) simulation using standardized patients in conjunction with human patient simulators with artificial intelligence that can carry on a conversation, as well as display behavioral characteristics; (2) plastic skin on a mannequin that feels like real skin—that is, warm, skin turgor, able to perspire; (3) simulation using standardized patients in conjunction with human robot or android that is ambulatory; and (4) simulation laboratories that depict all types of environments realistically such as the operating room, postanesthesia care unit, delivery room, community home, school environment, military field, and so on. The future may also yield the creation of objective-based clinical experiences and measurement of the standard skill sets of safe, competent practitioners. Finally, the future is here with respect to transitioning from passive lecture style instruction to active experiential and reflective instruction. The experiential classroom and laboratory of the future will promote adult active participation, clinically safe risk taking, and the facilitation of diverse learning styles.

In conclusion, simulation as a crucial learning strategy in nursing and health professions education is not only here to stay but is also changing and improving at lightning speed. It is no longer a matter of choice for faculty to embrace simulation; it is rather when and what type. A final thought regarding simulation in the future: "The problem is never how to get new innovative thoughts in your head but how to get the old ones out" (G. Donnelly, personal communication, March 10, 2011).

REFERENCE

CAN Insurance Company. (2009). *CAN HealthPro Nurse Claims Study: An analysis of claims with risk management recommendations 1997–2007.* Retrieved March 9, 2011, from at https://www.nso.com/pdfs/db/Nurse_SLCS_x-8540–510_final_web.pdf?fileName=Nurse_SLCS_x-8540–510_final_web.pdf&folder=pdfs/db&isLiveStr=Y

Index